Design, Evaluation, and Translation of Nursing Interventions

Souraya Sidani, PhD

Professor and Canada Research Chair
Health Intervention: Design and Evaluation
School of Nursing
Ryerson University
Toronto, Ontario, Canada

Carrie Jo Braden, PhD, RN, FAAN

Professor and Associate Dean for Research
Hugh Roy Cullen Professor of Nursing
School of Nursing
The University of Texas Health Science Center at San Antonio
San Antonio, Texas, US

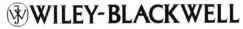

WILEY-BLACKWELL

A John Wiley & Sons, Ltd., Publication

Wiley-Blackwell is an imprint of John Wiley & Sons, formed by the merger of Wiley's global Scientific, Technical and Medical business with Blackwell Publishing.

Registered office: John Wiley & Sons Ltd, The Atrium, Southern Gate, Chichester, West Sussex, PO19 8SQ, UK

Editorial offices: 2121 State Avenue, Ames, Iowa 50014-8300, USA
The Atrium, Southern Gate, Chichester, West Sussex, PO19 8SQ, UK
9600 Garsington Road, Oxford, OX4 2DQ, UK

For details of our global editorial offices, for customer services and for information about how to apply for permission to reuse the copyright material in this book please see our website at www.wiley.com/wiley-blackwell.

Library of Congress Cataloging-in-Publication Data

Sidani, Souraya.
  Design, evaluation, and translation of nursing interventions / Souraya Sidani, Carrie Jo Braden.
       p. ; cm.
  Includes bibliographical references and index.
  ISBN-13: 978-0-8138-2032-3 (pbk. : alk. paper)
  ISBN-10: 0-8138-2032-4 (pbk. : alk. paper)
  1. Nursing–Research.   I. Braden, Carrie Jo, 1944–   II. Title.
   [DNLM: 1. Nursing Care.   2. Evaluation Studies as Topic.   3. Nursing Research.
  4. Research Design.   5. Translational Research.   WY 100.1]
   RT81.5.S56 2011
   610.73072–dc23
                                                                    2011014378

A catalogue record for this book is available from the British Library.

This book is published in the following electronic formats: ePDF 9780470961506; ePub 9780470961513; Mobi 9780470961520

Set in 9/12.5 pt Interstate Light by Aptara® Inc., New Delhi, India
Printed and bound in Malaysia by Vivar Printing Sdn Bhd

1 2011

Design, Evaluation, and Translation of Nursing Interventions

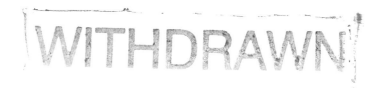

Contents

SECTION 5   TRANSLATION OF INTERVENTIONS

Preface

Provision of high-quality care to persons with different health problems rests on the delivery of interventions that are appropriate and effective in addressing the presenting problem. Interventions are subjected to a systematic process consisting of four phases, before making them available for use in the context of day-to-day practice.

The first phase relates to the careful design of interventions, which is based on a comprehensive understanding of the presenting problem and the development of interventions that target the problem. The acquired knowledge is synthesized into an intervention theory that clarifies the nature of the targeted problem; identifies the active ingredients, mode of delivery, and dose of the intervention; and explains the mechanisms underlying the intervention's effects on the intended outcomes. The second phase focuses on the operationalization of the intervention into an intervention manual. The manual details the human and material resources required to deliver the intervention, as well as the specific actions or steps undertaken to carry out the intervention. The manual directs the actual implementation and assessment of the fidelity of the intervention implementation. The third phase consists of a series of consecutive studies for investigating the acceptability, feasibility, efficacy, and effectiveness of the intervention. To be relevant to practice, the studies' results should indicate which clients, presenting with which personal and health or clinical characteristics, benefit, to what extent, from the intervention delivered in what mode and at what dose, under what context. The fourth phase involves the translation of the intervention. Translation entails the transformation of the studies' results into meaningful guidelines and the transfer of the guidelines to healthcare professionals who are ultimately responsible for providing the intervention in their day-to-day practice.

Although the systematic process has been delineated, there are limited resources available to inform nurses and other healthcare professionals of the general approaches and specific methods for designing, evaluating, and translating interventions. This book is concerned with describing the phases of the systematic process and clarifying what is to be achieved, and how, in each phase. It is intended to serve as a helpful "one-step" reference for healthcare professionals planning to engage in this process. The content of the book covers conceptual, methodological, and practical knowledge needed to carry out each phase. The conceptual knowledge clarifies the aspects of the problem that should be understood to guide the development of interventions; the active ingredients of the intervention that are responsible for inducing the desired changes in the presenting problem; the mechanisms underpinning the intervention effects on the intended outcomes; and the definition and indicators of the acceptability, feasibility, efficacy, and effectiveness of the intervention. The methodological knowledge presents different but complementary approaches for designing and evaluating interventions. The principles underlying each approach are explained and its strengths and limitations are discussed. The practical knowledge entails detailed description of the methods and procedures for carrying out the approaches in each phase of the process.

The goal is to support students, researchers, and healthcare professionals in the careful design, systematic evaluation, and meaningful translation of interventions, and, consequently, in the provision of high-quality care.

Acknowledgment

The authors gratefully acknowledge the informal feedback from colleagues, the constant challenge of students, and the instrumental support of staff (at the Health Intervention Research Center and the Office of Nursing Research and Scholarship), which contributed to the refinement of our thinking and continuous expansion and evaluation of our conceptual and methodological knowledge.

This work could not be accomplished without the love, encouragement, and unlimited support of our family (in particular Leila Sidani).

Section 1

Introduction

Chapter 1

Introduction to Intervention Research

In many countries around the world, nursing has achieved recognition as a scientific discipline (Lutzen, 2000). Nursing research is developing rapidly (Hallberg, 2009), evidenced by the quantity and quality of nurse-led studies reported in regional and international journals describing the health and/or illness experience and response to interventions of individuals residing in countries that vary in cultural beliefs and values, and in healthcare systems. To preserve recognition as a scientific discipline, nurses need to generate, expand, and refine the knowledge base that demonstrates the unique contribution of the discipline to meet the needs of individuals, families, groups, and society at large. Nursing's contribution is reflected in the provision of high-quality care that successfully promotes health, addresses clinical problems, and produces beneficial outcomes. Therefore, it is imperative to prioritize efforts to advance nursing science so that it supplies the theoretical and practical knowledge required for the provision of high-quality care (Evers, 2003; Hallberg, 2009).

The nursing process forms the foundation of high-quality nursing care. The nursing process consists of four steps: (1) assessment, (2) diagnosis, (3) intervention, and (4) evaluation, which nurses implement when caring for individuals, families, or communities (thereafter referred to as clients). Nurses assess the biophysiological, physical, psycho-behavioral, and sociocultural conditions of clients in order to identify their health needs, values, and preferences, and to formulate a diagnosis. A nursing diagnosis clearly delineates the nature of the actual or potential health-related problem with which clients present and requiring remediation. An in-depth and lucid understanding of the clients' condition and presenting problem is necessary for selecting appropriate and effective interventions to be implemented for, on behalf, or with the clients, with the goals of promoting and restoring health through resolution of the presenting problem. Evaluation refers to monitoring clients' status on a regular basis to determine the extent to which the interventions were successful in achieving the intended goals. This description of the nursing process

Design, Evaluation, and Translation of Nursing Interventions, First Edition.
Souraya Sidani and Carrie Jo Braden.
© 2011 John Wiley & Sons, Inc. Published 2011 by John Wiley & Sons, Inc.

highlights the centrality of interventions. Interventions constitute the essential element that characterizes nursing care (Tripp-Reimer et al., 1996).

Carrying out the nursing process in the context of day-to-day practice requires a sound knowledge base that informs nurses of interventions that are effective in addressing the clients' presenting problem and in promoting their health (Evers, 2003; Kim, 2002). Nursing interventions that are effective in producing the intended beneficial outcomes are carefully designed, systematically evaluated, and successfully translated into the day-to-day practice setting. The process of designing, evaluating, and translating interventions is conducted in a way that maintains rigor within a context characterized by evolving perspectives or paradigms underlying science and practice. This chapter begins with an overview of the paradigm shift, then highlights the steps of the process for designing and evaluating interventions prior to translating and using them in the day-to-day practice setting.

1.1 Overview of paradigm shift

The new millennium is witnessing a shift in paradigm of what constitutes high-quality care and of what comprises acceptable evidence to guide provision of high-quality care. Although evidence-based practice was introduced as an approach for delivering high-quality care (Guyatt et al., 2002), efforts to implement it in the day-to-day practice setting is raising many questions about the utility of available knowledge in guiding practice. For example, while evidence is becoming available about the effects of interventions on specific outcomes, there is much less evidence about the specific mechanisms underlying the intervention effects. There is even less evidence to guide intervention translation within specific practice settings. Insufficient evidence about mechanisms linking interventions to outcomes for specific clients, coupled with a growing demand of enlightened clients for a participatory role in health-related decision-making, is bringing the person or client-centered approach to the forefront of what defines high-quality care (American Nurses Association, 2003; Institute of Medicine, 2001; McCormack & McCance, 2006). Person- or client-centered care is congruent with the philosophical orientation underpinning nursing practice. In addition, it complements evidence-based practice in defining high-quality care (Sidani et al., 2006). The emergence of this conceptualization of high-quality care led some scholars in various disciplines, including nursing, to reflect on the methods used throughout the process of designing, evaluating, and translating interventions. There is a growing request to embrace alternative methods that have the potential to generate theoretical and practical knowledge to inform delivery of care (e.g., Gross & Fogg, 2001; Nallamothu et al., 2008; Sidani et al., 2003) and to plan effective knowledge translation and implementation strategies (Eccles et al., 2005) that are relevant to a variety of practice settings within and across countries (Hallberg, 2009).

1.1.1 Evidence-based practice: a review

Evidence-based practice was introduced as an approach for delivering high-quality care (Guyatt et al., 2002; Jennings & Loan, 2001). It is broadly defined as "the conscientious, explicit, and judicious use of current, best evidence in making decisions about the care of individual patients" (Sackett et al., 1997, p. 2). Proponents of evidence-based practice believe that interventions found effective and safe on the basis of best available evidence can be delivered in a consistent manner to produce the same effects in clients presenting with the same problem, under the conditions of day-to-day practice (Victora et al., 2004). They advocate the development of guidelines to inform practice. Guidelines are systematically developed statements of recommendations to assist health professionals in decision-making about client care (Lugtenberg et al., 2009). The guidelines specify the target population in terms of experience of the presenting problem, the intervention(s) to be used to address the problem, and the procedures for monitoring the intervention outcomes (Titler et al., 1999). The guidelines are disseminated to health professionals who are expected to implement them as recommended. The end results are provision of best available care and improvements in clients' condition.

The above definition of evidence-based practice underscores the importance of best evidence in guiding practice. Proponents of this approach to care place high value on research as compared to other sources of evidence. In particular, they consider most appropriate evidence derived from primary or meta-analytic studies that used the randomized controlled or clinical trial (RCT) design to investigate the effects of interventions. The RCT is deemed the gold standard for intervention evaluation research (Richardson, 2000). The features that characterize the RCT design include careful selection of participants on the basis of stringent eligibility criteria; random assignment of participants to the experimental and comparison groups; concealment of treatment allocation; manipulation and standardization of intervention delivery; blinding of research staff and participants to allocated treatment; and control of contextual factors. These features are believed to minimize the influence of potentially confounding factors, which is required for demonstrating the causal effects of the intervention on outcomes.

To date, experience with evidence-based practice raises concerns with the nature of the evidence forming the basis for developing guidelines for practice, with the emphasis on using and/or adhering to these guidelines in practice, and with the strategies for transferring the guidelines into the practice setting. The relevance of empirical evidence on intervention effects derived from RCT studies to the practice setting has been questioned. Recent critique of the RCT design highlights its limitations in maintaining internal and external validity. The limitations stem from the features of the RCT. The application of strictly defined inclusion and exclusion criteria confines the accrued sample to a very selective and homogeneous subgroup of the target population seen in the practice setting. Random assignment does not reflect the process of selecting and providing interventions within the context of practice. This method of treatment allocation is often not well received by clients participating in an RCT and the health professionals responsible for their care. It may contribute to self-selection into the trial, to attrition, and to dissatisfaction and nonadherence of participants with the allocated treatment and subsequent poor outcome achievement; these, in turn, result in inaccurate estimates of the intervention effects that may not be replicable in the practice setting. Manipulation and standardization of the intervention are not congruent with day-to-day practice, where treatment is not withheld from needy clients, and interventions are modified to fit the needs and values of clients, and/or given sequentially in response to changes in clients' condition. Therefore, interventions validated in RCT studies may not be transferable to and easily incorporated in the practice setting. The experimental control that characterizes the RCT is unrepresentative of the complexity of the practice context; thus, the intervention effects may not be reproduced in practice (Grapow et al., 2006; Huibers et al., 2004; Lindsay, 2004; Richardson, 2000; Robitaille et al., 2005; Valentine & McHugh, 2007).

The emphasis on using and/or adhering to guidelines has been criticized for reducing practice to a mechanistic application of empirically supported interventions that is informed by generic algorithms (Sehon & Stanley, 2003). The algorithms instruct health professionals which interventions to select and implement to address the clients' presenting problem. This mechanistic application of generic algorithms does not take into consideration the clients' experiences, needs, beliefs, and perceived acceptability of the intervention. Also, it disregards the health professionals' skills at critical thinking, and obligations to respond flexibly to the clients' needs. Further, the guidelines' recommendations are often stated in general terms that simply identify the interventions to be given. They do not clearly specify the conditions under which the interventions are most effective, and do not explain how the intervention effects are produced. Yet, knowledge of who benefit the most from the intervention given at what dose and in what mode is essential for guiding practice (Brown, 2002; Sidani & Braden, 1998).

Numerous projects have been undertaken to transfer, translate, and implement evidence into practice. Various strategies have been utilized in these endeavors, of which education is the most common. Typically, educational strategies are didactic, involving passive learning, where health professionals are informed of the evidence and expected to apply the intervention in their day-to-day practice. However, recent literature on knowledge translation indicates that overall, attempts to implement evidence-based practice in particular settings were not successful at sustaining changes in health professionals' practice and hence in improving the quality of client care (Sales et al., 2006). Considerable variation in success rate was observed within an individual intervention and across interventions (Eccles et al., 2005; Lugtenberg et al., 2009). Findings of relevant studies consistently pointed that health professionals, including nurses, do not depend on research as a source of evidence to guide practice. Rather, they rely on other sources, primarily clinical knowledge either gained personally or shared by colleagues, as well as patient experience (French, 2005; Spenceley et al., 2008).

This state of affairs has contributed to reconsideration of different sources of evidence as acceptable for generating the knowledge needed to guide practice, and the client-centered as an approach to provide high-quality care (see Section 1.1.2). Acceptable sources of evidence include local knowledge and client experience, as well as research. Local knowledge is embedded within particular practice settings and is accumulated in two ways. First, local knowledge is obtained through performance evaluation and/or quality improvement initiatives undertaken in the setting. The results of these initiatives represent valuable information about the practice area requiring change; unmet needs of clients and of health professionals working in the setting; and the type and impact of interventions delivered to address the health problems of the locally served population (Rycroft-Malone et al., 2004). Second, local knowledge is gained through health professionals' experience and is embedded in the human capital, that is, expert professionals available in the setting. Local knowledge is critical for translating evidence. It directs efforts at adapting guidelines to fit the contextual characteristics of a particular setting. Client experience is emerging as a useful source of evidence to guide the process of making decisions about care of individuals, families, and communities. Patient experience is not clearly defined in the literature on evidence-based practice; however, it appears to connote attendance to the clients' characteristics, needs, and preferences (Mykhalovskiy & Weir, 2004), as advocated in the implementation of client-centered care. Research evidence has been expanded to include quantitative and qualitative studies. Accumulating results suggested that non-RCT designs (e.g., quasi-experimental and cohort) provide meaningful evidence supporting the effectiveness of interventions delivered under usual conditions of day-to-day practice (Concato & Horwitz, 2004; Nallamothu et al., 2008; Vandenbroucke, 2004). Findings of non-RCT designs, in combination with those of studies investigating factors that moderate and/or mediate intervention effects, address questions of concern to health professionals. In other words, they enhance the clinical relevance of research findings, which can promote uptake and application of interventions in the practice setting.

1.1.2 Client-centered care

Client-centered care has been, and still is, highly valued in nursing (Lauver et al., 2002). It is resurging as an approach aimed to provide high-quality care (Naylor, 2003). Client-centered care is congruent with the philosophical orientation of nursing practice (Rolfe, 2009). Nurses are instructed, socialized, and expected to deliver client-centered care. Nurses recognize the multidimensionality of clients' experience, acknowledging the biophysiological, physical, psycho-behavioral, and sociocultural domains of health; respect the uniqueness of clients' needs; and individualize care to be consistent with the clients' needs. The description of client-centered care, available in the literature, has focused on characterizing this approach to care at the individual client level. The features that distinguish client-centered care are: (1) acknowledging the client as a unique person; (2) understanding the individual characteristics, needs, beliefs, values, and preferences of the person; and (3) responding flexibly to the persons' characteristics, needs, and preferences (McCormack, 2003; Radwin, 2003). Responding flexibly, also termed responsiveness (Radwin et al., 2009), involves participation of persons in decision-making and individualization of care (McCormack & McCance, 2006; Sidani, 2008). Participation of persons in the process of decision-making consists of a joint effort between the health professionals and the person to identify his or her needs and preferences, and to select the intervention that will address the person's needs and that the person views as acceptable (Sidani et al., 2006). Individualization of care involves customization of the intervention activities, dose, and/or mode of delivery so that they are mindful of the person's characteristics, resources, and/or context. The client-centered approach has also been applied to the care of families. Family-centered care encompasses similar features; however, the focus is on the family as a unit. The application of the client-centered approach to the care of communities is reflected in the collaborative participation of community members in identifying health needs and in developing, adapting, or selecting relevant interventions.

The implementation of client-centered care is expected to benefit the individuals, families, and communities. It is proposed that this approach promotes clients' sense of independence and control through their participation in treatment-related decisions (Reid Ponte et al., 2003); increases satisfaction with care related to the receipt of the intervention of choice; enhances adherence to treatment; and, subsequently, achievement of intended outcomes (Sidani et al., 2010). The limited number of studies that investigated the benefits of the client-centered approach to care have focused on either participation of clients in decision-making or individualization of educational interventions. The results of these studies were promising, showing improvement in health outcomes for clients who participated in decision-making and/or received client-centered care or individualized interventions (e.g., Fremont et al., 2001; Lauver et al., 2002; Sidani, 2008; Wensig & Grol, 2000).

Responding flexibly to clients' characteristics, needs, and preferences raised the issue of discrepancy between the selected intervention and the intervention considered most effective on the basis of the best available evidence. That is, clients may find acceptable, express a preference for, and choose interventions which may not be effective or may have been minimally effective in managing the presenting problem or producing the desired outcomes (Wensig & Grol, 2000). To address this issue, Coyler and Kamath (1999) proposed an integrated "patient-centered evidence-based" approach to care. Briefly, this approach entails identifying evidence-based interventions, incorporating only those interventions as alternatives from which clients can choose and/or nurses can individualize to be consistent with clients' characteristics and preferences (Sidani et al., 2006). The integrated client-centered evidence-based approach has implications for the definition of high-quality care.

1.1.3   High-quality care redefined

High-quality care refers to the delivery of interventions that are appropriate, acceptable, effective, safe, and efficient. Appropriate interventions are logical, reasonable, and sound treatments that specifically address the health problem with which clients present. This implies that the nature of such interventions is consistent with the nature of the presenting problem, where activities comprising the interventions should fit with the defining characteristics and/or the determinants of the presenting problem, and the dose with which the interventions are given is compatible with the severity with which the problem is experienced. For instance, educational interventions involving the provision of information about a chronic illness and its management is appropriate for increasing clients' knowledge but may not be adequate for changing their self-management behaviors. In the latter case, behavioral interventions focused on facilitating the initiation and maintenance of self-management behaviors are more appropriate.

Acceptable interventions are agreeable to clients expected to receive the interventions. Agreeable interventions are perceived favorably; that is, they are consistent with the clients' beliefs about health in general, about the presenting problem, and about treatment. They are deemed suitable to their lifestyle, convenient, and easy to apply in their daily life (Sidani et al., 2009). For instance, persons who ascribe to a holistic perspective to health that admits a strong body–mind connection find complementary and alternative interventions (e.g., meditation) more acceptable treatments than conventional medical treatments; the former interventions are congruent with their beliefs about health and treatments (Tataryn, 2002). Related to acceptability is the notion of cultural relevance of interventions. Within and across countries, clients identify with different ethnic or cultural groups who share common experience and hold particular beliefs, values, and norms. Cultural relevance refers to the extent to which the content and/or activities of the intervention, the format for delivering the intervention, and the outcomes expected of the intervention are consistent with the ethnic and cultural experiences, values, and beliefs of the group or community (Resnicow et al., 1999). For example, intervention targeting dietary habits are acceptable to clients of diverse cultural backgrounds if they take into account the typical dishes and way of cooking adopted by respective groups, and/or the food items available within a particular context and affordable by clients residing in that context.

Effective interventions produce the best outcomes for clients. When carefully implemented, effective interventions are successful in addressing the presenting problem, reducing its severity, and/or in improving the physical, psychological, and/or social domains of health. For instance, behavioral interventions are considered effective in managing insomnia if they assist individuals sleep efficiently, reduce daytime fatigue, improve cognitive performance related to poor sleep, and ultimately enhance physical and psychosocial functioning.

Safe interventions are associated with no or minimal negative conse-quences. Negative consequences encompass physical and/or psychological discomfort, as well as side effects or untoward reactions experienced with or as a result of the interventions. For example, adherence to behavioral in-terventions for managing insomnia may result in increased daytime fatigue within the first 2 weeks of treatment; however, the experience of this discom-fort does not exceed that suffered following a "bad night" sleep, is temporary, and is outweighed by the long-term benefit of the intervention manifested in adequate sleep quantity and quality.

Efficient interventions are those worth their cost. They produce the intended beneficial outcomes within the context of human and financial resources used to implement them. For instance, the costs of cognitive behavioral interven-tions for managing insomnia relates to those incurred by therapist and persons for delivering the sessions over a specified time period, whereas the costs of pharmacological treatment to address the same problem encompass the pur-chase of the pills over an extended period of time. The cost-efficiency of the cognitive behavioral interventions stems from their long-term improvement in sleep and daytime functions (Jacobs et al., 2004).

The provision of high-quality, client-centered evidence-based care consists of delivering appropriate, acceptable, effective, safe, and efficient interven-tions. Whereas evidence-based practice is concerned with identifying effec-tive, safe, and efficient interventions, client-centered care focuses on the appropriateness and acceptability of interventions to clients. Implementation of client-centered evidence-based care requires a sound knowledge base that informs health professionals of the following:

(1) The nature, severity, and determinants of the health problem with which clients present.
(2) The nature, dose, and mode of delivering interventions that are appro-priate for addressing the presenting problem and that are acceptable to clients holding different personal and cultural beliefs, values, and attitudes toward health and healthcare.
(3) The effectiveness, safety, and cost-efficiency of the interventions, as com-pared to no-treatment or to other available interventions for the same presenting problem.
(4) The personal and clinical profile of clients who benefit from the interven-tions to varying degree.
(5) The contextual factors that may interfere with the implementation and/or effectiveness of the interventions.
(6) The mechanisms through which the interventions produce their effects on the desired outcomes and/or side effects.

This type of knowledge is generated through the application of a process for designing and evaluating interventions. It forms the basis for developing guidelines that present specific recommendations for delivering the interven-tion in a manner that is responsive to clients' characteristics and preferences and that is mindful of the clients' resources and context, with the ultimate goal of producing the desired short- and long-term outcomes. The guidelines are then translated to fit the context of particular settings.

1.2 Process for designing, evaluating, and translating interventions

The process for designing, evaluating, and translating interventions is systematic, rigorous, yet flexible. It involves phases that are logically sequenced; however, the results of each phase drive the work forward toward the next phase or backward toward earlier phases. In the former case, appropriate interventions found acceptable to different subgroups of the target population are tested for efficacy; in the latter case, interventions that are not well received or deemed unacceptable to clients or health professionals should be reconceptualized (i.e., going back to the drawing board!) or refined. For example, initial evaluation of the Pro-Self Program revealed that patients with cancer were overwhelmed with its content that covered multiple symptoms and proposed to have different modules, each focusing on one symptom, provided on an as-needed basis (Dodd & Miaskowski, 2000; Larson et al., 1998). Each phase is carried out using research methods that are most pertinent to achieve the stated goals and objectives and to maintain the validity of findings. The phases of the process are consistent with those described by Whittemore and Grey (2002), Campbell et al. (2000), and the National Institutes of Health. The phases are briefly reviewed in the following sections relative to the design, evaluation, and translation of interventions.

1.2.1 Design of interventions

The first phase in the design of interventions focuses on gaining a clear and thorough understanding of the presenting problem requiring remediation. This understanding should clarify the nature of the problem, the specific indicators with which it is manifested, the range of severity with which it can present or be experienced, the determinants or factors that contribute to the problem, and possible consequences of the problem. Understanding of the problem is derived deductively from relevant middle range theory, and/or inductively from a systematic exploration of the problem as experienced by the target population. Knowledge about the presenting problem is critical as it points to the aspect(s) of the problem amenable to change or remediation; this, in turn, indicates the nature of the intervention activities that are most appropriate to address the presenting problem.

The second phase in the design of interventions is concerned with elaborating the intervention. This work is guided by relevant middle range and practice theories. The aim is to elucidate the essential, specific elements or active ingredients and the nonspecific elements of the intervention. These intervention elements are necessary to specify the components and activities comprising the intervention, the mode or format for delivering the intervention, and the dose with which the intervention should be given to attain the preset outcomes. This information then guides the development of the intervention protocol required for proper implementation of the intervention.

The third phase is the development of the intervention theory. The theory describes the conditions that influence the implementation of the interventions and the achievement of outcomes; it also clarifies the mechanisms responsible for its effects. The conditions relate to the characteristics of the clients receiving the intervention, the interventionist delivering the intervention, and the setting or environment in which the intervention is given. The mechanisms represent the changes that should take place in order to achieve the desired outcomes. The intervention theory guides the evaluation of the intervention.

Although the three phases rely on theoretical and empirical knowledge to design appropriate interventions, members of the target client population and health professionals (who will ultimately be involved in its implementation in practice) are invited to participate in these phases. These individuals help clarify the presenting problem and the activities and mode for delivering the interventions. Their involvement is crucial for enhancing the acceptability of interventions.

1.2.2 Evaluation of interventions

In general, evaluation of interventions proceeds in three consecutive phases. The first phase consists of a pilot test. The primary focus is on examining the acceptability and feasibility of the intervention. Acceptability refers to the clients' perception of the intervention in terms of its appropriateness, effectiveness, severity of side effects, and convenience of implementation (Sidani et al., 2009). Feasibility relates to the ease with which the intervention is delivered and the factors that facilitate or hinder its implementation. In addition, the pilot test explores the extent to which changes in the hypothesized mechanisms underlying its effects and outcomes occur following implementation of the intervention. The results of the pilot test guide the refinement of the intervention theory and/or any aspect of the intervention delivery, such as its elements or activities, mode of delivery, and dose. The refinement can be done in collaboration with the research staff (in particular, the interventionists) and the clients who participated in the pilot test. The revised intervention is then subjected to further evaluation.

The purpose of the second evaluation phase is to determine the efficacy of the intervention. Efficacy refers to the extent to which the intervention causes the intended effects. The focus is on examining the extent to which the intervention produces its effects under ideal conditions. The ideal conditions are those that minimize the potential influence of any factors, other than the intervention, that could contribute to the outcomes, and that maximize the power to detect the hypothesized effects. The features of the RCT design allow control for potential confounds. This experimental control is necessary to attribute, with confidence, the observed outcomes to the intervention, that is, to demonstrate the causal relationship between the intervention and the outcomes (Sidani & Braden, 1998; Victora et al., 2004). Results of the efficacy study inform the next step to be undertaken in the process of intervention evaluation. For interventions that do not show the expected effects, the next step entails exploratory work to identify what contributed to the unanticipated findings. The search is for conceptual and/or methodological factors that could account for the findings. Conceptual factors are illustrated with inadequate specification of the severity of the problem amenable to treatment by the intervention under evaluation, influence of a confounding client characteristic (e.g., age), and low intervention dose that did not induce the anticipated mechanisms responsible for producing the anticipated changes in the outcomes. Methodological factors are illustrated with issues with fidelity of intervention delivery and nonadherence to the intervention. For interventions that demonstrate the hypothesized causal effects, the next step is an evaluation of their effectiveness.

The main concern of the third evaluation phase is to investigate the effectiveness of interventions. Effectiveness refers to the extent to which the intervention produces the intended beneficial outcomes when delivered under the real world, or usual conditions of day-to-day practice. Under the latter conditions, the intervention is implemented (1) by health professionals with different levels of theoretical knowledge, practical experience, and skills in delivering the intervention; (2) to clients presenting with a range of personal and clinical characteristics representing different subgroups of the target population, and with varying levels of perceived acceptability of and/or motivation to apply the intervention; and (3) in practice settings with different contextual features that may affect the implementation of the intervention (Sidani & Braden, 1998; Tunis et al., 2003). Practical or pragmatic clinical trials are considered appropriate for evaluating the effectiveness of interventions (Thorpe et al., 2009). The results point to the characteristics of clients who benefit to different degrees from the intervention implemented in what format and at what dose; by health professionals with personal characteristics and professional qualifications; and in with what type of context. In other words, the findings of effectiveness studies provide the knowledge health professionals need to properly deliver the intervention in the context of day-to-day practice.

1.2.3 Translation of interventions

Translation involves the development of guidelines for implementing the intervention in day-to-day practice and the incorporation of the guidelines as part of usual practice. To be useful in informing practice, the guidelines should be specific, describing (1) the presenting problem amenable to treatment by the intervention, with a particular emphasis on the aspects of the problem targeted; (2) the active ingredients of the intervention and their operationalization in relevant components and actions that should be carried out to claim that the intervention is delivered, (3) the range of nonessential elements of the intervention and their operationalization in mode or format for delivering the intervention in a flexible way that is responsive to clients' preferences; and (4) the minimal and optimal dose associated with the beneficial outcomes and side effects. The guidelines should also explain the mechanisms underlying the intervention effects. Different strategies are used to assist healthcare professionals incorporate the guidelines in their practice.

1.3   Overview of the book

The development of the knowledge base needed to inform nurses of interventions deemed appropriate, acceptable, effective, and safe, and to direct the selection and implementation of interventions that are responsive to clients' characteristics and preferences, should rely on a combination of research methods. The different methods that can be used in the phases of the process for designing, evaluating, and translating interventions are the focus of this book. The methods are discussed relative to each step of the process for designing, evaluating, and translating interventions. The second section of the book (Designing Interventions) concentrates on the design of interventions. The content of this section is consistent with the perspective that interventions are rational, designed in response to a health problem and to achieve desired outcomes. Deductive and inductive strategies are presented to generate a thorough understanding of the problem amenable to intervention, to clarify elements of the intervention (i.e., active ingredients, components, activities, mode of delivery, dose), to develop an intervention theory that explains how the intervention produces the intended outcomes, in what groups of persons, and to design tailored interventions that are responsive to clients' characteristics. The third section of the book (Implementation of Interventions) addresses issues pertaining to the implementation of the intervention. The issues relate to the development of an intervention protocol that directs the delivery of the intervention; training of interventionists in providing the intervention; and the assessment of fidelity with which the intervention is implemented. In the fourth section (Evaluation of Interventions), conventional and alternative research designs and methods are presented for examining the feasibility, acceptability, efficacy, and effectiveness of interventions. The role of preferences for treatment and methods for examining their influence within a research context are discussed. The fifth and last section of the book (Translation of Interventions) covers issues and strategies for translating interventions into the day-to-day practice setting.

Section 2

Designing Interventions

Chapter 2

Overview of Designing Interventions

For interventions to be appropriate, acceptable, effective, safe, and efficient, they should be carefully designed. The process for developing interventions is systematic, beginning with gaining an understanding of the presenting problem requiring remediation, moving to clarifying the elements of the intervention and elaborating on the operationalization of the intervention elements, and ending with the generation of the intervention theory. The application of this process requires comprehensive knowledge of the topical or substantive area of interest, critical thinking, use of multiple research methods, and diligent work. To appreciate the importance of this systematic process, this chapter presents definitions of what constitutes an intervention and a presenting problem, and highlights the need for different approaches and methods in the process for designing interventions.

2.1 Nursing interventions defined

2.1.1 Definition of interventions

Interventions constitute the essential component of nursing, playing a pivotal role (Conn et al., 2001) in characterizing the discipline and distinguishing nursing practice from that of other health professionals. Although the term "intervention" is widely used in written (e.g., books, published research reports) and verbal (e.g., end of shift report in the practice setting) communications, only three formal definitions have been located in the nursing literature:

(1) Bulecheck and McCloskey (1992) defined a nursing intervention as an autonomous action based on a scientific rationale that is executed to benefit the client in a predicted way related to the nursing diagnosis and the stated goals.
(2) Sidani and Braden (1998) presented the following definition of interventions: Interventions refer to treatments, therapies, procedures, or actions

Design, Evaluation, and Translation of Nursing Interventions, First Edition.
Souraya Sidani and Carrie Jo Braden.
© 2011 John Wiley & Sons, Inc. Published 2011 by John Wiley & Sons, Inc.

implemented by health professionals to and with clients, in a particular situation, to move the clients' condition toward desired health outcomes that are beneficial to the clients.

(3) Burns and Grove (2005) stated that nursing interventions are defined as deliberate cognitive, physical, or verbal activities performed with, or on behalf of, individuals and their families, that are directed toward accomplishing particular therapeutic objectives relative to individuals' health and well-being.

A thorough examination of the three definitions points to two key attributes that define the term "intervention." The first attribute is that an intervention is essentially an action. It involves the application of functions that are cognitive, verbal, and/or physical in nature, or performance of behaviors. The second attribute is rationality. Rationality implies that an intervention is not provided haphazardly or mindlessly. Rather, an intervention is given in response to a problem, and the action is directed toward attainment of preset goals or achievement of beneficial outcomes. These attributes underscore the importance of carefully designing interventions that rests on an adequate understanding of the presenting health-related problem, a thorough delineation of the actions to be performed, and a clear specification of the outcomes to be achieved.

What distinguishes nursing interventions from those developed and/or implemented by other healthcare professionals is that the actions comprising nursing interventions are within the scope of nursing practice, as delineated by relevant regulatory professional organizations. The scope of nursing practice may differ across regions within a country and across countries, based on the values held in a particular society and the resources available for meeting the health needs of the population. For instance, in rural, remote areas, nurses' scope of practice may be extended, where they are ascribed responsibilities and functions that will allow them to triage and manage emergencies. Despite this variability, nursing actions encompass independent and interdependent functions (Evers, 2003). Independent functions consist of responsibilities for which only nurses are held accountable (Sidani & Irvine, 1999). The initiation and implementation of independent nursing interventions is under nurses' control. For example, client education and pressure ulcer management are independent interventions. Interdependent functions entail responsibilities that are dependent on the functions of other health professionals for their accomplishment (Sidani & Irvine). Accordingly, the implementation of interdependent nursing interventions requires collaboration between nurses and other professionals. These interventions are exemplified with blood products administration and case management.

Nursing interventions are given to, on behalf of, or with clients, depending on the nature of the actions to be performed. In some instances, nurses deliver the interventions to clients with minimal participation of the clients in carrying out the actions comprising the interventions such as administration of blood products. In other instances, nurses carry out the interventions with the agreement but on behalf of clients as may happen when arranging home care postdischarge from hospital. Last, and as is the case with many interventions, nurses perform the activities with the active participation of the clients, where clients assume responsibility and actually engage in some of these actions. Cognitive-behavioral interventions aimed at promoting self-management or engagement in healthy behaviors are examples of the latter type of nursing interventions.

In summary, nursing interventions are actions performed by nurses in response to health-related problems experienced by clients to achieve desired outcomes. The nurses' actions are undertaken independently or in collaboration with other professionals. They are carried out on behalf of or with clients. Clients include individual persons, families, or communities.

2.1.2 Characteristics of interventions

Interventions are generally characterized in relation to the overarching preset goal, the type of actions comprising them, and level of complexity. As explained in Section 2.1.1, nursing interventions are given, and therefore designed, in response to problems with which clients present that require remediation or prevention, with the ultimate goal of maintaining or promoting health.

The overarching preset goal refers to the overall direction of the actions constituting the intervention relative to the identified health-related problem. Interventions can be designed to either prevent or manage problems. For example, changing a nonambulatory patient's position in bed every 2 hours aims to prevent pressure ulcer, and instructing persons with asthma to avoid irritants such as dust and smoke is directed at preventing dyspnea. A program of physical activity is implemented to manage fatigue, whereas having a patient listen to relaxing music assists in managing pain. Health promotion and smoking cessation are directed at promoting engagement in healthy behaviors and overall health. Presetting the overarching goal of an intervention to prevent or manage a presenting problem is contingent on the nature of the problem, the seriousness of its consequences, and the aspect(s) of the problem amenable to change.

The type of actions comprising interventions relate to their nature relative to the domains of health they target. Thus, interventions can be physical, behavioral, psychological, cognitive, or social in nature. The Nursing Intervention Classification (Bulecheck & McCloskey, 2000) offers example of different specific actions within each type of interventions. Physical interventions are illustrated with performance of range-of-motion exercises for a bedridden person. Behavioral interventions are exemplified with provision of feedback on the appropriateness of activities performed by a person, whereas psychological interventions are exemplified by offering emotional support, and cognitive interventions by cognitive reframing of beliefs. Social interventions are illustrated with the initiation and facilitation of support group. In addition, most of the interdependent nursing interventions are founded on actions related to communication with other health professionals, and on coordination or management of services needed by clients. An example of communication action is relaying information on changes in clients' status to physicians, and an example of coordination action is making arrangements for blood work or physiotherapy. When designing nursing interventions, the type of actions selected to form the intervention is determined by the nature of the presenting problem the intervention targets.

The level of complexity reflects the number of components and respective actions within a component constituting an intervention. A component of an intervention is a set of interrelated actions that are directed toward addressing a particular aspect of the presenting problem and toward reaching a common objective. For example, psycho-educational interventions consist of two distinct components: (1) psychological and (2) educational. The psychological component includes specific actions such as exploration of feelings and provision of emotional support, geared at enhancing psychological well-being. The educational component encompasses provision of information on the illness and its treatment in writing (e.g., pamphlet) and verbal discussion of strategies to implement the treatment plan; these actions aim at increasing knowledge about illness and treatment. Nursing interventions vary in level of complexity. Interventions with low level of complexity are simple and entail one action or one component focused on addressing a specific aspect of a problem. Changing patients' position in bed is an example of simple interventions. Interventions with high level of complexity involve multiple components and their respective actions, targeting different aspects or determinants of the same problem or different interrelated problems. Behavioral therapy for insomnia is a complex intervention addressing the same presenting problem, insomnia. It includes (1) sleep education providing information on the functions of sleep and variability in sleep needs across individuals; (2) sleep hygiene, which consists of general strategies to promote sleep such as avoiding caffeine and nicotine before bedtime; and (3) stimulus control therapy, which comprises a set of recommendations for activities to avoid or to perform around bedtime and when awake after sleep onset with the goal of reassociating the bed and the bedroom with sleep. Strategies to promote adherence to behavioral therapy for insomnia also may be incorporated as part of intervention delivery. Diabetes self-management education is a complex intervention addressing different interrelated problems. This complex intervention is designed to assist persons with diabetes modify behaviors related to diet and physical activity that contribute to increased blood sugar and engage in new behaviors related to symptom monitoring and management that prevent complications of diabetes such as hypoglycemia. As implied in this discussion, the level of intervention complexity is consistent with the nature and number of problems to be addressed.

The design of nursing interventions should account for the three characteristics: (1) overarching preset goal, (2) type of actions, and (3) level of complexity. These characteristics vary with the number and nature of the presenting problem and the aspect of the problem amenable to change.

2.2   Presenting problems

2.2.1   Definition of problem

Generally speaking, a problem is a situation in need of a solution. Clients, including individuals, families, or communities, present with a wide range of problems that nursing professionals are expected to address independently or in collaboration with other healthcare professionals. In health-related disciplines, such as nursing, problems are termed "diagnoses." Each discipline, and specialty within a discipline, has identified a list of problems or diagnoses that its respective professionals are responsible or accountable to address. For example, psychiatry and psychology developed the Diagnostic and Statistical Manual of Mental Disorders (DSM). Similarly, in nursing, the North American Nursing Diagnosis Association generated a compendium of diagnoses or problems that nurses can address independently. The problems are categorized as actual or potential.

An actual problem is an existing condition with which clients present and that requires remediation. It reflects an alteration in functioning in any domain of health that clients actually experience at the moment. Examples of actual problems include symptoms such as pain and fatigue; difficulty performing activities of daily living; nonadherence to treatment; emotional stress; an epidemic or spread of an infectious disease in the community; and burden experienced by caregivers of persons with dementia. In these instances, nursing interventions aim at managing the presenting actual problem, that is, improving the problem experience, treating or resolving it, or assisting clients to manage it successfully.

A potential problem refers to a discrepancy between a current condition (i.e., the way things are) and an ideal condition (i.e., the way things ought to be). It reflects an inadequacy in the type or level of current functioning that increases the probability of resulting in an actual problem or dysfunction. Engagement in what has been considered "unhealthy" behaviors illustrates a potential problem. For instance, smoking increases the likelihood of shortness of breath or dyspnea and lung cancer, and physical inactivity is associated with high risks for fatigue and obesity. In these instances, nursing interventions are geared toward preventing the potential problem, that is, reducing the chances of its occurrence.

In summary, problems are conditions with which clients present that require improvement or remediation. Nursing interventions are designed and/or implemented to address presenting problems. The presentation of problems varies along different dimensions (discussed next).

2.2.2   Characteristics of problems

Problems, whether actual or potential, vary in nature, manifestations, causative factors or determinants, and level of severity among different client populations and/or under different circumstances. The nature of the problem reflects the domain of health in which the alteration or discrepancy in function takes place. Problems are experienced in any one or a combination of the following domains of health:

(1) Biophysiological
(2) Physical
(3) Psycho-behavioral
(4) Social

Examples of problems within each domain include: high blood pressure in the biophysiological domain; difficulty walking in the physical domain; alcohol or substance abuse in the psycho-behavioral domain; and lack of a social support network in the social domain. Some problems are conceptualized as experienced in more than one domain of health. Symptoms, for instance, encompass changes in usual function, feeling, or behavior (biophysiological domain); that are consciously sensed and cognitively interpreted by clients to ascribe it a meaning, which shapes the clients' response to the symptom (psycho-behavioral domain) (Dodd et al., 2001; University of California, San Francisco, School of Nursing Symptom Management Faculty Group, 1994).

Manifestations of a problem refer to the changes that reflect the problem. In other words, they are the specific attributes that indicate the presence of the problem. The manifestations are objectively observed or subjectively reported in any domain of health. Although the manifestations empirically define problems and distinguish a particular problem from others, they may differ within and across client populations. For instance, Middle Eastern and Asian persons tend to report somatic manifestations of stress, that is, they experience physiological or physical changes such as abdominal pain, in association with stress, more so than persons from a European descent; the latter group tends to express stress in the psychological domain such as anxiety.

Causative factors or determinants of a problem are circumstances or conditions that contribute to the problem. It is often the case that multiple factors conduce to the occurrence of a particular problem. The factors can co-occur simultaneously or interrelate interactively to produce the problem. The specific factors or combination of factors contributing to the problem could vary across client populations or within the same population over time. For example, dyspnea may be triggered by a host of factors related to weather conditions, environmental allergens, and emotional stress in clients with asthma.

Level of severity refers to the intensity with which the problem is experienced. It has to do with "how badly" the problem is perceived. Severe problems are often considered distressing, having serious consequences, and interfering with clients' well-being. The level of a problem's severity is subjectively perceived by clients. Thus, clients experiencing the same problem may rate it at different levels of severity. The obvious example is the experience of postoperative pain, where individuals subject to the same surgical procedure report varying levels of pain and respond to it differently; some prefer to endure severe pain whereas others demand immediate relief.

The design of nursing interventions should take into consideration the characteristics of the presenting problem. Actual or potential problems experienced in different domains of health and at different levels of severity and in relation to different causative factors demand interventions of different nature and dose.

2.3 Design of interventions

As mentioned previously, the design of interventions is based on a lucid, in-depth knowledge of the presenting health-related problem. This comprehensive understanding of the nature of the problem, its manifestations, causative factors or determinants, and level of severity is necessary to identify the specific characteristic or aspect of the problem that is amenable to change, improvement, or treatment. The identified aspect becomes the focus of attention and drives the generation, selection, and specification of the active ingredients that constitute the intervention. The basic principle is that the intervention actions that operationalize the active ingredients are responsive to and consistent with the aspect of the problem amenable to treatment. Specifically, the general category of the problem, that is, actual or potential, points to the overarching goal preset for the intervention. Interventions are designed to manage an actual problem or to prevent a potential problem. Some problems may not be addressed directly; however, it may be more appropriate and feasible to design interventions that target their causative factors. Therefore, acting upon determinants contributes to the prevention of the problem. The nature of the problem and its manifestations highlight the type and number of actions needed to remedy, resolve, or prevent the presenting problem, which determine the complexity of the intervention. The level of problem severity indicates the dose with which the intervention is to be given. Accordingly, the generation, selection, and specification of the intervention's active ingredients and respective actions demand a systematic process of critical analysis of the consistency between the presenting problem and the elements of the intervention.

The process for designing interventions involves deductive and/or inductive analytic approaches. Both approaches are applied to gain an understanding of the problem and to specify the active ingredients and respective actions of the intervention. However, each approach accomplishes these goals in a different way and yields variable but complementary knowledge on the problem and the intervention. Both approaches are needed to develop appropriate, acceptable, effective, safe, and efficient interventions.

The deductive approach is theory-based, relying on middle range and practice theories in the process of designing interventions. Middle range or explanatory theories describe the problem. They define the nature and manifestations of the problem; specify the factors contributing to the problem and explain the mechanisms linking the factors to the problem; depict the levels of severity with which the problem may be experienced; and identify the consequences of the problem. In addition, middle range theories point to the aspect of the problem amenable to change or treatment, actions that are useful to address the identified aspect of the problem, and the goal that the intervention is set to achieve. Practice or change theories provide information on mode, format, and strategies for successfully implementing the intervention actions, on the dose with which the intervention is to be given to achieve the preset goal, and on the human and material resources needed for delivering the intervention (National Institutes of Health-National Cancer Institute, 2000; Sidani & Braden, 1998).

The theoretical knowledge embedded in middle range and practice theories is critical for developing interventions that are appropriate, effective, and safe. The deductive approach yields theory-based interventions comprising of actions that are carefully carved to address the presenting problem; that is, the intervention actions are reasonable, sound, and consistent with the nature of the problem, capable of successfully managing or preventing the problem, with no or minimal side effects. Emerging empirical evidence indicates that, in the field of health behaviors, theoretically based interventions are more effective in changing the targeted health behaviors as compared to interventions that are not informed by theory (Painter et al., 2008). Even if found effective, theory-based interventions may not be acceptable to clients of diverse backgrounds or efficient when implemented in the practice setting. The inductive approach is proposed for enhancing the acceptability and efficiency of interventions.

The inductive approach is experiential, relying on input or feedback of clients who will receive the intervention and of health professionals who will deliver the intervention in the practice setting. The inductive approach consists of involving clients and health professionals in activities aimed at clarifying the presenting problem, identifying the aspect of the problem amenable to treatment, and specifying the goal and actions of the intervention. Participation of clients and professionals in this process is well illustrated in the collaborative approach to research (Bryman, 2001). A variety of strategies could be used to actively engage clients and professionals in this process. Some strategies focus on developing an understanding of the problem and related intervention actions that are grounded in the clients' and/or professionals' perspectives. Other strategies are devised to elicit the clients' and/or professionals' input regarding the problem and the intervention as conceptualized on the basis of relevant theories. The clients' and professionals' input guides the refinement of the intervention and/or adaptation of the intervention to be responsive to their preferences and to be feasible within particular settings. Accordingly, the interventions are acceptable and efficient, which are characteristics that facilitate their uptake and incorporation in day-to-day practice.

The strategies used to generate an understanding of the problem and to design interventions are discussed in the next chapter. Specific methods and procedures for applying the strategies within the deductive and inductive approaches are described and illustrated with examples taken from the literature where available, or our own work.

Chapter 3
Understanding the Problem

The development of a thorough and comprehensive understanding of the presenting problem requiring intervention is the first and critical step in the process of designing interventions (Campbell et al., 2007). This understanding entails clarification of the nature of the problem, its manifestations, causative factors or determinants, level of severity with which it may be experienced, and consequences. Different approaches can be utilized, independently or in combination, to gain an understanding of the problem. The described approaches reflect the use of top-down and bottom-up or empowerment approaches to the clarification of the problem and the design of interventions; however, they do not address the issue of the party (i.e., health professionals or clients) assuming the responsibility for naming the problem. Labonte (1993), Laverack and Labonte (2000), Braden (2002), and others (Kelly et al., 2010) provide information about involvement and participation of stakeholder groups in problem identification and naming.

The knowledge gained during the described approaches to understanding the problem is integrated into a theory of the problem. The theory of the problem guides the design of the intervention to address the presenting problem. The focus of this chapter is on the description of three general approaches for gaining an understanding of the problem: (1) theoretical, (2) empirical, and (3) experiential. A framework for combining approaches is presented.

3.1 Theoretical approach for understanding the problem

The theoretical approach relies on relevant theories to develop an understanding of the presenting problem requiring intervention. Generally speaking, a theory is a set of ideas that explain phenomena occurring in the world. Phenomena include events, behaviors, or situations encountered within particular contexts or circumstances. The theory consists of a group of statements, based on careful reasoning and/or evidence that present a systematic and logical view of the phenomena. The statements are logically organized to identify, define, and describe the phenomena and to explain the relationships among them. The relationships represent direct and indirect associations among the phenomena.

Design, Evaluation, and Translation of Nursing Interventions, First Edition.
Souraya Sidani and Carrie Jo Braden.
© 2011 John Wiley & Sons, Inc. Published 2011 by John Wiley & Sons, Inc.

A direct association reflects an immediate linkage between two phenomena, where one phenomenon flows straightforwardly from or is a function of the other. An indirect association can take either of two forms: (1) moderated or (2) mediated. A relationship between two phenomena is considered moderated when it is affected by another phenomenon, called moderator. Thus, the moderator is the condition under which the relationship exists whereby the occurrence, strength or magnitude, and/or direction of the relationship vary according to the value of the moderator (Holmbeck, 1997). A relationship between two phenomena is considered mediated when another phenomenon intervenes between the two. This mediating phenomenon provides an explanation of how or why the two phenomena are related. It specifies the mechanism underlying the relationship, whereby one phenomenon influences the mediator, which, in turn, affects the other phenomenon (MacKinnon & Fairchild, 2009).

The theories of relevance in the first step of the intervention design process are descriptive, explanatory theories providing a comprehensive view of the presenting problem. Middle range theories are explanatory and, therefore, considered appropriate and useful in generating an understanding of the problem. These theories (1) identify the problem, the factors that cause or contribute to the problem, and the consequences of the problem, that is, its impact on functioning and health-related quality of life; (2) define the problem at the conceptual level by clarifying its nature and essential attributes and at the operational level by specifying the manifestations of the problem; (3) delineate the relationships between the causative factors, the problem and/or the consequences by specifying the nature (i.e., whether they are direct, moderated, or mediated) and the direction (i.e., whether they are positive or negative) of the relationships; and (4) explain the mechanisms underlying the proposed relationships.

To be useful in generating an understanding of the presenting problem, middle range theories need to be relevant to the health-related problem of concern. This necessitates a clarification of the problem, the availability of middle range theories that present a systematic view of the problem, and consistency in the definition of the problem between the two. Clarification of the problem entails delineation of the nature of the problem with which clients present. This is done by addressing the question: What is the problem about? It may be related to the performance of a health behavior, a self-care activity, or a skill; or it may be a symptom or an alteration in physical, psychological, or social functioning; or it may be lack of knowledge about the health condition. Clarification also involves specification of the problem as experienced by a particular client population under particular contexts, which is necessary for generating a relevant understanding of the problem and subsequently for designing interventions that are responsive to the characteristics and contexts of the target client population.

Once the problem is clarified, the search is for middle range theories that explain the problem. The search covers a wide range of sources, including textbooks, published articles, or professional Web sites addressing the problem.

The attention is on theoretical literature for the purpose of identifying relevant theories that offer a systematic conceptualization of the problem. Presentations of the theories are reviewed carefully to generate a clear definition of the problem and each of the contributing factors, and a comprehensive account of the proposed relationships among them. Middle range theories are selected to generate an understanding of the presenting problem if they define it in a way that is consistent with its nature as clarified. The literature reporting results of studies that tested the selected theories is also reviewed to determine the extent to which the conceptual and operational definitions of the problem and the proposed relationships among them are supported empirically (Brug et al., 2005). Of special interest are studies that tested the middle range theories in the particular client population and the context of interest. The findings of the latter studies facilitate the adaptation, that is, the operationalization of the problem, causative factors, and propositions among them to the particular target population and/or context. Middle range theories with adequate empirical support in different populations and contexts, especially those of interest, are used to develop the theory of the problem (described later in the chapter).

To illustrate, let us assume that the presenting problem relates to engagement in physical activity. A clarification of its nature entails viewing it in terms of performance of a health behavior, and specifying it in terms of the action to be targeted and the context in which it is to be carried out (Fishbein & Yzer, 2003). Thus, the problem of engagement in physical activity can be specified as walking for 30 minutes three times a week for women with full-time employment. The literature review reveals several middle range theories of health behaviors that provide comprehensive views of the problem. Of those, the social cognitive theory and theory of reasoned action/planned behavior have been frequently used to generate an understanding of factors contributing to engagement in different health behaviors, including physical activity, in various client populations. The two theories focus on health behaviors; however, they propose different sets of determinants of health behavior performance. The social cognitive theory posits two main determinants: (1) beliefs in the benefits of the behavior and (2) the personal agency or self-efficacy regarding performance of the behavior. The theory of reasoned action/planned behavior explains the interrelationships among factors that influence behavior performance. Specifically, this theory proposes that behavior performance is directly determined by the intention to do the behavior; intention is a function of attitudes toward and subjective norms concerning behavior performance; attitudes and norms are influenced by the beliefs held by persons. Fishbein (2000) ascertained that these types of factors are relevant determinants of health behaviors in almost any client population. Therefore, it can be deduced that they also are applicable to the sedentary employed women targeted in the example. For instance, Vallance et al. (2008) based the development of a guidebook (i.e., the intervention) to promote physical activity in breast cancer survivors on the propositions of the theory of planned behavior. Specifically, the authors conceptualized the problem as a health behavior that is directly influenced by intention to engage in the behavior. Intention, in turn, is determined by attitudes toward the behavior, subjective norms, and behavioral control. Attitudes reflect the instrumental (i.e., perceived benefits) and affective (i.e., level of enjoyment) evaluations of behavior performance. Subjective norms represent social pressures to perform the behavior as perceived by the individual. Behavioral control is the degree of personal control the persons perceive they have over performing the behavior; it is operationalized into self-efficacy and controllability. Attitudes, subjective norms, and behavioral control are affected by underlying beliefs about the behavior and its benefits.

The use of the theoretical approach to generate an understanding of the presenting problem is advantageous in that theories provide a generalizable conceptualization of the problem and its determinants (Foy et al., 2007). By transcending individual cases, theories describe the nature of the problem, identify the causative factors that contribute to the problem, and offer an accurate account of how the causative factors affect the problem directly or indirectly. Thus, theories prevent the danger of relying on practical experience. They help understand the mechanisms or processes linking the causative factors with the presenting problem and the context under which the processes operate. This understanding of the problem guides the search for specific aspects of the problem or its causative factors to be targeted by the intervention, with the ultimate goal of successfully addressing the presenting problem (Green, 2000; Michie & Abraham, 2004; Michie et al., 2008; Pillemer et al., 2003; Rothman, 2004). For instance, conceptualizing engagement in physical activity, specifically walking for 30 minutes three times a week, within the perspective of the social cognitive theory highlights the need for interventions that target the sedentary employed women's beliefs about the benefits of walking and perceived self-efficacy regarding this behavior. Briefly, theories are powerful tools to make informed decisions when designing interventions (Fishbein & Yzer, 2003).

The theoretical approach has some limitations in gaining a comprehensive understanding of the presenting problem. The reliance on one single middle range theory constrains the perspectives on the nature and determinants of the problem to those identified in the theory. Therefore, additional causal factors that may contribute to the problem could be missed, thereby limiting the capacity to account for all possible factors pertinent to a complex problem experienced by particular client populations (Green, 2000). For instance, the social cognitive theory omits environmental influences on performance of health behaviors such as neighborhood safety that may prevent employed women to walk for 30 minutes after returning from work. Further, for many of the health-related problems with which clients present, there is a limited, if any, number of relevant middle range theories that are useful in generating an adequate understanding of the problem and all its possible determinants. In addition, of the available middle range theories, very few have been subjected to extensive empirical test across the range of client populations seen in practice (Brug et al., 2005). For example, nurses provide care to individual clients who experience specific physical (e.g., nausea and vomiting) or psychological (e.g., anxiety) symptoms. For almost all symptoms, there is no well-articulated theories that clearly define the symptom at the conceptual and operational levels and specify its key determinants within the physiological and psychological domains, in different client populations. In these instances, the empirical approach would be helpful in gaining a comprehensive and accurate understanding of the problem.

3.2   Empirical approach for understanding the problem

The empirical approach relies on systematically generated evidence to gain an understanding of the presenting problem requiring intervention. The evidence is obtained through a careful review of pertinent literature. The literature encompasses quantitative or qualitative studies that investigated the problem, as well as reviews that integrated or synthesized the evidence pertaining to the problem. Quantitative studies of interest are those that used nonexperimental, cross-sectional, or longitudinal designs to describe the presenting problem and examine its relationships with related concepts (i.e., determinants and consequences), in particular, client populations under particular contexts. Results of *descriptive* cross-sectional studies clarify the nature of the problem, its manifestations, and level of severity as reported by clients at one point in time, whereas those of longitudinal studies indicate changes in the manifestations and severity levels of the problem across occasions. Awareness of changes in the problem over time is informative as it guides the selection of the specific dose and timing for delivering the intervention and it directs the estimation of the magnitude of the intervention effects on the problem, anticipated following implementation of the intervention above and beyond natural recovery or resolution of the problem. Results of *correlational* cross-sectional studies delineate the nature of the association between the problem, and its determinants and consequences. Findings of correlational longitudinal studies provide evidence of the sustainability of these relationships, and have the potential to inform which factors preceded the problem; such temporal sequencing among concepts is required to support naturally occurring causal linkages. Qualitative studies involve those that focused on understanding the presenting problem from the clients' perspective. Of interest are studies that elicited clients' experience of the problem, inquired about factors that contributed to the problem and the impact of the problem on the clients' well-being, and generated a model or theory summarizing the intricate relations among factors, problem, and consequences.

All types of literature reviews are useful in developing a comprehensive understanding of the presenting problem: concept analysis, meta-analysis, and meta-synthesis. Concept analyses consist of reviewing theoretical, empirical, and gray literature pertaining to the problem of interest and synthesizing the literature for the purposes of clarifying the problem in terms of its essential attributes, defining it and distinguishing it from related concepts, and identifying its antecedents and consequences (Hupcey & Penrod, 2005; Walker &

Avant, 2001). Accordingly, results of concept analyses shed light on the nature, manifestations, determinants, and consequences of the presenting problem. Meta-analyses involve a critical appraisal and synthesis of empirical evidence related to the presenting problem. Of relevance are meta-analyses set to synthesize results of quantitative studies that examined the relationships between the problem and its determinants. Findings of these meta-analyses indicate the extent to which the relationships are replicated across populations and contexts, the expected direction and magnitude of the relationships, and the factors that moderate or mediate the relationships. Meta-syntheses entail a synthesis of findings obtained from qualitative studies that investigated the presenting problem (Sandelowski & Barraso, 2007). Although the application of this type of literature review has been limited to date, its findings can provide a comprehensive list of factors that contribute to the problem and a model of the interrelationships among them, as illustrated in Guruge et al. (2010).

The application of the empirical approach comprises the following steps:

(1) *Clarifying the problem:* This first step involves delineating the nature of the presenting problem and the characteristics of the client population experiencing the problem, as described in the previous section. This step is important for specifying the key words to be used in searching the literature and the criteria for selecting literature sources. The goal is to enhance relevance of the literature.

(2) *Specifying the key words:* The key words encompass the terms used to refer to the problem, including the specific words and its synonyms frequently appearing in the scientific literature and mentioned in lay conversation or documents. For instance, key words for searching the literature on fatigue include: fatigue, tiredness, exhaustion, weariness, weakness, lethargy, lassitude, and lack of energy. The terms referring to the problem are used independently or in combination with other key words representing the target client population, context, and/or determinants of the problem. In the example of fatigue, additional terms may include: breast cancer (for target population), cancer treatment-related fatigue (for context), and chemotherapy or insomnia (for determinant).

(3) *Specifying the selection criteria:* The criteria ensure literature sources that addressed any aspect of the problem (i.e., manifestations, levels of severity, determinants) are selected for review. Additional criteria are preset to include high-quality studies. Quality is defined in terms of appropriately preventing or addressing biases or threats to validity that are specific to each type of design.

(4) *Conducting the search:* The search for relevant literature is carried out using multiple databases such as CINAHL, MEDLINE, and PUBMED. The search may yield a large number of sources whose abstracts should be reviewed to determine if they meet the selection criteria. Having a list of the preset general criteria related to the problem, population, and context facilitates the review. The content of the abstract, specifically purpose, sample, and results are evaluated for its fit with the criteria. The results

of this evaluation are documented on the list and are used to report on the number of sources that did and did not meet the selection criteria and the reasons for excluding them from the review. Copies of the selected sources are obtained for full review.

(5) *Extracting data:* Selected sources are carefully reviewed to extract methodological and substantive data summarized in Table 3.1. The data extracted from all studies are incorporated in a table or database in preparation for integration or synthesis of findings. Based on the preset selection criteria, studies of high quality are included in the literature integration or synthesis.

(6) *Synthesizing data:* The synthesis is done at two levels, within and across types of research design. For quantitative studies, (1) descriptive results pertaining to the prevalence, manifestations, and severity of the problem are analyzed descriptively to determine the range and mean values reported across studies; (2) correlational results pertaining to the association between the problem and its determinants and/or consequences are synthesized using the vote counting method (Cooper, 1998) and/or the meta-analysis method. The vote counting method involves identifying the number of studies that found statistically nonsignificant relationship between the problem and a determinant, statistically significant relationship in the expected direction, or statistically significant relationship in the unexpected direction. A determinant is considered to contribute to the problem if it showed significant association in the expected direction in the majority of the studies (>50%) included in the synthesis. The meta-analytic method complements the vote counting method by providing an estimate of the magnitude of the relationship. This is accomplished by averaging the effect sizes obtained across studies. For qualitative studies, the emerging themes that reflect manifestations and consequences of the problem or that identify factors that contribute to the problem are integrated using the strategies suggested by Sandelowski and Barraso (2007). Alternatively, a modified vote counting method can be applied to determine the number of studies that reported the same theme.

Once the synthesis is completed within each category of research approach (i.e., quantitative and qualitative), the integration across approaches is carried out. Integration consists of comparing and contrasting the synthesized findings obtained with each approach, and identifying consistencies and discrepancies across approaches. Consistencies indicate convergence in recognizing manifestations, determinants, and consequences of the presenting problem commonly experienced by clients. Discrepancies reflect, in addition to differences in research approaches, variability in the problem experience among client populations and/or contexts. Literature reviews have been frequently used to understand the nature, manifestations, determinants, and consequences of symptoms experienced by a variety of client populations. For instance, Visovsky and Schneider (2003) synthesized what is known about cancer-related fatigue; Sidani (2003) conducted a concept analysis of

Table 3.1 Methodological and substantive data to be extracted for literature review

Methodological data	Substantive data

Research design:
 Quantitative: Descriptive, correlational, cross-sectional, longitudinal
 Qualitative: Grounded theory, phenomenology
	Target population
	Context or setting
	Presenting problem:
	
	    Conceptual definition
	
	    Operational definition

Sample size
Instruments for assessing the problem, determinants, consequences:
 Content covered
 Method of administration
 Reliability and validity
 Potential biases
Strategies used to minimize bias or to maintain rigor
	Factors contributing to problem:
	
	    Conceptual definition
	    Operational definition
	
	Results:
	 Manifestations of problem
	 Severity of problem
	 Impact of problem on well-being
	 Determinants or factors (1) demonstrating statistically significant relationship with problem, or (2) consistently reported by participants as affecting problem
	 Nature of the relationship between factors and problem: (1) direct or indirect, and specific variable that moderated or mediated relationship; (2) direction (positive or negative) and magnitude (effect size) of relationship

dyspnea; and Mahon et al. (2010) performed a meta-analysis to identify factors that predict anger in adolescents and that moderate the relationship between each predictor and anger.

The advantages of the empirical approach rest on grounding the understanding of the problem on actual or real world data obtained by multiple researchers, from a variety of clients under different contexts, using different methods. Results that are consistent across populations, contexts, and research methods provide a comprehensive and accurate conceptualization of the problem. Comprehensive lists of manifestations, determinants, and consequences of the problem are generated, reflecting different but complementary perspectives. These comprehensive lists reduce the likelihood of omitting a potentially significant indicator or determinant. The range of the severity level with which the problem is experienced by particular client populations or across populations and contexts is identified; further, factors contributing to different levels of problem severity could be revealed. This knowledge is useful in directing the development of interventions and/or the selection of intervention dose to appropriately address the problem presenting at different levels of severity. In contrast, discrepancies in findings point to variability in the problem presentation across client populations and contexts. This is critical to learn about in order to design relevant interventions that are consistent with the characteristics of different target populations and applicable within different contexts.

The limitations of the empirical approach relate to the availability of well-planned and executed studies that investigated the problem in the particular client population and context of interest. Therefore, the relevance and applicability of the integrated findings to the specific client population and context may be questionable. In this case, the experiential approach is appropriate for gaining an understanding of the problem that reflects the perspective of specific population.

3.3　Experiential approach for understanding the problem

The experiential approach relies on input from the target population to generate an understanding of the presenting problem requiring intervention. Using a collaborative participatory approach, researchers work closely with members of the target population to uncover the target population's view of the problem. The approach entails consulting with the members to formulate the target population's perception of the meaning, manifestations, determinants, and consequences of the problem. The consultation is done by holding group sessions. The group discussion offers more advantages than individual interviews to learn about the target population's perspective. Through group discussion, the members have the opportunity to respond to each other's comments; to question ideas; to clarify, elaborate, and explain points; and to reach agreement. This dynamic interaction elicits an in-depth and comprehensive discussion of the problem. Further, the group context promotes open and honest discussion of the problem, and prevents members from giving potentially misleading information. This, in turn, increases the likelihood of gaining collective knowledge of the problem that transcends individual idiosyncrasies and accurately captures the target population's perspective (Vogt et al., 2004). Participants in the group sessions are selected to represent a broad range of those who experience the problem, thereby ensuring that a variety of viewpoints are accounted for when describing the target population's perspective.

The group discussion should be carefully planned and executed in order to capture the target population's conceptualization of the problem. Concept mapping is a useful procedure to attain this goal. Concept mapping is a structured conceptualization process aimed at articulating thoughts or ideas related to a complex phenomenon or situation, and the relationships among them (Trochim, 1989). The process integrates a mix of quantitative and qualitative strategies for data collection and analysis, and involves members of the target population in all steps. As described by Trochim and colleagues (Burke et al., 2005; Trochim & Kane, 2005), the concept mapping process consists of six steps: (1) preparation, (2) generation of statements, (3) structuring of statement, (4) representation, (5) interpretation, and (6) utilization. The application and suggested adaptation of the steps to the generation of the presenting problem conceptualization are presented next.

Step 1: Preparation. In this planning step, decisions are made on the selection of participants and the focal questions to guide the group discussion. As mentioned earlier, participants are individuals who experience the presenting problem of interest and representative of various subgroups of the target population. The subgroups are defined in terms of relevant sociodemographic and/or clinical characteristics. Including a range of participants is necessary to reflect the variety of viewpoints prevalent in the target community. Accordingly, a large number of participants are invited to take part in the different steps of the concept mapping process. Several group sessions are planned to accommodate all participants, where each session includes up to 20 individuals. A series of questions is prepared to elicit participants' view of the features or manifestations of the presenting problem, the factors that contribute to the problem, the relative importance of these factors, and the mechanisms or pathways driving the relationships between the factors and the problem. Additional subquestions are generated to prompt for clarification of ideas or words (e.g., what do you mean?), for delineation of pathways among factors (e.g., can you explain how these factors are related? Which occurred first and brought/led to the other?), and for reaching agreement on points of discussion (e.g., does this reflect your thoughts?).

Step 2: Generation of statements. In this step, selected participants are invited to attend the group session. The session is facilitated by a moderator who is experienced in managing group dynamics, eliciting individual participants' view, and gearing the group toward reaching agreements. The moderator poses the focal questions prepared in Step 1, requests participants to generate statements or items that reflect their thoughts or ideas related to the problem, and prompts for additional information or clarification as needed. Rather than using one broadly stated focal question about the problem as suggested by Burke et al. (2005), such as "What are some characteristics of neighborhoods that could relate in any way, good or bad, to a woman's experience of intimate partner violence" (p. 1396), three questions are asked of participants to obtain their understanding of the problem. The first question focuses on the experience of the presenting problem, with a special attention to its manifestations (i.e., changes in any aspect of functioning or situation they consider as indicative of the presence or occurrence of the problem) and level of severity (i.e., manifestations experienced across the continuum of severity). The second question inquires about factors that contribute to the occurrence and/or severity of the problem (e.g., what happened that led to the problem or what brought this problem?), whereas the third question prompts participants' account of the impact of the problem (e.g., how did the problem affect you?). The moderator and his/her assistant record the participants' responses on resources (e.g., projected computer screen, board, flipchart) visible to all group members. The responses are recorded verbatim in the form of statements as expressed by the participants. Once all statements are documented, the moderator engages the group in a review of the statements to identify duplicates, to recognize irrelevant ones, and to confirm a final list of statements about the presenting problem. The investigators review the transcript of the group session to verify that the generated list of statements accurately and comprehensively reflects the discussion. When several group sessions are held, the investigators consolidate the statements obtained in each session into a final list that consists of an exhaustive nonoverlapping account of all ideas or thoughts about the problem expressed by participants.

Step 3: Structuring of statements. The goal of this step is to gain an understanding of the interrelationships among the ideas or thoughts generated in Step 2 that depict the target population's conceptualization of the problem. This is accomplished by having the group members sort the statements into piles and rate the importance of statements in reflecting the problem. The sorting exercise is done individually by each member of the group. Each statement is printed on a card; each member is given the cards for all statements and instructed to put the cards into piles where each pile contains statements representing similar ideas, as perceived by the individual. No specific directions are given to do the sorting; rather, group members are given the freedom to arrange the statements in a way that is meaningful to them. However, they are requested to place each statement into one pile only, and not to put all statements into one pile. There is no restriction on the number of piles that can be generated. The data obtained with the sorting exercise are entered into a database for analysis. The database consists of a similarity matrix. The rows and columns of the matrix represent the statements, and the data in the cells represent the number of group members who place the pair of statements into the same pile. The similarity matrix is then subjected to multivariate analysis using multidimensional scaling technique and hierarchical cluster analysis. The analysis produces a map that locates nonoverlapping clusters of statements reflecting similar ideas (Trochim & Kane, 2005). In addition to sorting, the group members are asked to rate each statement in terms of its importance or relevance to the problem, on a five-point rating scale. These data are also entered in a database and analyzed descriptively. The Concept System software can integrate the importance rating with the sorting data to indicate clusters of statements with varying levels of importance (Burke et al., 2005). The map is presented to the group members for discussion.

Step 4: Representation. The aim of this step is to choose a final set of clusters that best captures the target population's conceptualization of the problem. To this end, the same or another group of members representative of the target population are invited to a session that proceeds:

(1) By reading the statements generated in Step 2 to familiarize the group members with the ideas or thoughts about the problem.

(2) By showing the map of clusters and explaining that it illustrates the groupings of statements obtained with quantitative data analysis performed in Step 3.

(3) By reviewing the statements grouped into each cluster and eliciting the group members' feedback about the cluster. Specifically, their agreement is sought on the extent to which the statements organized in a cluster reflect a common idea. The members are given the freedom to challenge the presented clusters and to regroup the statements into clusters that are meaningful to them.

(4) By reviewing all clusters located on the map to determine the total number of clusters that reflect conceptually distinct ideas about the problem.

(5) By reviewing the statements within and across clusters that were rated most important to identify the ideas of relevance to the problem.

If more than one session is held, then the investigators reconcile the results and integrate them into one comprehensive set of clusters, which is discussed with the group members in the next step of concept mapping.

Step 5: Interpretation. This step focuses on labeling the clusters and exploring the pathways delineating the relationships among the clusters, as conceived by members of the target population. Again, the members are invited to a session and requested, as a whole group or as small groups of 4–5, to carefully review the statements organized into a cluster in Step 4; to discuss the ideas captured in the statements; to identify the common theme underlying the ideas; and to come up with a label (i.e., short phrase or word) that best describes the theme. The labeling may be based on statements, within a cluster, rated as most important in Step 4. Once all themes are labeled, the moderator engages the group in a cognitive exercise to identify themes that reflect determinants, manifestations, and consequences of the problem, and to diagram relationships among them. Specifically, group members are asked to indicate (1) what each labeled cluster or theme represents: a determinant of the problem, that is, something that takes place before and leads to the problem; a manifestation of the problem, that is, a change in functioning that indicates the presence of the problem; or a consequence of the problem, that is, the impact of the problem on well-being or quality of life; and (2) which determinants are related to each other and to the problem and in what way. Burke et al. (2005) suggested to instruct participants to "create a story" that would share their ideas about how the clusters relate to each other. This exercise results in a concept map that includes concepts emerging from the labeled clusters and linking lines that delineate which concepts are related and in what way (illustrated with arrows linking related concepts), and a set of phrases that describe the proposed linkages among concepts.

Step 6: Utilization. In this step, the investigators involve members of the target population in making decisions on the use of the concept map to design a program, refine services, or guide program evaluation. Within the context of generating an understanding of the presenting problem, the concept map guides the development of the theory of the problem and subsequently the design of interventions.

Burke et al.'s (2005) work illustrates the application of concept mapping to explore women's perception of residential neighborhood factors that contribute to the experience of partner violence.

Concept mapping is a useful procedure for clarifying and accurately reflecting the target population's conceptualization of the presenting problem. The integration of quantitative and qualitative methods for data collection and analysis allows exploration of complex phenomena and enhances the credibility of the results. Obtaining data from individual participants and from the group enhances the richness of, and the likelihood of reaching collective agreement on the resulting conceptualization. The involvement of representatives of the target population in the six steps of the procedure ensures the relevance of the concept map to the population of interest. This point is critical when dealing with specific populations having beliefs and values or perspective on the presenting problem that may not be consistent with what is known about it.

The implementation of concept mapping is challenging. It is resource and labor intensive. The conduct of the group sessions requires availability of suitable location for holding the meetings, of well-trained and experienced group moderators, of skilled research assistants for entering and analyzing data, of appropriate software for analyzing the data, of materials for documenting the statements and for sorting and rating them, and of equipment/technology for visually presenting the clusters/map to the group. In addition, the group sessions are long (about 3–4 hours) and involve intensive cognitive work (Burke et al., 2005). In particular, the statement sorting exercise is burdensome. Cognitive mapping (mentioned by Jackson & Trochim, 2002) is an alternative procedure that can be used to clarify a population's conceptualization of the problem while minimizing burden on participants. Cognitive mapping consists of having group members generate ideas reflecting determinants, manifestations, and consequences of the problem; group similar ideas capturing a common theme; and delineating the relationships among themes. This procedure uses qualitative methods only, applied in a group format, to develop a concept map linking the determinants, manifestations, and consequences of the problem into a cohesive and comprehensive picture. Accordingly, it is appropriate to elicit the perspective on the problem of clients of diverse ethnic or cultural background.

Concept mapping, the procedure recommended for use in experiential approaches to understanding the problem, has some limitations related to the selection of the target population members and the size of the group participating in the six steps. These limitations may lead to biased results that are not applicable to all subgroups of the target population.

Each of the three approaches has advantages and limitations. The implementation of a combination of approaches is effective in generating an understanding of the presenting problem. With such a combination, the limitations inherent in one approach are counter-balanced by those of other approaches. The resulting problem conceptualization is comprehensive, accurate, and relevant to the target population.

3.4 Combined approach for understanding the problem

Intervention mapping is a process to guide intervention planning (Bartholomew et al., 1998; Kok et al., 2004). The process will be described in more details in Chapter 4. The preliminary step of the intervention mapping process is discussed here. This step focuses on the specification of the problem requiring treatment and of its causative factors. This is accomplished by incorporating theory, empirical evidence, and experiential data related to the problem of interest. Once the problem in need of remediation is identified, the literature is searched for empirical evidence about the prevalence, manifestations, and level of severity with which the problem is experienced by the target population or populations with similar characteristics, as well as about determinants or factors associated with the problem. The search is for different categories of factors including behavioral, educational, social, environment or ecological, organizational or health system-related factors, as suggested by the PRECEDE-PROCEED model (Hale, 1998; Mirtz et al., 2005). Once identified, the factors are further classified into: (1) predisposing factors that render clients susceptible or increase their tendency to experience the problem; (2) enabling or precipitating factors that bring about the problem; and (3) reinforcing or perpetuating factors that serve to maintain the problem. The literature search results in a provisional list of causative factors that is confined to what has been traditionally investigated, is limited in scope, and does not offer adequate explanations of the mechanisms linking the factors to the problem. Therefore, theories are identified to provide a broader view of the problem and its determinants. Relevant literature is reviewed to determine the applicability of the theories to the problem of interest. One or more theories may be selected to enlighten the conceptualization of the problem and its determinants, and explain the linkages among them. The integration of empirical evidence and theoretical concepts yields a comprehensive list of factors contributing to the problem and of manifestations of the problem, and a set of propositions describing and clarifying the relationships. Experiential data are sought to determine the target population's view of the problem. This can be done with an inductive approach based on the modified concept mapping procedure, or a deductive approach based on semistructured group interview technique. When the concept mapping procedure is applied, the resulting concept map is integrated with the problem conceptualization derived from empirical evidence and theories in order to enhance the relevance of the problem conceptualization to the target population. The semistructured group interview technique is applied to explore the relevance of the problem conceptualization derived from empirical evidence and theory to the target population. The group interview is conducted with members of the target population. The group moderator (1) informs the members of the presenting problem to be discussed; (2) presents the conceptualization of the problem by identifying its nature, manifestations, and determinants; (3) elicit the

Table 3.2 Theory of insomnia

Nature	Insomnia is conceptualized as a learned behavior. It refers to self-reported disturbed sleep in the presence of adequate opportunity and circumstances for sleep.
Manifestations	Insomnia is manifested in any or a combination of difficulty falling asleep, difficulty staying asleep, and early morning awakening.
Severity	Severity of insomnia is operationalized in terms of the time to fall asleep, the time awake during the night, the number of nights it is experienced, and the score on the insomnia severity index. Insomnia is considered severe if it takes clients more than 30 minutes to fall asleep and/or the clients are awake for more than 30 minutes during the night on at least 3 nights per week. Insomnia Severity Index scores in the range of 15–21 reflect clinical insomnia of moderate severity, and in the range of 22–28 indicate clinical insomnia of high severity.
Determinants	Three categories of factors contribute to insomnia: 1. Predisposing factors, which increase clients' vulnerability to develop insomnia, including arousability, familial or genetic tendency, age, and gender. 2. Precipitating factors (e.g., onset of illness and stress related events) disrupt sleep. Clients begin to sleep poorly. 3. Perpetuating factors represent strategies clients use in an attempt to deal with poor sleep but they serve to fuel or maintain the sleep problem. These include: extended time in bed, irregular sleep schedules, and engaging in activities in bed that are incompatible with falling asleep or back to sleep (e.g., reading, eating, watching TV, listening to music, reviewing the day's events and/or problem-solving).
Consequences	The consequences of insomnia include daytime fatigue, irritability, difficulty concentrating, and difficulty performing activities of daily living.

members' perception of the relevance of the conceptualization by inquiring about the individual members' personal or vicarious experience of the problem; (4) asks the members about additional determinants and manifestations of the problem frequently encountered by the target population but not represented in the conceptualization; and (5) engages them in discussion to reach agreement on most important and relevant determinants and manifestations of the problem and to clarify their understanding of the proposed linkages among the problem and its determinants.

The utility of the combined approach rests on the triangulation of information that yields a comprehensive, broad, yet validated conceptualization of the presenting problem that is relevant to the target population. However, its implementation is time consuming and labor intensive.

3.5   Theory of the problem

Whether derived using the theoretical, empirical, experiential, or combined approach, the resulting understanding of the problem is integrated into a theory. The theory presents a coherent conceptualization of the nature of the problem, its manifestations, level of severity, and causative factors or determinants, as well as consequences. The nature of the problem is the domain of health, functioning, or well-being in which the problem occurs. The manifestations are the changes experienced by clients that indicate the presence of the problem. Level of severity is the gravity or intensity with which the problem is experienced, and/or the perceived distress induced by the problem. Causative factors or determinants are factors that contribute to or cause the problem. Consequences are the sequels or effects or impact of the problem on the clients' health and well-being. Table 3.2 summarizes the theory of a commonly experienced problem, insomnia, derived through a combination of the theoretical and empirical approaches. The theory of the problem guides the design of interventions.

Chapter 4

Clarifying Elements of the Intervention

Once an understanding of the presenting problem requiring remediation is gained, the second step in the process of designing interventions involves the selection of intervention and the clarification of its elements. To be effective in managing the problem, interventions must be consistent with the aspects of the problem amenable to change; also, they need to be relevant to the client population experiencing the problem. Therefore, selection of interventions is done carefully, whereby the aspects of the problem amenable to change are identified and intervention strategies or activities that target the identified aspects are delineated. Three general approaches can guide the selection of interventions and are discussed in this chapter: the theory-based approach, the empirical approach operationalized into intervention mapping, and the experiential approach eliciting input of the target client population. Following selection, the interventions are specified in terms of their goals, components, and activities that capture the active ingredients and nonspecific elements of the intervention, mode of delivery, and dose.

4.1 Theory-based approach for designing interventions

The theory-based approach rests on the propositions of the middle range theory underlying the problem for developing interventions. As explained in the previous chapter, the middle range theory provides a conceptualization of the problem that (1) defines the problem at the conceptual and operational levels, (2) identifies its causative factors and consequences, and (3) delineates the direct and indirect relationships among the causative factors, the problem experience, and the consequences. In addition, the middle range theory points to aspects of the problem that are amenable to change (i.e., "where" we can intervene) and the strategies that can be used to effectively manage them (i.e., "what we can do") (Brug et al., 2005; Campbell et al., 2007; Lippke & Ziegelman, 2008). Aspects of the problem that could be modified include

Design, Evaluation, and Translation of Nursing Interventions, First Edition.
Souraya Sidani and Carrie Jo Braden.
© 2011 John Wiley & Sons, Inc. Published 2011 by John Wiley & Sons, Inc.

the problem experience (i.e., manifestations) and the causative factors. The middle range theory highlights the particular manifestations and/or determinants that the intervention can target to manage the problem directly and/or indirectly, respectively. Also, the middle range theory indicates the nature of the strategies, which should be consistent with the nature of the manifestations and determinants to be modified. For instance, dyspnea is conceptually defined as the experience of difficulty in breathing and operationalized as the subjective sensation of shortness of breath and the objective indicator of rapid and irregular respiration. Emotional disturbances, particularly anxiety, trigger dyspnea. The experience of dyspnea interferes with physical and psychological functioning. This conceptualization suggests the possibility to intervene in two aspects of dyspnea: (1) its objective manifestation and (2) its emotional determinant. Strategies can be used to (1) promote slow and regular respiration such as breathing control exercises, which directly address this presenting problem, or (2) alleviate anxiety such as progressive muscle relaxation, which indirectly addresses the presenting problem by managing its determinant.

The application of the theory-based approach entails the following steps:

Step 1: Clarify the conceptualization of the problem advanced by the middle range theory. The first step focuses on gaining an understanding of the presenting problem derived from relevant middle range theory. The understanding encompasses the nature of the problem, its manifestations, level of severity, causative factors, and consequences, as experienced by the client population of concern. Special attention is given to the manifestations and causative factors, and the explanation of the pathways linking the causative factors to the problem. The pathways can be represented in a causal model where direct and indirect relationships among factors and the problem are illustrated with arrows. This illustrative model ensures an accurate depiction of all propositions of the middle range theory, which facilitates understanding of the complex interrelationships. Figure 4.1 exemplifies the relationships among the determinants of engagement in physical activity and this health behavior, which were derived from the theory of planned behavior and guided the development of the guidebook by Vallance et al. (2008), as an intervention to promote performance of physical activity in breast cancer survivors.

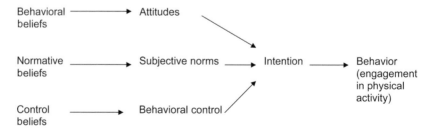

Figure 4.1 Pictorial depiction of theory of planned behavior.

Step 2: Determine aspects of the problem to be targeted for intervention.
The second step is concerned with identifying the aspects of the problem
amenable to change and, hence, to be targeted for intervention. A careful
review of the middle range theory can shed light on what specific mani-
festation(s) and/or causative factor(s) can be modified. This information
can be either clearly stated in pertinent propositions of the theory or inferred from the description of the manifestations and/or causative factors.
For instance, the theory of reasoned action/planned behavior identifies
the beliefs underlying attitudes, subjective norms, and behavioral control
as target for intervention (Fishbein & Yzer, 2003; Vallance et al., 2008).
In situations when the middle range theory does not provide explicit indication of the target for intervention, a thorough and systematic analysis
of the problem conceptualization is implemented. The analysis involves a
meticulous review of each aspect (i.e., determinant, manifestations) of the
problem to judge the extent to which it can be modified. The judgment is
based on an understanding of the nature of the problem's aspect and on
logical thinking relative to its amenability for change. The conceptualization
of insomnia presented in the previous chapter is used here to illustrate the
application of the systematic analysis. In this conceptualization, insomnia is
viewed as a learned behavior, manifested in difficulty falling asleep and/or
difficulty staying asleep. Three categories of factors contribute to insomnia:
predisposing, precipitating, and perpetuating. The analysis begins by questioning the extent to which insomnia, as a learned behavior, can be altered
directly. Logically, this may not be possible. However, the characterization
of insomnia as a learned behavior suggests that it can be "unlearned" and
substituted with other behaviors that promote sleep. This, in turn, points
to the need for behaviorally based interventions to manage this problem,
but it does not indicate the specific behavior(s) to be changed. The analysis
then moves to other aspects of insomnia to determine their amenability to
change. The second aspect to review is the manifestations of insomnia (i.e.,
difficulty falling and/or staying asleep). There is no theoretical proposition
that suggests these manifestations can be manipulated. The third aspect
to analyze is the set of factors contributing to insomnia. Predisposing factors are innate characteristics of people, such as genetic tendency, age,
and gender that increase the tendency to experience insomnia; therefore,
they cannot be modified. Precipitating factors, such as illness onset and
stress, are often out of the individual's control and cannot be changed. Perpetuating factors representing strategies clients use in an attempt to deal
with poor sleep fuel or maintain the sleep problem. Accordingly, these factors are amenable to change. They can be unlearned and substituted with
sleep-promoting strategies.

Step 3: Delineate the intervention strategies. The third step involves the delineation of intervention strategies that target the aspects of the presenting problem identified as amenable to change. The strategies form the
active ingredients of the intervention and are derived from the propositions of the middle range theory, if available, or from logical reasoning.

Middle range theories are descriptive explanatory in that they clarify the nature of the problem and its determinants, and elucidate the interrelationships among them. Although some of these theories propose targets for intervention, a scant number of theories explicitly identify intervention strategies to manage the problem (Michie et al., 2008). The social cognitive theory is an example of theory that indicates intervention strategies. It specifies ways to manage self-efficacy, which is posited as the key determinant of health behavior. Four techniques are recommended to change self-efficacy: (1) mastery experiences, (2) modeling or vicarious experience, (3) persuasion, and (4) giving physiologically compatible experiences (Bandura, 1997).

Logical reasoning is used to generate intervention strategies that target aspects of the problem amenable to change, as identified by a middle range theory. Logical reasoning is based on a thorough understanding of the nature of the problem aspect and critical thinking of how it can be modified. Maintaining consistency between the nature of problem aspect and the nature of the intervention strategy is essential for designing treatments that directly, effectively, and efficiently manage the presenting problem. In the example described above, the theory of planned behavior identifies beliefs underlying attitudes, subjective norms, and behavioral control as target for intervention to promote physical activity. Beliefs are cognitive structures that can be modified by providing information. The information should be relevant to each of the three determinants of intention and engagement in physical activity, where (1) the physical (e.g., improved muscle strength) and psychosocial (e.g., sense of enjoyment) benefits of exercise are presented to promote favorable attitudes toward this health behavior, (2) the opinions of healthcare professionals about exercise are shared to clarify subjective norms and the role that significant others can play to help in performing exercise is described to encourage clients to solicit their advice and support, and (3) the steps in preparing for and performing exercise, and ways to overcome common barriers are discussed to enhance clients' sense of behavioral control (Vallance et al., 2008). In the example of insomnia, the perpetuating factors are classified into engagement in activities in bed that are incompatible with sleep (e.g., eating, watching TV, reading, reviewing the day's events in bed) and irregular sleep patterns (e.g., having inconsistent sleep-wake schedule and spending extended time in bed). The first type of factors contributes to the development of insomnia through the following pathway: with repeated performance of the activities in bed, clients learn to associate the bed and the bedroom with wakefulness rather than sleep. The goal of intervention strategies to address this type of determinants is to strengthen the bed and bedroom as cues for sleep and weaken them as cues for activities that interfere with sleep. The intervention then consists of instructions for activities to do and/or avoid around bedtime and when awaken during the night (Epstein & Bootzin, 2002). The second type of factors contributes to insomnia by disrupting the biologic sleep rhythm.

The goal of intervention strategies to address this type of determinants is to develop a consistent sleep-wake schedule. The intervention involves assessing the clients' total sleep time and setting regular times to go to bed and to wake up that allow clients to stay in bed for the identified total sleep time only (Spielman et al., 1987).

Step 4: Selecting the mode of delivery and dose of the intervention. Interventions are not delivered in the void; rather, they are implemented through a particular medium such as face-to-face individual or group sessions, computer-assisted programs, or booklets. The medium is carefully selected to be consistent with the nature of the intervention strategies, and to facilitate the delivery of the intervention's active ingredients in a "pure" form, "untainted" by any element inherent in the selected medium. Continuing with the examples presented above, a guidebook is considered an appropriate medium to relay information relevant to beliefs underlying attitudes, subjective norms, and behavioral control for physical activity. The guidebook is disseminated to a large number of clients who would read it at their convenience. Only information pertaining to the three types of beliefs is presented in the guidebook, as a way for maintaining the purity of the intervention. Further, to be useful to a wide range of clients, the information is written in simple, nontechnical language, at the sixth grade level, which minimizes the potential for misunderstanding. Group sessions led by a sleep therapist is selected as the medium for delivering the intervention strategies to manage insomnia. This medium facilitates interactions between the therapist and clients, which are required to clarify the instructions, to set the sleep-wake schedule, and to discuss strategies to overcome barriers clients may encounter when implementing the instructions and the sleep-wake schedule in their day-to-day lives.

In addition to mode of delivery, the dose of the intervention is specified. In general, dose refers to the level at which the intervention should be given in order to achieve the changes in the outcomes. It is operationalized in terms of amount (i.e., how much of the intervention), frequency (i.e., how many times is the intervention given over a specified period of time), and duration (i.e., how long is the intervention given). The nature, complexity (i.e., type and number of components and activities), and mode of delivery of the intervention guide the specification of the intervention dose. For instance, the guidebook containing relevant beliefs information to promote physical activity is administered once; however, clients may read it at their own pace and as frequently as needed. The intervention for managing insomnia is given in at least two sessions allowing clients to implement the instructions and sleep-wake schedule in their daily lives and to discuss any challenges encountered in this endeavor. The sessions are 90 minutes each and offered once a week, providing ample opportunity for clarifying the instructions and discussing challenges.

Practice, prescriptive theories are useful sources for specifying the intervention mode of delivery and dose (Sidani & Braden, 1998). These theories guide the organization of the intervention strategies, the description of the procedures to be followed when implementing the strategies and the identification of human and material resources needed to carry out the strategies (Sidani & Sechrest, 1999). Examples of practice, prescriptive theories include theories of communication and principles of adult education. For instance, Thompson et al. (2007) developed an Internet program for promoting maintenance of healthy diet and physical activity behaviors in children, on the basis of elements of the elaboration likelihood model. The model proposes that messages are processed centrally or peripherally. Central processing of messages involves conscious attention to and evaluation of the messages (i.e., elaboration) and, therefore, the messages are likely to induce lasting change in information. As a cognitive process, elaboration is enhanced if the message is perceived as relevant. Accordingly, Thompson et al. included strategies to promote relevance of the messages contained in the Internet program to children. The strategies were: use of graphics, key short messages, and story telling by characters familiar to the target children.

Step 5: Specify elements of the intervention. This last step consists of integrating information on the intervention active ingredients, mode of delivery, and dose in a comprehensive and meaningful description. The description serves to define the intervention at the conceptual level and to guide its operationalization into an intervention manual. The description of the intervention elements is discussed in more details in the last section of this chapter.

The theory-based approach for designing interventions has advantages and limitations. The advantages relate to the specificity, effectiveness, and generalizability of theory-based interventions. Middle range theories point to the aspects of the presenting problem that can be modified and to the intervention strategies that target these aspects, which maintains the specificity of the intervention. This, in turn, enhances our understanding of the mechanisms underlying the intervention effects and improves the effectiveness of the intervention in addressing the problem (Conn et al., 2001; Lippke & Ziegelman, 2008; Michie et al., 2008; Thompson et al., 2007). Effectiveness of the intervention is improved because the aspects contributing most significantly to the problem are appropriately addressed and not inadvertently missed (Green, 2000; Michie & Abraham, 2004). Preliminary empirical evidence indicates that theory-based interventions are more effective than interventions that are not informed by theory in producing beneficial outcomes related to health behaviors (Painter et al., 2008). Reliance on theory is critical for delineating the active ingredients of the intervention and for distinguishing those from nonessential intervention elements. The clarification of active ingredients or specific elements and nonspecific or common elements improves the accurate implementation of the intervention and its correct replication across clients and contexts, which is the core of generalizability (Foy et al., 2007; Pillemer et al., 2003).

The limitations of the theory-based approach for designing interventions include the following:

(1) Middle range theories offer a unique conceptualization of the presenting problem, specifying a particular set of causative factors and manifestations that can be modified. This set may not be comprehensive and may not account for all relevant factors and manifestations operating in complex situations (Green, 2000) and in client populations of diverse ethnic or cultural backgrounds.

(2) Middle range theories may not have adequate and sufficient empirical support that enables identification of the relative importance of different factors and manifestations requiring remediation (Lippke & Ziegelman, 2008; Rothman, 2004).

(3) Middle range theories fall short of providing enough information of how to modify the identified aspects of the presenting problem as target for intervention; in other words, the theories do not explicitly propose specific intervention strategies (Brug et al., 2005; Rothman, 2004). The latter limitation is addressed in the empirical approach for designing interventions.

4.2 Empirical approach for designing interventions

The empirical approach recommends the use of empirical evidence to generate a conceptualization of the presenting problem, to identify aspects of the problem that can be modified, and to guide the selection of interventions aimed at inducing change in the identified aspects of the problem. Overall, the empirical approach follows steps similar to those described for the theory-based approach. The difference lies in the source of information used in each step, which is highlighted next.

In Step 1, the conceptualization of the problem is derived from a systematic review of quantitative and qualitative studies that investigated the problem. The results of the review are integrated into a conceptualization of the problem that delineates its determinants, manifestations, and consequences, as described in Chapter 3. In addition, literature pertaining to interventions implemented to address the presenting problem is systematically reviewed, using the meta-analytic technique or integrative review approach (Whittemore & Knafl, 2005). The results point to intervention strategies that have been applied to manage the presenting problem or any of its specific determinants or manifestations, to strategies consistently found to be effective or ineffective, and to the magnitude of the intervention strategies' effects on the outcomes reported for different client populations or contexts. A list of effective strategies is derived. For instance, Michie et al. (2008) and Abraham and Michie (2008) identified and validated a list of techniques to change various determinants of health behaviors such as self-efficacy, intention, and environmental constraints, through a review of relevant literature. Similarly, Ryan (2009) identified three general approaches related to knowledge and beliefs, self-regulation skills and ability, and social facilitation that contribute to engagement in self-management behaviors. Each approach is comprises specific strategies exemplified by goal setting, self-monitoring, and managing emotional response.

In Step 2, the aspects of the problem to be targeted for intervention are identified through any or a combination of (1) results of correlational studies that identify factors consistently and significantly predicting the problem; (2) findings of quantitative or qualitative studies that aimed at prioritizing factors for change; and (3) results of intervention evaluation studies that reported significant change in the factors following implementation of specific intervention strategies. The latter results confirm that the factors are amenable to change (Bartholomew et al., 1998).

In Step 3, intervention strategies found effective in managing aspects of the problem amenable to change are selected. If more than one intervention demonstrated effectiveness in changing a particular factor, then the one with the most significant and large effects is chosen. In Step 4, the mode of delivery and dose of the interventions that showed a significant impact are adopted as reported in relevant literature or adapted. In Step 5, the information about the selected strategies is integrated to describe the intervention. For instance, Blue and Black (2005) conducted a descriptive integrative literature review to identify components and dose (i.e., strength) that constitute interventions aimed at improving both physical activity and dietary behaviors in adults. The researchers categorized the intervention components into (1) education to change knowledge and attitudes, (2) behavior change strategies to overcome barriers, (3) social strategies to promote an environment supportive of behavior change, and (4) organizational strategies related to modification of policy. The dose of the interventions varied between 42 and 52 contacts made in group or individual sessions. The contacts were offered more frequently early in the course of intervention delivery.

A variant of the empirical approach is intervention mapping (Kok et al., 2004). Intervention mapping is described as a systematic process for developing health education programs aimed at promoting engagement in healthy behaviors. The process integrates theory, empirical findings, and input from the target population at different steps. It begins with the development of an understanding of the presenting problem derived from relevant theory, empirical evidence, and the target population's view, as described in Chapter 3. The remaining steps of intervention mapping that focus on the development of the intervention are detailed next and illustrated with the work of Fernández et al. (2005).

Step 1: Definition of the proximal intervention objectives. This step consists of sequential activities aimed at specifying the objectives to be achieved as a result of the health education intervention. The first activity consists of reviewing the conceptualization of the problem to clarify the health behavior of concern and identify specific determinants of the behavior that are most important and amenable to change. For example, Fernández et al. (2005)

determined low uptake of breast and cervical cancer screening as the problem of concern among Hispanic farmworkers. They found that personal (e.g., language barriers) and environmental (e.g., inadequate healthcare coverage) factors influence the women's screening behavior, based on a review of literature and consultation with community partners. Guided by health behavior theories, the researchers categorized the personal factors into those representing knowledge, attitudes, outcome expectation, perceived barriers, and benefits, and the environmental factors into perceived social norms, peer or family support, availability and accessibility of screening services, and self-efficacy. The second activity in the first step of intervention mapping is to specify proximal objectives for the health education intervention. Proximal objectives refer to changes that should take place at the individual, organization, and/or community levels as a result of the intervention. They explain who and what will change following the intervention. For instance, Fernandez et al. specified proximal objectives at individual and contextual levels. Examples of objectives for individual women were: call to schedule an appointment for screening and to obtain a mammogram, and examples of objectives at the organizational context level were: clinic directors will seek funds for screening programs, and physicians and other healthcare providers will make referral for mammograms. The third activity in the first step consists of developing matrices to cross-link the category of determinants and specific factors within each category, with the proximal objectives. The fourth activity involves the development of performance or change objectives that specify exactly what should be changed relative to a particular determinant of health behavior and to achieve the respective proximal objective. The performance or change objectives are stated clearly and concisely to reflect what is to be done to bring about the desired changes in the determinant of the problem. The performance or change objectives are incorporated into the cells of the matrices. Table 4.1 is an example of a matrix adapted from Fernández et al. (2005).

Table 4.1 Matrix linking determinants, proximal objectives, and change objectives

Level	Proximal objective	Determinant 1: knowledge	Determinant 2: attitude
Individual	Women will call to schedule an appointment	Women describes where to call and where to go	Women believe her role is to request mammography if her doctor had not recommended it
Organization	Physicians and other healthcare providers will make referral for mammograms	Providers describe excess morbidity and mortality from breast cancer in the target population	Providers believe that giving recommendations are an important part of care

Step 2: Selection of theoretical methods and practical strategies. Bartholomew et al. (1998) distinguish between theoretical methods and practical strategies in the development of health education interventions. Methods are general theoretical techniques that directly target determinants of health behaviors and strategies are practical ways to organize and apply the method. The second step of intervention mapping consists of generating a list of methods and strategies that match the proximal and performance or change objectives set for each determinant of health behavior identified in the matrix. Two complementary approaches are used to select intervention methods. The first is brainstorming, aimed at coming up with a provisional list of methods thought to influence the determinants. The second involves a review of theoretical and empirical literature searching for intervention methods that have been found effective in changing each determinant. For example, Fernández et al. (2005) identified modeling as an intervention method to change self-efficacy, based on social cognitive theory, and education as an intervention method to increase knowledge of health-related issues in different populations, based on empirical findings. For each of these methods, strategies are specified to operationalize them. Role-model stories of women who underwent screening and detected early cancer is a strategy operationalizing modeling, and presentation of information and question-and-answer sessions between lay health workers and clients are strategies operationalizing education. Methods and strategies are generated for each determinant listed in the matrix.

Step 3: Design of the intervention. This step of intervention mapping entails the actual design of the health education intervention by delineating the intervention strategies and mode of delivery, integrating the strategies and organizing them into a coherent and meaningful sequence of activities to be applied, and specifying the resources needed to implement the intervention. An intervention manual (discussed in Chapter 8) is prepared to guide the delivery of the intervention. This third step of intervention mapping also entails a pilot test of the intervention, which along with the remaining steps (i.e., implementation and evaluation) form the content of other chapters in this book.

The empirical approach, and in particular intervention mapping, has the following advantages:

(1) The content of the intervention is grounded in relevant theory and empirical evidence.
(2) The product of intervention mapping is a framework that clearly delineates the relationships among determinants, objectives, and strategies, which will guide the specification of outcomes expected of the intervention.
(3) Intervention mapping offers an opportunity to incorporate the views of the target population into the identification of determinants to be modified.

The weakness of the empirical, as well as the theory-based, approaches is the minimal involvement of the target population in developing and/or selecting interventions; yet such involvement would enhance the acceptability and relevance of interventions to client populations, specifically those of different cultural or ethnic backgrounds. The experiential approach overcomes this limitation.

4.3   Experiential approach for designing interventions

The experiential approach is characterized by the active participation of the target population in the design of interventions. Three techniques can be used to elicit views of the target population on aspects of the presenting problem that can be modified and on intervention strategies to address them: (1) focus group, (2) concept mapping, and (3) assessment of treatment preferences.

4.3.1   Focus group

Semistructured group sessions are held with representatives of the target population to inquire about intervention strategies they could use to address the presenting problem. Members of the target population are carefully selected to represent a range of the population subgroups defined by socio-demographic and clinical characteristics such as the experience of the problem at different levels of severity and of various determinants of the problem. The group session is facilitated by a skilled moderator. The session proceeds by introducing the nature of the presenting problem and clarifying the task at hand, which is to learn about strategies to manage the problem. The moderator describes the problem in more details, explaining its manifestations, and identifies determinants of the problem based on what is already known. The moderator than asks participants to indicate the determinants they frequently encounter, they consider to contribute most significantly to the experience of the problem, and they view as modifiable. The moderator engages participants in a discussion of strategies they have learned about and/or are applying to manage the problem in general, and the determinants identified as important in specific. The general question to be posed is: What do you or other members of your community do to manage/control/cope with the problem/specific determinants? Additional questions are used to probe for clarification of specific strategies and for extent of their perceived effectiveness. The moderator then requests participants to review the list of strategies; determine the strategies that are relevant to various subgroups of the target population and are feasible within their contexts; and reach an agreement on the strategies to be selected for integration into a comprehensive intervention. Similar semistructured focus group sessions can be held with professional and lay health workers providing services to the target population. The input of these workers complements that of the target population in determining relevant, effective, and feasible interventions to manage the presenting problem. The application of this technique is useful in eliciting the perspective on the problem and the identification of relevant interventions, of different ethnic or cultural groups, as illustrated by Villarruel et al.'s (2005) and Tanjasiri et al.'s (2007) work.

4.3.2 Concept mapping

As described in Chapter 3, concept mapping is a systematic technique to generate an understanding of the target population's conceptualization of the presenting problem. The product of this technique is a concept map that identifies factors contributing to the problem and clarifies the interrelationships among the factors and the problem. In the last step of concept mapping, the investigators involve members of the target population in decisions regarding the use of the map. One such use relates to the generation of intervention strategies to address each factor influencing the members' experience of the problem. This can be done in a group session, where the moderator engages representatives of the target population in a brainstorming exercise to come up with services offered within the community and/or ways or specific strategies applied by individual clients to manage the factors. The resulting list of services and strategies is subjected to further analysis, where participants in the group session are requested to eliminate redundancies, refine the list accordingly, and rate the importance of each listed service and strategy in successfully addressing the factors and/or problem. In addition, participants are asked to comment on the feasibility of the listed service and strategy. The quantitative analysis of these ratings point to strategies perceived as important and feasible that can be incorporated into a comprehensive intervention. Kelly et al. (2007) implemented the concept mapping technique within a community-based participatory research project to explore the views of the African American community on factors affecting engagement in physical activity. For each factor, participants identified an action plan and recommended specific strategies. For example, neighborhood safety was of concern to the community; in particular, the need to improve parks was considered of importance. The suggested action plan was to clean up the parks, and respective strategies included: identify parks in most need of cleaning and organize clean up events in partnership with service organization and schools in the neighborhood.

4.3.3 Assessment of treatment preferences

This technique aims at determining intervention and/or mode of delivery perceived favorably by the target population. The implementation of this technique begins by identifying interventions to address the presenting problem and/or its determinants, as well as modes for delivering them. The interventions and modes of delivery may be derived from any or a combination of approaches described previously, that is, theory-based, empirical, and experiential. A description is prepared for each intervention. The description presents information related to the name of the intervention, its goal, and the activities to be performed by health professionals and clients when applying the intervention strategy. Similarly, possible modes of and doses for delivering the intervention are detailed in a written format, as explained by Sidani et al. (2006). Persons representing the target population are invited to either an individual or group interview session. During the session, persons (1) are informed of the presenting problem and its modifiable aspects, (2) are told that a range of interventions are available to address the problem, (3) are asked to read the description of each intervention carefully, (4) rate the extent to which they perceive the intervention appropriate and feasible within their community or personal life context, (5) indicate the interventions they prefer to use to manage the presenting problem, (6) review the presented modes and doses for implementing the interventions, and (7) choose the one mode and dose they most prefer. The ratings are obtained in individual interviews or from individual participants in a group session, and are analyzed descriptively to determine the intervention, mode of delivery, and dose preferred by the majority or particular subgroups of the target population. In addition, participants in a group session engage in a discussion aimed at reaching an agreement on interventions, modes of delivery, and dose that are most appropriate to the target population; understanding the rationale for the group choice; and exploring the feasibility of implementing the selected intervention by the target population.

A variant of this technique was used by Rosal et al. (2004) to explore the preferences of low literate Hispanic adults for diabetes education. Participants were presented with intervention materials (i.e., poster depicting food items approved for persons with diabetes, items to limit and items to avoid) and were engaged in a discussion of their utility. In addition, the researchers elicited the participants' view on strategies to enhance management of type 2 diabetes. Participants expressed preferences for topics they wanted to learn more about (e.g., food they should not eat, consequences of not following healthy diet, stress management) and for modes for giving diabetes education (e.g., live demonstration and small interactive talk).

The advantages of the experiential approach relate to the involvement of the target population in the design of interventions for managing the presenting problem. The interventions, whether suggested through brainstorming or selected from what is already known, are consistent with the beliefs, values, and/or preferences of the target population, and feasible within the community and/or individual client context. Accordingly, the experiential approach is highly valuable in developing interventions that are relevant to clients of different ethnic or cultural backgrounds. Perception of interventions as relevant enhances uptake of, engagement in, and adherence to treatment, which, in turn, promotes achievement of beneficial outcomes (Kiesler & Auerbach, 2006; Mills et al., 2006). The limitations of the experiential approach relate to its implementation: it is time consuming particularly in terms of eliciting participation of representatives of the target population. Further, its findings may be biased by participants representing specific subgroups of the target population.

As presented, each approach has strengths and limitations. It may be useful to combine approaches to design appropriate interventions that are effective in managing the presenting problem, yet relevant to the target population. A sequential application of the three approaches, beginning with the theory-based approach, followed by the empirical approach, and ending with the experiential approach (specifically, assessment of treatment preferences) is a logical combination recommended for the development and testing of interventions (Campbell et al., 2007; Whittemore & Grey, 2002). Regardless of the approach used to design it, the intervention should be well specified and clearly described.

4.4 Specification of interventions

The application of any or a combination of approaches for designing interventions results in a list of specific strategies to address the presenting problem and the mode and dose for delivering them. This information should be organized in a meaningful way to specify what the intervention is all about, to characterize it, and to distinguish it from other interventions available to manage the same problem. The information is best organized into the intervention goals, components and activities, mode of delivery, and dose.

4.4.1 Intervention goals

The goals that the intervention is set to achieve are specified. An intervention may have two types of goals, (1) ultimate and (2) immediate. The ultimate goal reflects the resolution of the presenting problem and/or the prevention of its unfavorable consequences. The immediate goals relate to specific aspects of the problem that is, determinants and/or manifestations that should be changed in order to manage the presenting problem. At least one immediate goal is stated relative to each aspect. In the example of the behavioral intervention for managing insomnia, stimulus control therapy, the ultimate goals are to reduce the severity of insomnia and to promote sleep, and the immediate goals are to improve understanding of sleep and factors that influence sleep, to increase awareness of behaviors that promote sleep and that interfere with sleep, to assist persons with insomnia reassociate the bed and the bedroom with sleepiness, and to acquire a consistent sleep pattern.

4.4.2 Intervention components and activities

The intervention components and activities specify the strategies identified through the process of designing the intervention. The strategies are of two types: (1) specific and (2) nonspecific. The specific strategies reflect the active ingredients or specific elements that characterize the intervention. They are theoretically hypothesized to bring about the intended changes in the presenting problem and/or its determinants or manifestations. They are unique to and distinctive of the intervention. The nonspecific strategies are those that accompany the intervention and/or its implementation; however, they are theoretically inert as they are not hypothesized to produce the expected changes (Kazdin, 2003; Stein et al., 2007). The nonspecific strategies may be considered those used to facilitate the delivery of the active ingredients of the intervention. In the example of stimulus control therapy for managing insomnia, the specific active ingredients include: (1) increasing awareness about sleep, factors that influence sleep, and factors that perpetuate poor sleep, and general behaviors to promote sleep; (2) discussing instructions for activities to do and/or avoid around bedtime and when awaken during the night; and (3) setting a regular wake-up time. The nonspecific strategies include: (1) problem-solving that is, identifying barriers to the implementation of the instructions and solutions to overcome them, (2) reinforcing the implementation of the instructions, and (3) promoting a sense of trust and support. The identified strategies, whether specific or nonspecific, are organized in a meaningful way that would facilitate the development of the intervention manual (discussed in Chapter 8) and the actual delivery of the intervention in a logical sequence. The intervention strategies may be organized into components. A component is a set of interrelated specific and nonspecific elements and respective activities that are directed toward achieving a common goal (Sidani & Braden, 1998). Thus, an intervention component, and its respective activities, is specified for each of the intermediate goal. Structuring the intervention into components that are consistent with the stated intermediate goals ensures that all aspects of the presenting problem are specifically targeted. This, in turn, enhances the appropriateness of the intervention and subsequently its effectiveness in reaching the preset ultimate goals; however, it increases the complexity of the intervention. Table 4.2 illustrates the components and activities of the stimulus control therapy.

4.4.3   Intervention mode of delivery

The mode of intervention delivery is specified in terms of medium, format, and approach. Medium is the means through which the intervention strategies are implemented and the respective activities are carried out. Two media are usually available: (1) written and (2) verbal. Format refers to the specific technique used, within the selected medium, to offer the intervention. Within the written medium, specific techniques include: pamphlet or booklet, poster, or computer-based. Within the verbal medium, specific techniques include: face-to-face meetings with individual clients or a group of clients, telephone sessions, and audiotaped or videotaped presentations. It is important to note that the healthcare professionals offering an intervention becomes the medium through which the active ingredients are delivered. Thus, their characteristics and behaviors could influence the implementation of the intervention. Approach represents the manner in which the intervention is given. It can be standardized or tailored. The standardized approach consists of giving the same intervention components and activities, at the same dose, to all

Table 4.2 Components and activities of stimulus control therapy

Immediate goal	Component	Activities

To improve understanding of sleep and of factors that influence sleep	Sleep education	Specific activities:
		  Provide information on:
		    What is sleep and why we sleep
		    What is insomnia and what keeps insomnia going
		    What factors influence sleep
		Nonspecific activities:
		  Have clients reflect on their beliefs and behaviors related to sleep

To increase awareness of behaviors that promote sleep and that interfere with sleep	Sleep hygiene	Specific activities:
		  Discuss behaviors that influence sleep:
		    Physical activities
		    Sleep environment
		    Fluid and food intake
		    Alcohol, caffeine, nicotine
		    Exposure to daylight
		    Napping
		Nonspecific activities:
		  Have clients reflect on the behaviors they engage in and determine the behaviors to modify

To reassociate the bed and bedroom with sleepiness and acquire a consistent sleep pattern	Stimulus control instructions	Specific activities:
		  Discuss stimulus control instructions:
		    Going to bed only when sleepy
		    Using bed only for sleep
		    Getting out of bed if cannot sleep
		    When out of bed, engaging in quiet activity until sleepy
		    Waking up at the same time every day
		Nonspecific activities:
		  Assign homework: implementation of all stimulus control instructions
		  Monitor sleep daily
		  Resolve problems with nonadherence to instructions
		  Reinforce changes in sleep behaviors and improvement in sleep (monitored with sleep diary)

clients, regardless of the relevance and appropriateness of the intervention's components, activities, medium, format, and dose to the needs and characteristics of the clients. The tailored approach involves customizing the intervention to the needs, characteristics, and/or preferences of individual clients seeking treatment for the presenting problem (Lauver et al., 2002; Radwin, 2003).

It is important to clarify that the mode should be specified for each component of the intervention and that more than one medium and/or format could
be selected to deliver each component. Further, it is conceivable to provide
some intervention components and activities in a standardized approach and
others in an individualized approach. For example, the mode for delivering the
stimulus control therapy consisted of a combination of medium, format, and
approach. Overall, the intervention is given in a verbal, group format. In addition, a booklet is distributed to clients for future reference related to the sleep
education and hygiene component. Whereas most stimulus control instructions are standardized and applicable to all clients, negotiation for setting
regular wake-up time and discussion of adherence issue are individualized.
The sleep therapist addresses these points with individual clients attending
the group sessions as well as in individual contacts with clients made over the
telephone.

4.4.4 Intervention dose

Dose refers to the level at which the intervention is delivered in order to produce the intended changes in the targeted aspect of the presenting problem.
Similar to the dose of medications, the dose of nonpharmacological interventions is operationalized into four elements: (1) purity, (2) amount, (3) frequency, and (4) duration (Scott & Sechrest, 1989). Purity reflects the "concen-
tration of the active ingredients" of the intervention, which can be quantified
as the ratio of specific to nonspecific strategies constituting the intervention.
Amount, frequency, and duration reflect exposure to the intervention. Specifically, amount refers to the quantity with which the intervention is to be given,
which is often operationalized as the number of sessions needed to deliver
the intervention and the length of each session. For intervention components
given in a written medium, amount is the length of time it takes client to read
the information presented. Frequency is the number of times the intervention
sessions are to be given over a specified period of time such as a week or
month. Duration is the total length of time during which the intervention is
to be given. Of these elements amount, frequency, and duration have been
commonly reported to specify the dose of nonpharmacological interventions
(Manojlovich & Sidani, 2008). For instance, the stimulus control therapy is
offered in a total of six sessions, of which four are group sessions and two
are individual telephone contacts. Each group session is 90 minutes and each
individual contact is 20 minutes in length (amount). The sessions are given
once a week (frequency), over a 6-week period (duration).

Specification of the intervention in terms of its goals, components, activities, mode of delivery, and dose serves several purposes. First, it clarifies
the specific active ingredients of the intervention, which is critical for distinguishing it from other treatments targeting the same presenting problem and
form the basis for developing instruments to assess and monitor the fidelity of
its implementation in the context of research and/or practice. Second, specification of the intervention provides guidance for preparing the treatment

manual, which describes what is to be done, how, and in what sequence when implementing the intervention. The treatment manual directs the training of interventionists or healthcare professionals in the delivery of the intervention. Third, specification of the intervention is the backbone for generating the materials used to assess clients' preferences for treatment and for describing the intervention in publications.

Chapter 5
Intervention Theory

Developing an understanding of the presenting problem and identifying aspects of the problem amenable to change are critical for designing interventions that appropriately target the problem. Specifying the intervention in terms of goals, components, activities, mode of delivery, and dose is important for clarifying what it is about and characterizing its distinctive targets. The remaining step in the design of interventions is the delineation of the outcomes expected of the intervention and the mechanisms underlying the intervention effects. The information on the presenting problem, the intervention, and the outcomes is then integrated into the intervention theory. The intervention theory guides the development of the treatment manual, the plan and conduct of studies aimed at evaluating the intervention effects, and the translation and transfer of the intervention to the practice setting. This chapter describes the step for delineating the intervention outcomes, as well as the elements of the intervention theory.

5.1 Delineation of intervention outcomes

Overall, outcomes represent the intended responses to the intervention, operationalized in changes in clients' condition. As such, outcomes are derived from the goals preset for the intervention. As explained in the previous chapter, interventions have two types of goals: (1) immediate and (2) ultimate. Accordingly, two categories of outcomes may be delineated for intervention. First, immediate outcomes reflect changes in the specific aspects of the presenting problem (i.e., determinants and/or manifestations) that are targeted by the intervention. Therefore, several immediate outcomes may be specified for a multicomponent intervention. Changes in immediate outcomes are expected to occur directly as a result of, and within a short time period following the implementation of, the intervention. Second, ultimate outcomes encompass resolution of the problem or alterations in its level of severity, as well as prevention of its unfavorable consequences. Changes in ultimate outcomes are anticipated to take place once the immediate outcomes are achieved, and within a long period following the implementation of the intervention.

Design, Evaluation, and Translation of Nursing Interventions, First Edition.
Souraya Sidani and Carrie Jo Braden.
© 2011 John Wiley & Sons, Inc. Published 2011 by John Wiley & Sons, Inc.

Therefore, the ultimate outcomes serve as the criteria for determining the success of the intervention. This description of the categories of outcomes depicts a sequential order, where the intervention is hypothesized to have direct effects on the immediate outcomes, which, in turn, affect the achievement of the ultimate outcomes; thus, the immediate outcomes mediate the effects of the intervention on the ultimate outcomes.

The mechanisms underlying the intervention effects, also referred to as mediating processes, are the "links, phases, or parameters of the transformation process that the treatment brings about" (Lipsey, 1993, p. 11). The mediating processes represent the series of changes that occur in clients following the implementation of the intervention and are responsible for the achievement of the ultimate outcomes (Sidani & Sechrest, 1999). They explain the "why" and the "how" of the intervention effects. The processes can be depicted in the form of a causal model that delineates the interrelationships among intervention components, mediators, and ultimate outcomes (Nock, 2007; Pawson & Tilley, 1997).

Mediators encompass clients' reactions to treatment, enactment and adherence to treatment, and immediate outcomes. Clients' reactions to treatment are common to all components of an intervention and to a variety of interventions. They are operationalized as understanding and perception of the intervention. Understanding refers to clients' awareness of the intervention goals and comprehension of the specific activities or treatment recommendations they are expected to carry out in everyday life (Borelli et al., 2005; Sidani & Braden, 1998). Perception entails clients' views of the intervention components, activities, mode of delivery, and dose. The views relate to the satisfaction with the intervention (i.e., helpfulness in resolving the presenting problem). Clients' reactions to treatment are the instigators for the processes underlying the intervention effects. Interventions that are not well understood by clients are not properly enacted (Crano & Messe, 1985), whereas those that are not perceived favorably are not enacted or adhered to in everyday life (Bakas et al., 2009; Vincent & Lionberg, 2001). Accumulating evidence indicates that participants in intervention evaluation research, who receive a treatment they view favorably, show high levels of satisfaction and adherence to outcomes, and consequently the intended improvement in outcomes (Kiesler & Auberch, 2006; Preference Collaborative Review Group, 2009; Swift & Callahan, 2009). Enactment and adherence to treatment refers to the clients' correct performance of the specific activities or treatment recommendations they are expected to carry out in day-to-day life, and engagement in these activities at the recommended dose (Bellg et al., 2004; Carroll et al., 2007). Enactment of and adherence to the intervention activities and dose facilitate the attainment of the immediate outcomes, which, in turn, contribute to the achievement of the ultimate outcomes. The relationships among intervention, mediators, and ultimate outcomes are described in Figure 5.1.

The following illustrates the delineation of the mechanisms underlying the effects of stimulus control therapy. The therapy comprises three

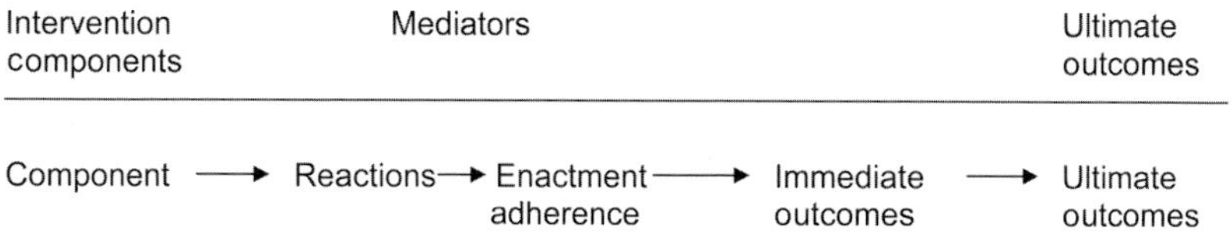

Intervention components	Mediators			Ultimate outcomes

Component ⟶ Reactions⟶ Enactment ⟶ Immediate ⟶ Ultimate
                           adherence   outcomes   outcomes

Figure 5.1 Relationships among intervention components, mediators, and ultimate outcomes.

components: (1) sleep education, (2) sleep hygiene, and (3) stimulus control instructions. In addition to clients' reactions and enactment and adherence to the components, the relationships among the components, mediators, and ultimate outcomes include the following:

Component 1: Sleep education. With the discussion of factors influencing sleep, such as biologic rhythms, clients develop understanding of the rationale for the stimulus control instructions related to waking up at the same time every day. Similarly, discussion of factors that keep insomnia going (i.e., perpetuating factors) increases clients' awareness of how sleep-related behaviors contribute to insomnia, which motivates them to initiate change. Knowledge of the nature of and reasons for sleep clarifies misbeliefs clients may have about sleep.

Component 2: Sleep hygiene. Informing clients of behaviors that promote sleep in general facilitates their correct performance, which creates internal (e.g., low levels of caffeine and nicotine in the body) and external (e.g., dark room) environments that are conducive to sleep.

Component 3: Stimulus control instructions. Bootzin, Franzen, and Shapiro (2004) clearly laid out the rationale for these instructions:

Instruction 1: Go to bed only when sleepy.
Rationale: This instruction assists clients to become sensitive to cues for sleepiness and likely to fall asleep quickly when they go to bed.

Instruction 2: Use the bed only for sleep and avoid doing other activities such as watching TV and reviewing the day's events in bed.
Rationale: With this instruction, clients break up behaviors associated with arousal in bed and strengthen the bed and bedroom as cues for sleep.

Instruction 3: Get out of bed if unable to sleep, engage in a quiet activity, and return to bed only when sleepy.
Rationale: Like the previous one, this instruction contributes to the association of the bed and bedroom with sleep and their dissociation from arousal. Further, instruction 3 promotes clients' sense of control and ability to manage insomnia.

Instruction 4: Set a regular wake-up time and get out of bed at the preset time irrespective of the duration of sleep.

Rationale: This instruction facilitates the development of a consistent sleep rhythm and builds some level of sleep drive; these are factors that influence sleep and increase the likelihood of falling asleep quickly.

Instruction 5: Do not nap during the day, if possible.

Rationale: Naps disrupt the sleep rhythm and reduce the advantage of increased sleep drive in inducing sleep faster.

In summary, the mediators of the stimulus control instructions are: beliefs and attitudes about sleep, self-efficacy about sleep, performance of sleep-promoting behaviors, and development of consistent sleep rhythm. These contribute to the ultimate outcomes of decreased levels of insomnia severity and improved daytime functioning.

5.2 Intervention theory

The intervention theory integrates information on the presenting problem, the intervention, and the outcomes into a unified whole. It provides understanding of the intervention in terms of (1) its active ingredients and respective components, mode of delivery, and dose; (2) the conditions for which it is given (i.e., determinants or manifestations of the problem that are modifiable); (3) its effects (i.e., ultimate outcomes); (4) the mechanisms underlying its effects (i.e., mediators); and (5) the conditions under which the mechanisms are initiated and the outcomes occur. The elements of the intervention theory can be organized into the structure–process–outcome framework to procure a logical sequence, familiar to healthcare professionals, for delineating the relationships among the elements.

5.2.1 Structure

Structure incorporates elements or concepts that influence the intervention's implementation, mediators, and outcomes. The concepts include the characteristics of clients receiving the intervention, the characteristics of interventionists or healthcare professionals providing the intervention, and the characteristics of the context (i.e., setting and environment) in which the intervention is offered.

5.2.1.1 Client characteristics

These consist of clients' personal profile, general health status, experience of the presenting problem, and resources available to clients. Client characteristics can influence uptake and adherence to the intervention, serve as the foundation for tailoring the intervention and its implementation, affect directly the mediators and/or outcomes, or moderate the effectiveness of the intervention in achieving the ultimate outcomes.

Personal profile. Clients' personal profile encompasses socio-demographic attributes and personal beliefs. Socio-demographic attributes include age, gender, level of education, marital status, employment, income, and ethnicity. Personal beliefs relate to clients' views and attitudes about health in general and about the presenting problem. There is emerging evidence supporting the direct and indirect influence of personal characteristics on the intervention and its outcomes. For instance, Janevic et al. (2003) found that as compared to unemployed, employed persons chose a self-directed program for the management of heart diseases. The self-directed program does not interfere with the person's work schedule. Givens et al. (2007) reported that African American, Asian American, and Hispanic participants did not believe in the biological causes of depression; hence, they did not view medications as a particularly useful treatment. Artieta-Pinedo et al. (2010) found that Spanish women who attended antenatal classes experienced lower level of anxiety upon admission for childbirth (ultimate outcome) than immigrant women.

General health status. General health status is operationalized into clients' physical and psychological domains of functioning that can interfere with the uptake, implementation, and effectiveness of the intervention. Poor physical health entails limitations in physical function and the presence of comorbidity. Limitations in physical functioning, such as difficulty in walking, may prevent clients from (1) fulfilling participation in the intervention activities like attending face-to-face intervention sessions and engaging in a physical activity program, and (2) experiencing improvement in the ultimate outcomes such as reduced fatigue as a result of a physical activity program. The presence of comorbid conditions can (1) alter the experience of the presenting problem or operate as a determinant of the problem, thereby making the intervention irrelevant or inappropriate to address the problem, (2) interfere with the implementation of the intervention components at the recommended dose, or (3) be directly associated with mediators and/or ultimate outcomes. For instance, clients with diabetes are encouraged to engage in physical activity to maintain their blood glucose level within acceptable range; however, the intensity and/or type of physical activity will have to be modified for clients with diabetes who also have cardiac diseases. Similarly, psychological impairments, such as limited cognition and depressed mood, may affect understanding of the intervention activities or treatment recommendations to be performed and initiation of and adherence to treatment, and/or may be directly correlated with mediators and outcomes.

Experience of the presenting problem. The uniqueness of clients contributes to variability in their experience of the presenting problem. The specific determinants of the problem may not be the same across all clients, or the magnitude of the determinants' influence on the problem may vary across determinants and across clients, where some clients are more affected by a particular determinant than others. Similarly, clients may not present with the same set of manifestations and with the same level of severity. Variability in the presentation of the problem has implications for the following:

(1) The appropriateness of the intervention components to all clients, suggesting the importance of considering the tailored approach for delivering

the intervention, where clients are offered different sets of components that correspond with the determinants and/or manifestations of the problem they actually experience. For example, the content of an educational intervention could cover only those topics identified by clients as important to learn about.

(2) The suitability of the intervention dose to clients presenting with different levels of problem severity, indicating the need to examine the effectiveness of different dose levels and/or to match the levels of intervention dose with the levels of problem severity. For instance, clients with cancer and receiving high doses of adjuvant therapy experience severe side effects. A one-session educational intervention providing information on symptom management strategies may not be adequate; rather, additional sessions are necessary to provide clients opportunities to carry out the strategies, to receive feedback on performance of strategies, and to discuss issues with the performance of strategies, which are critical to enhance their self-efficacy in symptom management.

(3) The clients' reaction to treatment in that emerging findings show that clients experiencing the problem at high levels of severity view intense interventions more favorably than those of low dose, having a strong impact on resolving their problem. For instance, Gum et al. (2006) reported that participants with severe depression selected medications (intense treatment) over behavioral therapy.

(4) The clients' response to the intervention, where those presenting with high levels of problem severity may not fully benefit from the intervention or may experience limited improvement in the outcomes. For instance, clients with severe acute pain may not be relieved from this symptom following listening to music; the latter intervention could be given in conjunction with pain medications.

Resources available to clients. Resources are often needed to carry out the intervention activities or treatment recommendations in day-to-day life. Availability of such resources and clients' ability to access them are contextual factors that impact the uptake, reactions, adherence, and subsequently effectiveness of interventions. For instance, clients with limited income cannot purchase healthy foods, which tend to be expensive, and frail older persons with diabetes living on their own may not have the support needed to prepare special meals.

5.2.1.2 Interventionist or healthcare professional characteristics

As mentioned in the previous chapter, healthcare professionals represent the medium through which interventions are delivered, specifically those given through face-to-face or telephone sessions, whether in an individual or group format. Hence, the active ingredients of the intervention are given through the interactions between the professionals and clients. Accordingly, the healthcare professionals' personal and professional characteristics play a role in the implementation and consequently the effectiveness of the intervention.

Personal attributes. Personal attributes include socio-demographic characteristics (such as age, sex, and ethnicity), communication skills, and demeanor.
Of the socio-demographic characteristics, sex and ethnicity have been mentioned as affecting the interactions between clients receiving the intervention
and the interventionists or healthcare professionals delivering the intervention. For instance, compatibility in sex is considered important when sensitive
topics are discussed, as clients may feel more comfortable discussing such topics with interventionists of the same sex. Compatibility in ethnicity is believed
to facilitate development of trust and rapport. Interventionists' demeanor also
contributes to the establishment of trust and rapport, which form the basis
of the relationship between the interventionist and clients. Recent analyses
indicate that such a relationship (formerly considered "placebo") promotes
clients' satisfaction with and adherence to treatment, and therefore effectiveness of the intervention (Baskin et al., 2000; Bowers & Clum, 1988). Interventionists' communication skills are essential for relaying intervention-related
information in a clear way that enhances clients' understanding of the activities or treatment recommendations they are to carry out. Such understanding
forms the basis for correct performance of the specific intervention activities
or treatment recommendations.

Professional qualities. Professional qualities that are of concern include educational background, experience, beliefs and attitudes toward the presenting
problem and toward the intervention, and level of competence or expertise
in providing the intervention. These professional qualities can influence the
extent to which the interventionists implement the intervention as originally
designed. For instance, Project MATCH Research Group (1998) reported differences in therapy implementation and outcomes across therapists. Crits-
Christoph and Mintz (1991) conducted a systematic review of studies evaluating psychotherapy. They found that novice psychologists implemented the
therapy under investigation as designed, whereas experienced psychologists
did not exactly follow the intervention protocol all the time. The latter group
of psychologists may have relied on their experience and expertise to modify
some aspects of the therapy to fit with the study participants' context, as
they usually do in their practice. Differences in the delivery of psychotherapy were associated with the achievement of better outcomes in participants
cared for by novice psychologists. The influence of interventionists' beliefs
about the problem and its treatment has not been investigated systematically. However, there is anecdotal evidence suggesting that these beliefs
shape the prescription of treatment (e.g., differences in perception of complementary, alternative therapies between physicians and clients) as well as its
implementation (e.g., a therapist who attributes insomnia to stress and anxiety
may focus cognitive behavior therapy on the management of anxiety rather
than on the discussion of stimulus control instructions as originally planned).
Fuertes et al. (2007) found moderate-to-strong relationships between the
therapeutic alliance that clients develop with their treating physicians and the
clients' perceived usefulness, adherence, and satisfaction with the prescribed
treatment.

5.2.1.3 Context characteristics

Context refers to the environment or setting in which the intervention is implemented. Context should have the physical and psychosocial features necessary to facilitate the delivery of the intervention and, hence, to achieve the intended outcomes. These features should be clearly delineated as they will guide the transfer and the application of the intervention in different settings.

Physical features. The physical features to consider include the availability of resources required for delivering the intervention, the physical layout of the environment and its attractiveness, and the convenience of the setting location to clients. For example, the implementation of group educational intervention requires the availability of a private room that has adequate lighting and ventilation, and a seating arrangement that promotes interactions among clients and with the healthcare professional, and that is easily accessible to clients; in addition, it demands the availability of equipment (e.g., laptop, projector, and screen) to deliver the content in the originally selected format. Similarly, the following are needed to have clients listen to music, with the ultimate outcome of reduced anxiety: private room, a comfortable chair, control over room light to dim it while clients listen to music and temperature to adjust it according to clients' comfort level, and equipment to play music (CD, CD player, or iPod, and earphones).

Psychosocial features. The psychosocial features relate to the culture of the organization in which the intervention is implemented, the working relationship among healthcare professionals employed in the organization and the interventionist responsible for delivering the intervention, and the norms and policies that guide care delivery in the organization. The psychosocial features affect the uptake and actual delivery of the intervention particularly at the stage of transfer and application in day-to-day practice. Some organizations or settings may refuse the intervention if it is not consistent with the prevailing culture and norms. For example, instituting sex education as a means to promote safe sex and to prevent HIV may not be accepted in private schools supported by religious groups.

5.2.2 Process

The process element of the intervention theory operationalizes the intervention. It encompasses the intervention components and dose. The intervention components operationalize the active ingredients of the intervention, which are theoretically hypothesized to bring about the intended changes in the mediators and/or the outcomes. Each component should be clearly labeled to reflect the active ingredients it captures. Also, it is described in terms of the goal it is set to achieve, the specific activities that constitute the component, and the mode selected for its delivery. The intervention dose is specified in terms of amount, frequency, and duration, as explained in the previous chapter.

5.2.3 Outcome

The outcome element of the intervention theory reflects the mechanisms mediating the intervention effects on the ultimate outcomes. As explained in

Section 5.1, the mediators entail clients' reactions to treatment, enactment and adherence to treatment, and immediate outcomes. The mediators are specified for each intervention component. The ultimate outcomes are also identified in terms of decreased severity or resolution of the presenting problem, and prevention of the consequences of the problem or promotion of general health, overall functioning and/or quality of life, if applicable. In addition to clarifying the nature of the expected mediators and ultimate outcomes, the timing and the pattern of change in the mediators, especially immediate outcomes, as well as pattern of change in the ultimate outcomes have to be specified. Timing of occurrence of change is the point in time at which the changes in the immediate and ultimate outcomes are hypothesized to take place during or after implementation of the intervention. Pattern of change is the trajectory illustrating the direction and rate of change anticipated for the immediate and the ultimate outcomes to demonstrate during and following delivery of the intervention, and reflecting the intended beneficial effects of the intervention. The timing and pattern of change in the immediate and ultimate outcomes vary across interventions. They are often a function of the nature and dose of the intervention, as well as the clients' reactions to and enactment and adherence to treatment. For instance, some interventions (e.g., self-management education) may induce small but incremental changes in the immediate (e.g., beliefs about presenting problem) and ultimate (e.g., self-care behaviors) outcomes. The changes are first observed after completing treatment and continue to increase in magnitude over the follow-up period. Other interventions (e.g., those focusing on behavior modification) may result in moderate-to-high changes in the immediate outcomes (e.g., self-efficacy) and small-to-moderate changes in the ultimate outcomes (e.g., level of anxiety) within a short time period following treatment delivery; however, the rate of change in the ultimate outcomes increases over time. Still, some interventions, if strictly adhered to, lead to significant changes in immediate and ultimate outcomes within a short time period after treatment delivery. Listening to music for dyspnea and behavioral therapy for insomnia illustrate the latter type of interventions. Listening to slow tempo calming music reduces respiratory and heart rates within the first 5 minutes of implementing this intervention because these body rates synchronize with the music tempo. Recent empirical evidence indicates that appropriate and consistent performance of the instructions constituting cognitive behavior therapy for insomnia within the first 1-2 weeks of treatment is associated with significant improvement in sleep onset latency, wake after sleep onset, total sleep time, and sleep efficiency (Sidani et al., 2007). This pattern of change in sleep-related outcomes led to modification of the intervention dose to include one session only (Edinger et al., 2007; Germain et al., 2006).

In addition to specifying the elements of the intervention theory, the relationships among them, as organized into structure, process, and outcomes, are delineated. As depicted in Figure 5.2, the relationships include direct and indirect ones, where the structure element have direct association with process and outcomes, and indirect relationships with outcomes. The latter relationships are of two types: (1) mediated, where the process elements mediate the

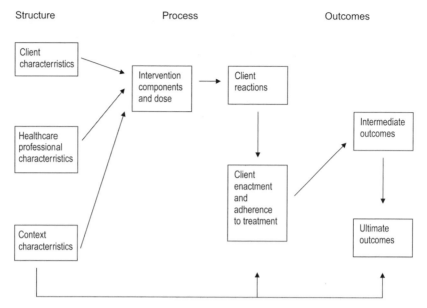

Figure 5.2 Propositions of the intervention theory.

association between structure and outcomes, and (2) moderated, where the structure elements serve as the conditions under which the effects of the intervention on the outcomes are observed. The process element is proposed to have a direct impact on the mediators and the ultimate outcomes, and the mediators link the process element and the ultimate outcome. The following specific propositions are advanced:

(1) Client characteristics influence the implementation of the intervention, reactions to treatment, enactment and adherence to treatment, immediate outcomes, and ultimate outcomes.

(2) Interventionist or healthcare professional characteristics influence the implementation of the intervention and clients' reactions to treatment, specifically understanding of and satisfaction with the intervention.

(3) Context or setting characteristics influence the implementation of the intervention.

(4) Client, interventionist, and context characteristics can also moderate the effectiveness of the intervention in inducing the intended changes in the immediate and ultimate outcomes.

(5) The intervention components and dose affect clients' reactions to treatment, enactment and adherence to treatment, and changes in immediate outcomes.

(6) Clients' reactions to treatment, enactment and adherence to treatment influence achievement of immediate outcomes.

(7) Changes in immediate outcomes induce changes in ultimate outcomes.

The above listed direct and indirect relationships among specific structure, process, and outcome elements of the intervention theory represents a comprehensive and complex set of interrelationships among factors, inherent in the real world, that contribute to the achievement of the intended ultimate outcomes. These interrelationships provide understanding of how best to address the presenting problem, using which intervention components, given at what dose, for clients with which characteristics and under what conditions, and why and how the intervention works in managing the presenting problem. Such understanding is the foundation for appropriate implementation, evaluation, translation, and transfer of the intervention into different practice contexts.

5.3 Utility of intervention theory

A well-developed and clearly delineated intervention theory guides the following:

(1) *The design of a research study to evaluate the effects of the intervention.* Overall, the intervention theory forms the basis for designing the research study. Its specific elements direct decision-making for different aspects of the study. Client characteristics help in prespecifying participants' eligibility criteria, which ensures that those experiencing the presenting problem and its aspects (i.e., determinants or manifestations) targeted by the intervention are included, and those possessing attributes that interfere with the implementation of the intervention and/or the achievement of immediate and ultimate outcomes are excluded. Healthcare professional characteristics are useful in selecting and training interventionists responsible for implementing the intervention. Context characteristics guide the identification of settings that facilitate the delivery of the intervention as designed. The intervention components and dose are critical for (1) preparing the treatment manual, which directs training of interventionists and monitoring fidelity of treatment implementation; (2) developing tools to assess and monitor fidelity of intervention implementation by interventionists and adherence to treatment by participating clients; (3) specifying the comparison treatment, which should not incorporate the active ingredients of the intervention under evaluation. The delineation of mediators and outcomes is required for the generation of their conceptual and operational definitions, the selection of appropriate measures, and the specification of the most opportune points in time for measuring them; the time points coincide with those at which the changes in mediators and ultimate outcomes are expected to take place.

(2) *The interpretation of a research study's results.* The propositions of the intervention theory assist in planning for data analysis and in clarifying factors that contribute to the observed intervention effects. Specifically, propositions of the theory regarding (1) the direct impact of the

intervention on the mediators and ultimate outcomes and the timing and pattern of change in the mediators and outcomes provide directions for the post hoc comparisons to be made, thereby reducing the likelihood of type I error; (2) the indirect effects of the intervention on the ultimate outcomes not only indicate the relationships to be tested but also give an explanation for the observed magnitude of the effect sizes, where the effect sizes (using Cohen's *d*) of the ultimate outcomes are anticipated to be smaller than those of the mediators; (3) the indirect effects of the intervention explain how and why the intervention produces its effects on the ultimate outcomes; (4) the direct and moderating influence of client, interventionist, and context characteristics identify the conditions that facilitate or hinder the effectiveness of the intervention, which offers possible explanations for non-significant intervention effects (Green, 2000; Rothman, 2004; Sales et al., 2006; Thompson et al., 2007).

(3) *The translation and transfer of the intervention.* The intervention theory identifies the client, healthcare professional, and context characteristics that influence implementation of the intervention. These characteristics inform those interested in offering the intervention in day-to-day practice of the conditions necessary for its delivery. The process and outcome elements of the intervention theory explain the how and why of the intervention, which is essential for proper delivery of the intervention and/or for guiding its modification to fit the features and needs of the local client population, healthcare professionals, and context, without altering the application of its active ingredients (Eccles et al., 2005; Foy et al., 2007) and, hence, its effectiveness in producing the intended beneficial outcomes.

Chapter 6
Tailored Intervention

The approaches for designing interventions discussed so far yield standardized interventions. Standardized interventions comprise the same set of components and specific activities or treatment recommendations that are delivered in their entirety, in a consistent manner, using the same mode of delivery and at the same dose, to all clients regardless of their personal characteristics and of their unique experience of the presenting problem. Standardized interventions may not be easily translated and incorporated into day-to-day practice, where the emphasis is on the individualization of nursing care so that it is responsive to clients' characteristics, needs, and preferences (McCormack & McCance, 2006; Radwin, 2003; Radwin et al., 2009). Tailored interventions represent a means for operationalizing the provision of individualized nursing care. In general, tailored interventions refer to those that are customized to individual clients. Customization involves the selection and implementation of specific intervention activities or treatment recommendations that are relevant to, and consistent with, the clients' unique characteristics. The selection and implementation of treatment activities or recommendations are guided by the results of a careful assessment of clients' characteristics and a sound algorithm. The algorithm consists of a set of decision rules that indicates which intervention activities or strategies, out of a preestablished library of strategies, are to be used for particular clients (Gerrish, 2000).

In the nursing literature, the terms "tailored interventions" and "individualized interventions" have been used interchangeably, as both types of interventions are customized to the characteristics of clients. Lauver et al. (2002) clarified the distinction between the two on the basis of the level of customization. Tailored interventions have predetermined goal and a preestablished set of specific strategies; they are characterized by a finite level of customization operationalized in terms of careful selection of specific strategies that are responsive to a number of client characteristics taking a range of possible values. Individualized interventions are highly customized in that very specific strategies are used to closely fit with the clients' personal characteristics and situation; the intervention strategies can be modified to be responsive to individual clients' characteristics and situation. Tailored and individualized

Design, Evaluation, and Translation of Nursing Interventions, First Edition.
Souraya Sidani and Carrie Jo Braden.

interventions should be well designed to clearly delineate the process of customization (also called tailoring process). Although the customization process is similar for tailored and individualized interventions, it has been more clearly explained for tailored interventions. In this chapter, the steps for designing tailored interventions are described. The effectiveness of tailored interventions is reviewed briefly, and the mechanisms underlying the effects of tailored interventions are highlighted.

6.1   Design of tailored interventions

The design of tailored interventions rests on the identification of the client characteristics on which to tailor the intervention and on clear delineation of the customization or tailoring process. Delineation of this process requires (1) development or selection of measures to assess clients' characteristics, (2) construction of a list of specific intervention strategies to be delivered to address the presenting problem in a way that is responsive to clients' characteristics, and (3) development of an algorithm specifying the rules that link the specific intervention strategies to the clients' characteristics (De Vries & Brug, 1999; Dijkstra & DeVries, 1999; Kreuter et al., 1999b). The intervention theory is useful in guiding the tailoring process. Overall, it identifies the client characteristics on which to tailor the intervention and direct the generation of rules that link the specific intervention strategy or activity to client characteristics.

6.1.1   Intervention theory

The intervention theory identifies the aspects of the presenting problem (i.e., determinants or manifestations) amenable to change, client characteristics that influence the uptake, reaction to, and adherence to the intervention, and the components, activities or specific strategies, and dose of the intervention that address the problem. These elements of the intervention theory are of importance in the design of tailored interventions. Knowledge of clients' experience of the presenting problem, personal profile, general health status, and resources points to the characteristics that would serve as the foundation for tailoring the intervention. Awareness of the intervention components, activities, and dose forms the basis for generating the list of preestablished intervention activities from which to select the most appropriate strategies. Understanding the linkages between the intervention components and activities on one hand, and the aspects of the problem they address and/or the client characteristics that influence the intervention on the other hand, guides the development of the tailoring algorithm. For instance, a very simple tailoring algorithm suggests offering the intervention component aimed at addressing the specific aspect of the problem, experienced by individual clients.

The literature on health behavior interventions exemplifies the use of theories for designing tailored interventions. Several theories, independently or in combination, guided the development of tailored interventions for promoting the adoption of health behaviors such as smoking cessation, reducing dietary fat intake, increasing fruit and vegetable consumption, and providing physical activity (Stretcher et al., 2005). Commonly used theories are the transtheoretical model of change, health beliefs model, and social cognitive theories (Revere & Dunbar, 2001). Each theory proposes a set of factors that influence clients' performance of health behaviors and suggest specific health information or intervention strategies to promote the adoption and/or maintenance of the behaviors.

6.1.2 Identification of client characteristics for tailoring

As explained in the previous section, the client characteristics identified for tailoring include the aspects of the presenting problem amenable to change, and the clients' personal profile, general health status, and resources. The specific characteristics known to vary across clients and to influence the intervention are considered for tailoring. Variation in the client characteristics is indicated by either of the following:

(1) Their presence or absence in different subgroups of the target population or in individual clients. For example, adoption and/or maintenance of regular physical activity are determined by a host of factors encompassing physical status (e.g., pain), psychological qualities (e.g., self-efficacy, motivation), socio-demographic characteristics (e.g., employment status, cultural values), and environmental resources (e.g., neighborhood safety). However, not all these factors operate to affect engagement in regular physical activity in all clients. Pain is a more prominent determinant in those with comorbid conditions and neighborhood safety is an issue for those residing in particular areas of a city.
(2) Their experience at different levels. For instance, clients experiencing severe levels of fatigue may not be able to perform high-intensity, high-dose exercise, as compared to those with low levels of fatigue severity.

When anticipated, such variation in client characteristics points to the needs for different intervention strategies, and/or modification of the intervention's specific activities, mode of delivery, or dose to effectively address the presenting problem in clients having different personal and/or clinical characteristics.

Available literature points to the application of tailoring in the design and implementation of interventions primarily targeting health behavior. The theories guiding the design of tailored interventions for promoting the adoption of health behaviors specify the client characteristics for tailoring. For example, the transtheoretical model is concerned with an individual's readiness for change; the health beliefs model focuses on the perceived threat of a problem; and social cognitive theory highlights knowledge, perceived self-efficacy, and social support as determinants of health behaviors. Accordingly, each theory considers particular determinants of the presenting problem for customization of the interventions aimed at adopting a health behavior of interest. Clients' personal profile, general health status, and resources are not to be ignored as characteristics on which to tailor these interventions' activities, mode of delivery, and/or dose. For example, awareness that employment on a full-time basis interferes with engagement in physical activity demands (1) additional intervention strategies aimed at exploring work-related activities that can be performed at a level to be counted toward daily recommendations, or (2) modification of mode of intervention delivery in the form of self-guided booklet (for clients unable to attend intervention sessions) or finding a "buddy system" comprising coworkers to promote engagement in physical activity within the work setting (e.g., taking a walk at lunch break). Further, understanding the cultural beliefs and values held by clients clarifies the types of physical activities, such as dancing, that are acceptable to and consistent with their beliefs and values; these types of activities are added to the list of preestablished strategies for promoting engagement in physical activity.

6.1.3 Assessment of client characteristics

Customization of interventions relies on assessment of client characteristics identified for tailoring (Dijkstra, 2005; Kreuter et al., 1999b). The results of assessment direct the selection of specific intervention strategies, mode of delivery, or dose that are relevant and consistent with the identified characteristics. Accordingly, assessment of these characteristics should be accurate if it is to guide the tailoring process. The instruments measuring the characteristics should be precise in capturing the essential attributes that define each characteristic and the clients' level on the characteristic. Therefore, the instruments should demonstrate reliability and validity. In particular, the instruments need to show content validity, sensitivity, and specificity. Sensitivity and specificity are critical for the identification of clients possessing the characteristics being assessed at the particular level specified for selecting relevant intervention strategies, mode of delivery, or dose. Consequently, the instruments used for assessment must have established normative values or cutoff scores to facilitate the interpretation of clients' responses and subsequently linkage to relevant intervention strategies, mode of delivery, or dose. For instance, tailoring of interventions for promoting physical activity demands assessment of self-efficacy, which is a client characteristic expected to influence this health behavior and forms the basis for customization. A validated measure of self-efficacy, with clear scoring instructions and interpretation of scores is needed to determine clients' levels on this characteristic. Invalid measures result in inaccurate assessment of the characteristic and/or clients' level on the characteristic, which contribute to the selection of irrelevant or inappropriate intervention strategies or activities.

6.1.4 Construction of a list of intervention strategies

The tailoring process demands the availability of a list of intervention components and/or specific treatment activities or recommendations to be selected and delivered in a manner that is responsive to clients' identified characteristics (Eakin et al., 2001). This implies that tailoring can take place at the level of the components of which the intervention is comprised; the specific activities or treatment recommendations that constitute each component; the mode for delivering the intervention components or activities; and the dose at which the intervention is provided. Therefore, the list can contain the following:

(1) The intervention components that target the different aspects of the presenting problem amenable to change, where the relevant component is given if the client experiences a particular aspect.
(2) Specific treatment activities or recommendations within each component, where the activities may vary in nature, providing alternative means to address the same aspect of the presenting problem.
(3) Different modes for delivering the components and/or specific strategies that are attractive or appropriate to clients with varying characteristics.
(4) The dose range at which the intervention can be implemented yet still produce the intended effects on the outcomes in clients presenting with varying levels of the identified characteristic or the health-related problem.

The list is derived from the intervention theory and related empirical and/or experiential evidence. The intervention theory clarifies the nature of the goals and active ingredients for the components, the type of alternative specific activities, the minimal and optimal dose required for effectively achieving the outcomes, and the different modes for implementing the intervention. Empirical evidence supports the comparative effectiveness of the range of components, activities, mode of delivery, and dose as specified in the intervention theory. Experiential evidence reveals alternative activities and modes for intervention delivery that are relevant to clients having different characteristics, or means for appropriately modifying the intervention while maintaining fidelity of implementing its active ingredients.

The literature on tailored interventions targeting health behaviors provides good illustration of an intervention list. The theories guiding the design of tailored interventions for promoting the adoption of health behaviors suggest specific health information or intervention components to achieve the intended outcomes. For example, the transtheoretical model delineates different types of information to give to clients at various levels of readiness (or stages) of change for the purpose of moving them closer toward adoption or maintenance of the targeted behavior. According to the health beliefs model, tailored interventions are directed at informing clients of their individual risks for a health problem and of appropriate strategies to minimize these risks. The social cognitive theory recommends psycho-educational and behavioral interventions for enhancing performance of targeted behaviors, where specific intervention components are delivered on the basis of individual clients' status on relevant determinants of the behavior. In particular, clients with limited knowledge are provided information to help understand the consequences of their behaviors, whereas those with low self-efficacy are instructed in the performance of the behavior. A tailored psycho-educational intervention aimed at assisting clients to manage pain requires the availability of a list of specific nonpharmacological interventions found to be equally effective in relieving the severity of this symptom. The list is generated from a systematic review of empirical evidence and/or guidelines. Examples of such interventions for pain are: listening to music (the music is nonvocal, slow tempo, and consistent with clients' preferences), relaxation (progressive muscle relaxation, breathing exercises), cutaneous stimulation (massage, electric muscle stimulation), and guided imagery. Recommendations for physical activity illustrate variability in some aspects of intervention dose. Clients are encouraged to engage in a total of 30 minutes of moderate intensity physical activity per day; however, the type of activity and the frequency of performing it is tailored, where clients select the type of activity they enjoy and can perform for 30 minutes all at once in one session or spread in three sessions of 10 minutes each over the day. Emerging empirical evidence supports the comparable effectiveness of Web-based and non-Web-based delivery of interventions in improving behavioral outcomes and suggests client subgroups who can benefit from Web-based delivery of the intervention to include: increase access to treatment for a large number of clients, particularly those who are isolated geographically (e.g., living in rural areas) or socially (i.e., unable to get out due to physical immobility or social role constraints for caregivers), and those who feel embarrassed or stigmatized by the presenting problem they experience (e.g., mental health issues) (Griffiths & Christensen, 2006).

6.1.5 Development of algorithm

The customization process involves the application of an algorithm which specifies the decision rules linking the intervention components, activities, mode of delivery, or dose with the client characteristic identified for tailoring (Dijkstra & DeVries, 1999; Eakin et al., 2001). The decision rules reflect the logic that underpins the selection of the intervention components, activities, mode of delivery, or dose in response to the results of assessing client characteristics. The rules are operationalized in a series of "if-then" statements (Kreuter et al., 1999b), which take the following form: "If the client presents with a particular characteristic at a specified level, then this specific component, activity, mode or dose is recommended as appropriate"; in this context, appropriateness implies responsiveness to the client's characteristic and contribution to the achievement of the intended intervention goal. The decision rule can be (1) simple, where the tailoring is done for one element of the intervention (i.e., component, activity, mode of delivery, or dose) and on the basis of a single client characteristic (e.g., one determinant of the presenting problem such as readiness for change); or (2) complex, where the tailoring is done for two or more elements of the intervention and on the basis of two or more client characteristics (e.g., one determinant of the problem and one personal quality such as cultural background). The level of complexity of the decision rule is a function of the specificity of the theoretical, empirical, and experiential knowledge about the linkages among the client characteristics and the intervention elements. For example, a tailored intervention aimed at assisting community-dwelling persons in the adoption of physical activity and guided by the transtheoretical model would incorporate an algorithm linking the person's readiness for change to specific types of interventions. Specifically, information pertaining to the consequences of inactivity and the benefits of physical activity is provided to persons at the precontemplation stage of change, whereas recommendations for physical activity and strategies for implementing the recommendations are discussed with persons at the contemplation stage of change. The algorithm has to be modified to account for other characteristics with which persons present, where recommendations for physical activity will have to be adapted before discussing them with persons at different age groups and the type of physical activity in which persons are encouraged to engage may differ to improve its consistency with the person's sex or culture, because the beliefs and values of certain cultural groups (e.g., South Asian) discourage women to participate in highly competitive exercise or sports (e.g., soccer) traditionally associated with men. Accordingly, the algorithm will have to specify the intervention activities to be offered for persons presenting with various profiles.

The algorithm underlying the tailoring process must be tested prior to its use within a research context. Offering inappropriate interventions that are not consistent with clients' characteristics could be potentially harmful (Kreuter et al., 1999b) in that clients may not receive relevant interventions that are acceptable to them; they may decide to withdraw from treatment, or if they complete treatment, then they may not experience improvement in the presenting problem. Such unfavorable experience with the intervention could prevent clients from seeking alternative treatment. The tailoring algorithm should be carefully derived from pertinent theoretical, empirical, and/or experiential evidence, and subjected to validation with experts. A group of experts in the theoretical underpinning of the intervention and in the clinical area of concern collaborate in this analytic exercise for the purpose of establishing the content validity of the tailoring algorithm. The experts review (1) the client characteristics for relevance as the basis for customization, (2) the instruments for measuring the characteristics for content validity and accuracy of score interpretation, (3) the list of alternative intervention elements (i.e., components, activities, modes of delivery, and dose range) for appropriateness and effectiveness in addressing the respective aspects of the presenting problem, as well as for comprehensiveness, and (4) the decision rules for clarity and accuracy in linking the intervention elements with the client characteristics. The experts engage in a discussion of what to change and how to refine the algorithm.

Once validated, the tailoring process is specified in terms of the following:

(1) The client characteristics (personal profile, general health status, resources, experience of the presenting problem) considered for tailoring.

(2) The instruments measuring the characteristics and the interpretation of responses or scores to determine their status or level on the characteristics.

(3) The list of alternative intervention elements (components, activities, modes of delivery, dose range).

(4) The decision rules for selecting the alternatives of intervention elements that are consistent with different client characteristics. The decision rules are delineated in "if-then" statements and illustrated in a matrix linking the combination of characteristics to be considered and the relevant intervention elements to be offered.

The following illustrates the description of a tailored cognitive behavioral intervention for promoting physical activity. The health beliefs model is the theory underlying the intervention, which focuses on exploring factors that interfere with clients' participation in physical activity and on assisting clients in overcoming perceived barriers to engagement in physical activity. Two possible barriers to physical activity are of concern to the target population of older women with arthritis: (1) pain and (2) limited social resources. The tailoring is done for these barriers and only relative to the specific intervention strategies to address them:

Characteristic 1: Client experiences pain (indicated by a score ≥ 5 on a 10-point numeric rating scale)

Strategy:

(1) Explore strategies used by client to manage pain and client's perception of the extent to which the strategies used are effective.
- If client is using pain medication prescribed by healthcare provider or if client is using nonprescribed nonpharmacological techniques, and if client perceives these strategies effective, then reinforce continued use of these effective strategies.
- If client expresses desire to not use pain medication, then explore reason for the desire.
  - If reasons relate to misbeliefs about medications, then clarify them by providing correct information on the way the medication works and on the issue of dependence.
  - If reasons relate to side effects of medications, then discuss interventions to manage the side effects.
  - If reasons relate to beliefs about pain and values for nonpharmacological interventions, then suggest alternative, nonpharmacological interventions from the prespecified list. The list includes: relaxation techniques, listening to music, heat and cold, and cutaneous stimulation (i.e., rubbing or massaging affected area).
- If client is using a nonpharmacological strategy and if client perceives the strategy of limited effectiveness, then suggest alternative nonpharmacological interventions from the prespecified list.

(2) Discuss the appropriate time for implementing the selected pain management strategy so that engagement in physical activity takes place when pain relief is at its peak.

Characteristic 2: Limited social resources indicated by partnering status (i.e., married or cohabitating)

Strategy:

(1) The specific intervention strategy differs on the basis of partnering status.
  - If client is nonpartnered, then inform him/her of community-based groups that organize physical activity events such as walking in malls.
  - If client is partnered, then encourage client to negotiate engagement in a type of physical activity, at a schedule that is convenient to both client and partner, and to recognize the possible favorable impact of participation in physical activity on the relationship with the partner.

6.2 Effectiveness of tailored interventions

Tailored interventions have gained acceptance in the field of health promotion. These interventions usually entail provision, through individual contact(s) with healthcare professionals, printed materials, and computer-assisted or Web-based program, of health information that is customized to selected clients' characteristics. The information is given to improve adoption of health behaviors. Results of several individual studies, integrated systematic reviews, and meta-analytic studies supported the effectiveness of tailored interventions in performance of targeted health behaviors, including smoking cessation (Fernandez et al., 2006), physical activity (Bock et al., 2001; Spittaels et al., 2007; Van Sluijs et al., 2005), and dietary behaviors (Kroezer et al., 2006). The long-term effectiveness of tailored interventions, particularly those addressing physical activity, was reported to be limited; the effect size was small at follow-up of greater than 3-month duration. This finding could be related to the tailoring algorithm that focused on only one characteristic, stage of change, in most studies. Considering additional client characteristics as the basis for customizing interventions could enhance their effectiveness. For instance, Kreuter et al. (2005) accounted for behavioral and cultural characteristics to tailor cancer prevention messages related to mammography, and fruit and vegetable intake. Behavioral characteristics included beliefs, perceived barriers, readiness for change, self-efficacy and past behavior performance. Four cultural constructs, prevalent among African Americans, namely (1) religiosity, (2) collectivism, (3) racial pride, and (4) time orientation guided the presentation of the tailored messages. Empirical evidence indicated that African American women who received the behaviorally and culturally tailored messages were more likely to adhere to the targeted health behaviors than those who received either behaviorally or culturally tailored messages.

6.3 Mechanisms underlying effects of tailored interventions

The mechanism thought to be responsible for producing the beneficial effects of tailored interventions has been summarized in the elaboration model (Kreuter et al., 1999a). The basic premise of this model states that persons tend to process information thoughtfully if they perceive it as personally relevant (Dijkstra, 2005). Through tailoring, the information presented to clients is highly personally relevant. Individuals pay attention to information perceived to be personally relevant and consistent with their characteristics and experiences. When attended to, such information is retained, and helps clients become motivated to acquire, enact, and sustain the skills desired for health behavior changes. Empirical evidence indicates that participants who received tailored health messages rated them favorably (i.e., interesting and relevant); they also reported that exposure to these messages generated positive thoughts which led them to thoroughly consider taking action toward changing their health behaviors (Dijkstra, 2005). Although this mechanism explains the effectiveness of tailored health messages, it also is applicable to other types of tailored interventions, where the perceived relevance of the intervention strategies, delivered to be consistent with or responsive to the individuals' characteristics, mediates their effectiveness in producing the intended intermediate and ultimate outcomes.

Section 3

Implementation of Interventions

Chapter 7

Overview of Implementation of Interventions

After carefully designing interventions, the next logical step in the process for designing, evaluating, and translating interventions is evaluating the effects of intervention on the intended intermediate and ultimate outcomes. Any evaluation endeavor involves the implementation of the intervention. Implementation or delivery of the intervention consists of carrying out the components and specific activities of which it is comprised through the selected mode and at the specified dose. The intervention should be implemented with integrity, that is, as planned in order to claim that it is successfully delivered and to validly determine its effects on the intended immediate and ultimate outcomes. Variations or drifts in the implementation raise questions about what is actually provided to clients and what is exactly responsible for producing the observed outcomes. The validity of conclusions regarding the efficacy or effectiveness of the intervention is at stake.

7.1   Variations in intervention implementation

The chances for variations in the implementation of interventions, in the context of either research or day-to-day practice, are rather high (Spillnane et al., 2007; Waller, 2009). The variations occur at different levels and for several reasons.

First, variations could happen at the level of operationalizing the intervention theory, when developing and specifying the intervention components and activities. Such variations are reflected in some discrepancy between the goals and/or active ingredients identified for the intervention and the components and/or activities operationalizing them. Thus, the specific activities constituting the intervention are not consistent with the goals or are not fully congruent or in alignment with the active ingredients of the intervention. This lack of correspondence between the conceptualization and operationalization of the intervention poses a major threat to construct validity of the intervention. Keller et al. (2009) reviewed reports of studies that evaluated interventions

Design, Evaluation, and Translation of Nursing Interventions, First Edition.
Souraya Sidani and Carrie Jo Braden.
© 2011 John Wiley & Sons, Inc. Published 2011 by John Wiley & Sons, Inc.

to promote physical activity. They found examples of interventions that fell short of specifying components and activities to address goals stated in relation to key mediators (i.e., immediate outcomes) such as self-efficacy. Possible reasons for inadequate operationalization of the intervention include: unclear conceptualization of the presenting problem and of the respective intervention, resulting in misspecification of the active ingredients of the intervention; limited time available for theorizing and analyzing the correspondence between the conceptualization and operationalization of the intervention due to social or other types of pressure to find solutions to emerging problems; and limited experience in the application of the systematic process for designing interventions.

Second, variations often take place at the level of implementing the intervention, when interventionists actually carry it out. Such variations are observed in drifts or deviations in the intervention components, activities, mode of delivery, and dose that are provided from those that are originally planned. These deviations can take two forms. The first form entails delivery of components and specific activities in a mode and dose that differ from those originally designed, by all interventionists, to all clients, across settings. Therefore, the intervention as a whole or some of its elements are not implemented as intended or as planned. This form of deviation is a major threat to construct validity (Cook & Campbell, 1979; Shadish et al., 2002) because there is lack of clarity about what the interventionists carried out and, hence, what produced the observed changes in the immediate and/or ultimate outcomes. This form of deviation in intervention implementation tends to be encountered in the following situations:

(1) When the intervention, whether simple or complex, is not well defined, that is, its active ingredients are not well specified, leaving much room for variability in the interpretation of what the intervention comprises. Thus, interventionists may use their own frame of reference and schema in articulating the elements of the intervention and in delivering them, resulting in variations in what different interventionists provide to clients in different contexts or settings. For example, the intervention "provide psychological support" could be interpreted as: listen to the client, encourage the client to ventilate his or her feelings, or give positive feedback (Sidani & Braden, 1998). Similarly, the intervention "teach patient" is broadly defined in terms of information to give to clients. The information can vary widely encompassing topics related to factors that contribute to the presenting condition, pharmacological, and/or nonpharmacological treatments for managing particular manifestations or symptoms that clients experience, or general strategies for self-management.

(2) When the intervention manual is either not available or its content is not presented in a lucid way to guide the implementation of the intervention. Thus, interventionists do not have a clear description of the step-by-step process to use as a reference when carrying out the intervention. Therefore, they may drift from what is intended.

(3) When the interventionists received inadequate training in the theoretical underpinnings of the intervention and/or in the process for implementing correctly all elements of the intervention. Thus, they may not have the cognitive knowledge and the practical skills to successfully deliver the intervention as planned.

The second form in which deviations in the implementation of the intervention are manifested involves inconsistency in carrying out some elements of the intervention by some interventionists, across clients, within the same or different settings. Therefore, clients supposed to receive the intervention under evaluation are given a select set of components or specific activities, at different dose levels, deviating from what is originally planned. This form of deviation, which is more commonly encountered than the first form, affects the reliability of the intervention implementation (Cook & Campbell, 1979; Shadish et al., 2002). Two factors may contribute to inconsistency in the delivery of the intervention. The first factor operates when providing standardized interventions; it relates to the interventionists' perception of the importance of individualizing some elements of the intervention to the personal needs and context or situation of clients. In general, interventionists are socialized to value client-centered care and trained to view clients as-a-whole and unique persons. They drift away from the planned intervention, modifying the nature of some intervention activities and the dose at which they are offered in an attempt to be responsive to clients' characteristics and context. Interventionists view such modifications as critical to demonstrate understanding and sensitivity to clients, which is the building block for initiating and maintaining a trusting relationship and a working alliance with clients. The relationship is the foundation for clients' satisfaction with, adherence to, and effectiveness of treatment (Fuertes et al., 2007; Johnson & Remien, 2003; Waller, 2009). The second factor operates when providing tailored interventions; it relates to lack of clarity in the customization process. In this type of interventions, interventionists are allowed to individualize elements of the intervention to be consistent with or responsive to clients' characteristics based on a well-delineated process and rules. When the process and rules for tailoring the intervention components, activities, mode of delivery, and/or dose are not well delineated and described, the interventionists are left with minimal guidance to select the specific aspect of the intervention for tailoring and to structure the customization process. As a result, what is tailored and how it is tailored vary across clients expected to receive the intervention under evaluation.

Third, variations in intervention implementation are observed at the level of the settings in which the intervention is delivered, within the context of research or day-to-day practice. Such variations are illustrated with differences in the components, activities, modes of delivery, and/or dose levels actually carried out by interventionists working at different sites (e.g., organizations, clinics). These variations affect the reliability of treatment implementation across settings. Characteristics of the sites are factors that may explain variations in intervention implementation. In particular, the prevailing culture and normative beliefs about the presenting problem and its treatment influence the acceptability of the intervention and/or some of its elements. Interventions that are not considered acceptable are not implemented. Alternatively, some of their elements are modified to fit the local context. In addition, the human and material resources contribute to the extent to which the intervention is delivered as planned. Human resources relate to the availability of well-trained interventionists with the required academic preparation, experience, and perspective on treatment in an adequate number to provide all planned intervention components and activities in the selected mode, and at the specified dose. Material resources relate to the availability of space and equipment needed to carry out the intervention components and activities in the selected mode. Where human and material resources are not available at the level needed for the delivery of the intervention as planned, modifications in pertinent elements of the intervention are made to be consistent with what is present or can be afforded locally, in particular settings. For instance, listening to calm, relaxing music, although found effective in reducing the severity of pain in different client populations, may not be perceived favorably as a complementary intervention for pain relief in some institutions dominated by strong beliefs in and support of nonstream medicine; small, nonprofit nursing homes located in rural areas may not have the staff mix or the right type and amount of equipment to provide this intervention to all clients who may need it.

Last, variations in intervention implementation occur at the level of clients who receive the intervention and are expected to carry out the treatment recommendations in their day-to-day life. These variations are exemplified in situations when clients engage in some, but not all, components, activities, or recommendations at dose levels that may deviate from what is recommended. These variations reflect differences in the extent to which clients adhere to the intervention, which influences the reliability of intervention implementation across clients. Several reasons may explain variations in clients' implementation of the intervention, including but not limited to the following:

(1) Misunderstanding of the nature of the intervention activities and/or the dose at which they are to be performed, which may be observed in situations where the intervention is complex or when the information is not relayed clearly to clients in a manner that is meaningful to them. To illustrate, Crano and Messe (1985) found that consumers' comprehension of the intervention was directly associated with the outcomes. The intervention consisted of varying the cost of electricity as a function of the time of the day at which it was used, whereby the cost was highest during peak hours. Consumers were informed of the changes in electricity cost in a letter sent to households. Clients differed in their understanding of the intervention and hence in its implementation, resulting in nonsignificant impact of the intervention on the outcome of electricity usage.

(2) Limited acquisition and sustainability of the skills, whether cognitive or behavioral, required to carry out the intervention activities correctly. This may occur when the skills to be learned are complex, demanding, and/or not well delineated, and when limited opportunities are provided to demonstrate, apply, and rectify, as needed, their enactment. For example, clients with chronic conditions are expected to learn and apply self-management skills related to monitoring and managing symptoms; taking a complex regimen of multiple treatments; coping with psychosocial consequences of illness; and making changes in their lifestyle (Barlow et al., 2002). Clients may not be able to grasp what these skills exactly entail and how best to perform them, all at once. Therefore, clients may not gain the skills, not apply them as taught, and lose the ability or will to perform them as recommended over time, which interfere with the achievement of the expected outcomes.

(3) Unfavorable attitudes or views toward the intervention, manifested in the perception that the intervention as-a-whole or some of its components or activities is/are inconsistent with the clients' beliefs and values, unacceptable to them, and/or unsuitable to their lifestyle. Unfavorable views influence satisfaction with the intervention, which, in turn, affects the degree of adherence to treatment. For instance, sleep restriction therapy aims at consolidating sleep by restricting the amount of time spent in bed to the individual client's sleep time and developing a consistent sleep-wake schedule. Sleep restriction therapy may not be appealing to persons with chronic insomnia because it appears to be at odds with common beliefs about sleep that a person needs 8 hours of sleep per night (Vincent & Lionberg, 2001). Clients of some cultural backgrounds (e.g., Chinese, Indian, African American) may express difficulty adhering to a low-fat diet that recommends avoiding deep fried food, which is a common and valued food choice in these groups.

(4) Unavailability of resources needed to implement the intervention activities. Obviously, when the resources are not present, clients cannot engage in the intervention activities or apply treatment recommendations. For instance, instructing clients residing in arid regions of the world characterized by hot, dry weather, and in the North or South Pole covered with snow and ice to increase the intake of fruit and vegetable is almost futile. Fruit and vegetables do not grow in these parts of the world, and importing them increases their costs, which is not affordable to the majority of the residents.

Regardless of the level at which they occur and of the reasons for their occurrence, variations in the implementation of the intervention have dire consequences on the validity of conclusions regarding the effects of the interventions on the intended outcomes. The consequences are of concern whether the intervention is implemented within the context of research or day-to-day practice.

7.2 Consequences of variations in intervention implementation

Variations in the implementation of the intervention, by either interventionists or clients, result in differences in what clients, expected to receive the intervention, are exposed to and actually enact. The differences present threats to construct, internal, and external validity of conclusions about the impact of the intervention on outcomes.

Deviations in the nature of the intervention elements (i.e., components, specific activities, mode of delivery) that are actually carried out, compared to the intervention elements that are originally designed threaten the construct validity of the intervention. Specifically, deviations in the delivery of the intervention components and activities, where those to which clients are exposed or those clients enact are dissimilar to those specified as operationalizing the active ingredients of the intervention, raise the question of what intervention was exactly implemented. Thus, clients may not receive or enact the intended intervention, and consequently may not demonstrate the anticipated changes in the outcomes. Deviations in the mode of intervention delivery may be associated with differences in the nonspecific elements of the intervention actually implemented relative to those delineated for the intervention. Of particular concern are the working alliance between the interventionist and the clients, and the supportive relationship among clients receiving the intervention in a group format. Accumulating evidence indicates that the interventionist-client alliance influences satisfaction with, adherence to, and outcomes of treatment (e.g., Fuertes et al., 2007; van Dam et al., 2003) and that the psychosocial and instrumental support that clients provide to each other in group sessions is beneficial, contributing to positive changes in the outcomes (Dirksen & Epstein, 2008). Accordingly, deviations in the nonspecific elements of the intervention associated with the achievement of the intended outcomes present an alternative competing explanation of the observed intervention effects. They weaken the confidence in attributing the observed effects, solely and uniquely, to the intervention active ingredients (Borrelli et al., 2005).

Variations in the implementation of the intervention across clients yield differences in the components, activities, mode of delivery, and/or dose received. Clients are exposed to and/or enact a select set of components and activities, in variable modes and at variable doses, so that not all clients receive the same active ingredients, nonspecific elements, and dose. The inconsistent delivery of the intervention dilutes the effects of the intervention on the intended outcomes, resulting in variability in the levels of outcomes observed following implementation of the intervention. Clients who receive the full intervention at the optimal dose demonstrate the expected pattern (i.e., duration and magnitude) of change in the outcomes; clients who receive some components and activities of the intervention at less than optimal dose show limited amount of change in the outcomes; clients who receive few, if any, components and activities, in various modes, and at a minimal dose level exhibit no change in the outcomes. Increased variability in the outcome levels decreases the statistical power to detect significant intervention effects, when comparing the group of clients who receive and the group of clients who do not receive the intervention; it also reduces the magnitude of the observed effect sizes (Bellg et al., 2004; Resnick et al., 2005). Consequently, the likelihood of committing type III error is increased. Type III error involves reaching erroneous conclusions about the effects of an intervention that has not been implemented appropriately and consistently (Carroll et al., 2007; Leventhal & Friedman, 2004; Sidani & Braden, 1998).

Inappropriate and inconsistent implementation of the intervention limits the extent to which the intervention can be replicated in different contexts (Bellg et al., 2004; Resnick et al., 2005) and can produce the intended outcomes. This issue of external validity relates to the ability to (1) determine the critical elements that define the intervention and should be delivered when replicating the intervention by different interventionists, with different clients and in different settings; (2) identify the intervention elements that could be modified and the most appropriate way to modify them in order to fit with the characteristics of different settings; and (3) specify the dose range that is associated with the achievement of the intended outcomes. Yet, such information is required for translating the intervention and applying it in a way that fits local contexts.

In summary, variations in implementation of the intervention can lead to inaccurate conclusions about its effects. Inaccurate conclusions contribute to the rejection of a potentially effective intervention (Bellg et al., 2004; Resnick et al., 2005). Strategies are needed to enhance treatment implementation and maintain validity of conclusions.

7.3   Strategies to enhance intervention implementation

Variations in the implementation of the interventions are to be minimized, if the goal is to reach correct conclusions about the effects of the intervention on the intended outcomes. The following are generic strategies used to limit variations and enhance the integrity of intervention implementation:

(1) *Development of an intervention manual:* The manual clearly delineates the goals and elements of the intervention, the techniques for carrying out the intervention, and the resources required for proper delivery of the intervention. As such, the manual is a means for operationalizing the intervention in a manner that maintains consistency with its conceptualization. The manual serves as a reference for training interventionists, for generating tools to assess the implementation of the intervention, and for continuous monitoring of intervention delivery.

(2) *Careful recruitment, training, and supervision of interventionists:* Recruitment and selection of interventionists are guided by the personal and professional characteristics of healthcare professionals identified in the intervention theory as influencing the implementation of the intervention. Interventionists possessing the identified attributes are

likely to understand the conceptualization underlying the intervention and to have the skills that facilitate the application of the active ingredients and the nonspecific elements of the intervention. Intensive training of the interventionists in the conceptualization and the operationalization of the intervention is critical to enhance their ability to deliver the intervention. Continuous supervision of interventionists' performance and provision of constructive feedback maintain integrity of treatment implementation.

(3) *Monitoring of integrity:* This entails assessment of the extent to which interventionists deliver the intervention as planned and specified in the manual, and the extent to which clients understand the intervention, perform the activities correctly, and adhere to the intervention. The assessment is done using various methods and at regular intervals throughout the intervention implementation. Monitoring integrity of treatment delivery provides the empirical evidence that helps in explaining the observed changes in the outcomes, whether significant or nonsignificant.

In this third section of the book, the generic strategies are described in detail. Issues in their application are also discussed.

Chapter 8

Development of Intervention Manual

Just like the research design is the blueprint for conducting a study, and the theoretical and operational definitions of concepts form the schema for developing respective measures, the specification of the intervention elements provides the framework for implementing the intervention. The intervention elements (i.e., goals, components, activities, mode of delivery, dose) define its nature, characterize its active ingredients that distinguish it from other interventions available to address the presenting problem, and delineate the general strategies for delivering the intervention. Similar to the need for operationalizing the research design into a study protocol that details the procedure for carrying out the study, and the concepts' definitions into a measure that captures the essential attributes, there is a need to describe the steps that are to be undertaken to implement the intervention. The intervention manual is a document that details what exactly is done, how, and when to deliver the intervention. As such, the intervention manual clarifies the logistics for implementing the intervention as planned, thereby maintaining integrity or congruence between the conceptualization and operationalization of the intervention. In addition, the intervention manual serves as a reference for training interventionists, for consistent implementation of the intervention across clients, and for monitoring integrity of treatment delivery. In this chapter, the procedure for developing and the content of the intervention manual are described and illustrated with examples from our own work. The importance and use of the intervention manual within the context of research and day-to-day practice are discussed.

8.1 Procedure for developing the intervention manual

The intervention theory (discussed in Chapter 4, Section 2 of the book) guides the development of the intervention manual. In particular, two element of the intervention theory are instrumental in this endeavor: (1) context and (2) process.

Design, Evaluation, and Translation of Nursing Interventions, First Edition.
Souraya Sidani and Carrie Jo Braden.
© 2011 John Wiley & Sons, Inc. Published 2011 by John Wiley & Sons, Inc.

8.1.1 Contextual characteristics

The contextual element of the intervention theory specifies the human and material resources required for delivering the intervention. Human resources involve the personnel that have the appropriate knowledge and skills to prepare for and actually engage in the implementation of the intervention. Some personnel assist in the preparation of the intervention, such as IT staff that assist in developing audiovisual materials required for treatment delivery, selecting audiovisual equipment, checking regularly its proper functioning, and making it available for use during the intervention implementation. The personnel involved in the implementation of the intervention include the interventionists assuming primary responsibility for delivering the intervention, as well as other professionals or laypersons who take part in providing some aspects of the intervention. For example, laypersons may be invited to a psycho-educational intervention to share their experience with the presenting problem, its treatment, and strategies to manage it, thereby serving as role models to participating clients. Material resources entail all items needed to implement the intervention. The items relate to the environment in which the intervention is offered (e.g., physical space) and the specific objects required for its delivery (e.g., equipment and forms). The specification of contextual characteristics in the intervention theory assists in generating a list of individual items that should be available to implement the intervention smoothly and as planned. The list is incorporated in the intervention manual.

8.1.2 Process

The process element of the intervention theory specifies the active ingredients of the intervention that are hypothesized to bring about the indented changes in the outcomes. The active ingredients are operationalized into the intervention components and respective specific activities to be performed to produce the changes in outcomes. The mode for delivering the intervention is identified to facilitate the implementation of the active ingredients in a "pure" form. The intervention dose is also determined. This information about the intervention is integrated into a plan that outlines what is to be done, how, and when. The "what" represents the specific activities to be carried out; the "how" reflects the selected mode of delivery; and the "when" illustrates the dose. The plan points to the sequence for carrying out the activities within and across the planned intervention sessions, as applicable. The plan is organized by intervention session. For each session, the component to be provided is indicated, and the respective activities to be performed in the selected mode are specified. The list of activities guides the generation of the step-by-step procedure, which is to be followed when offering each session of the intervention. The step-by-step procedure forms the main part of the intervention manual, as described in the next section.

8.2   Content of the intervention manual

In general, the intervention manual provides specific directions for implementing the intervention components and activities, in the selected mode, and at the specified dose. It describes the step-by-step procedure for doing so. As such, the content of the intervention manual is similar to the content of the "procedure book" available on inpatient units or outpatient clinics as a reference for the performance of particular procedures such as tracheostomy care. The procedure book gives information on the human and material resources that are needed to perform the procedure, and on the steps to be undertaken in preparing clients, applying the procedure, and documenting what was done. Similarly, the intervention manual contains separate sections covering the following content: overview of the intervention, resources required for providing the intervention, and procedure for carrying out the intervention. It is highly recommended to develop an intervention manual for any intervention, whether considered simple or complex consisting of multiple components, and whether using a standardized or tailored/individualized approach to delivery. Although the sections of the manual are the same for simple and complex interventions, the procedure section is more elaborate for complex than simple interventions in that it describes the steps for carrying out each component within each of the planned sessions. The content of the manual sections is detailed next, and illustrated with examples of a simple (i.e., listening to relaxing music) and a complex (i.e., stimulus control therapy) intervention.

8.2.1   Section 1: overview of the intervention

The first section of the manual gives an overview of the intervention to be implemented. The overview clarifies to interventionists planning on delivering the intervention, what the intervention is about and what it is set to achieve. This information serves as a general orientation about the intervention and as a reminder of its active ingredients that should be implemented under any circumstances, including those requiring attendance to clients' individual needs and contexts. The overview section of the manual reiterates the goals set for the intervention, the components (if applicable) constituting the intervention, and its mode of delivery and dose, as specified in the intervention theory.

The overview section of the manual for the simple intervention, listening to music, may include the following:

(1) *Name of intervention:* Listening to music.
(2) *Goal of intervention:* To alleviate state anxiety experienced by clients presenting with various acute or chronic conditions requiring medical or surgical treatment.
(3) *Mode of delivery—Individual session:* Clients select music of preference and listen to it using earphones.
(4) *Dose:* Session is of 20-minute duration; repeated as needed (i.e., when client experiences anxiety).

As noted, this overview does not identify the intervention components. This is typical for simple interventions that comprise one component only. Also, the overview hints that some aspects of the intervention are individualized: clients are given opportunity to select the music of their preference and to apply the intervention as needed.

The overview section of the manual for the complex intervention, stimulus control therapy, contains the following:

(1) *Name of intervention:* Stimulus control therapy
(2) *Goals of intervention:*
    (a) Ultimate goal: To reduce the severity of insomnia and promote sleep in clients presenting with chronic insomnia
    (b) Immediate goals:
        i. To improve understanding of sleep and of factors that influence sleep
        ii. To increase awareness of behaviors that promote sleep and that interfere with sleep
        iii. To reassociate the bed and the bedroom with sleepiness
        iv. To acquire a consistent sleep pattern
(3) *Components and activities:*
    (a) Component 1: Sleep education
        i. Goal: Inform clients about sleep and about factors that influence sleep.
        ii. Activities: Discuss the following topics:
            ○ What is sleep and why do we sleep?
            ○ What is insomnia and what keeps insomnia going?
            ○ What factors influence sleep?
    (b) Component 2: Sleep hygiene
        i. Goal: Discuss behaviors that promote or interfere with sleep.
        ii. Activities: Discuss and encourage clients to reflect on personal performance of general behaviors that affect sleep and related to physical activity, fluid and food intake, and use of caffeine and nicotine.
    (c) Component 3: Stimulus control instructions
        i. Goal: Reassociate the bed and bedroom with sleepiness and ac-quire a consistent sleep-wake pattern.
        ii. Activities: Present the instructions related to going to bed only when sleepy, using the bed only for sleep, getting out of bed if cannot sleep and engaging in a quiet activity until sleepy, and waking up at the same time every day; explain reasons for these instructions; and involve clients in finding ways to carry out the instructions.
(4) *Mode of delivery:*
    (a) Group format involving 4-6 persons.
    (b) Use combination of written and verbal presentation and group discussion.

      i. Written presentation: Distribute booklet summarizing content per-
      taining to sleep education and hygiene and stimulus control in-
      structions, for clients to follow through during verbal presentation
      and for future reference.

      ii. Verbal presentation: Use simple terms to relay information on
      sleep education and hygiene and stimulus control instructions.

      iii. Discussion: Ask questions to get clients to reflect on their beliefs
      and behaviors, how they relate to insomnia, and what they can
      do to change habits; assist clients in tailoring instructions to their
      personal context; explore issues of adherence; involve all clients
      in responding; and provide feedback to reinforce changes in sleep-
      related behaviors.

(5) *Dose:* Two sessions; each session is of 90-minute duration; given once
every other week, over a 4-week treatment period.

8.2.2 Section 2: human and material resources

The second section of the intervention manual presents a list of the human
and material resources required to carry out the specific intervention activities, in the selected mode. Human resources relate to persons other than
the interventionists assuming primary responsibility for implementing the intervention, who are involved in providing some aspects of the intervention
and/or assist the interventionists in carrying out some of the intervention activities. For instance, some interventions aimed at improving self-management
in clients with chronic disease, are designed to address multiple domains of
health, including medications, diet, exercise, and psychological adjustment.
Such interventions consist of multiple components, each focusing on a particular domain, and are delivered by different members of the healthcare team.
The team members are assigned to give the intervention component commensurate with their field of specialization, whereby the pharmacist discusses
medications, nutritionist discusses diet, physiotherapist discuses exercise, and
psychologist discusses psychological adjustment. Other interventions focusing on enhancing self-efficacy as mediator of self-management, may involve
laypersons or clients who demonstrate high levels of self-efficacy and effective
self-management. The clients are requested to share their experience, thereby
serving as role models. Role modeling is proposed as a strategy for enhancing
self-efficacy (Bandura, 1997). Additional human resources include technicians
who assist in setting up and ensuring proper operation of equipment to be used
when implementing computer-based interventions. By specifying the required
human resources in the intervention manual, interventionists responsible for
implementing the intervention are informed of the personnel assigned to deliver particular components or activities, and are cued to contact them and
collaborate with them to organize for the appropriate and timely delivery of
the intervention.

    Material resources consist of all items necessary for carrying out the in-
tervention as planned. The items relate to the environment in which the

intervention is offered and to objects required for its delivery. Whether offered in a laboratory setting, a clinical setting (i.e., inpatient unit or outpatient clinic), or a community setting (e.g., client home, neighborhood at large, community center), it is essential to clarify those aspects of the environment that should be available to facilitate the implementation of the intervention. These aspects are identified as context characteristics in the intervention theory that can potentially affect the delivery of particular interventions. They include the following:

(1) Physical space, such as availability of a room that is of the appropriate size (e.g., medium-sized room to hold group sessions, small room for individual session), that minimizes distraction by external noise or events, and/or that ensures privacy.
(2) Furniture, such as availability of round table to promote group discussion, comfortable recliner to facilitate listening to music, fridge to store perishable food items to be used for demonstration.
(3) Ambience or physical features, such as room temperature and lighting, and arrangement of items that allow uninterrupted performance of intervention activities (e.g., having patient rooms at equal distance from the nursing station in an inpatient unit to permit close surveillance of their condition by their primary nurse).

The objects required for intervention delivery are derived from its elements, in particular activities and mode of delivery, specified in the intervention theory. The objects encompass the following:

(1) Equipment through which the intervention is given, such as laptop or desktop needed to provide computer-assisted, standardized or individualized, educational programs; laptop or DVD player, projector, and screen to show a video demonstrating the performance of a task or skill; CD player and earphone to listen to music, weight scale, sphygmomanometer, or pulse oximeter to monitor and give immediate feedback on changes in the respective parameters; and cycling machine to perform recommended exercises under interventionist's supervision.
(2) Written materials, such as pamphlets or booklets, presenting key information guiding clients' application of intervention activities or treatment recommendations, on their own, within the context of their daily life.
(3) Forms to be completed by clients and/or interventionists during the implementation of the intervention, such as measures of the manifestations or determinants of the presenting problem which are completed prior to tailoring interventions, or sheets to document the individual client's goals and action plans.
(4) Forms graphing individual clients' progress toward achieving the agreed upon goals.
(5) Specific supplies needed to carry out the intervention activities, such as DVD, tapes, pens, and food items or menu.

Obviously, the human and material resources required for the implementation of the intervention vary with the nature of the intervention. The type of resources mentioned above is by no means exhaustive; however, they reflect the categories of items to be listed in the intervention manual. The list then serves as a reminder for the interventionists to ensure the availability of all items, in the right amount or number (i.e., number of clients expected to receive the intervention at the same time). For complex interventions given in several sessions, it may be useful to list the human and material resources needed for each session, particularly if the specific items differ across the sessions, where some items are given only in one session (e.g., educational booklets are distributed to clients attending the first session) and other items are necessary to facilitate the remaining sessions (e.g., forms graphing progress which are often given in subsequent sessions as means to reinforce performance of recommended behaviors).

The resources section of the manual for the simple intervention, listening to music, includes the following:

Resources needed:

- *Environment:* Private room with capability to dim light while listening to music and to control room temperature maintained at 20°C for comfort across all clients; recliner for clients to assume a comfortable position while listening to music.
- *Equipment:* CD player, earphones.
- *Objects:* CDs with different types of relaxing, instrumental music (e.g., classical, light jazz) for clients to choose from; form to record types of activities that clients performed while listening to music such as reading, unstructured imagery, sleeping/dozing off, and closing eyes.

The resources section of the manual for the complex intervention, stimulus control therapy, includes the following:

Resources needed:

(1) Session 1:
  (a) Environment: Medium-sized room allowing
      i. seating of a group of 4–8 clients in a roundtable format to promote group discussion;
      ii. good lighting to make it easy to read written information;
      iii. comfortable temperature; and
      iv. good acoustics and minimal external noise to make it easy to hear, particularly for clients with hearing problem, and to reduce distraction.
  (b) Objects:
      i. Folders to distribute to clients containing sleep education and hygiene booklet, list of stimulus control instructions, list of activities to be completed by clients once they identify quiet activities in which to engage when they cannot sleep; daily sleep diary forms

for clients to document the wake-up time agreed upon and to be followed consistently, schedule for the remaining intervention sessions

ii. Form graphing the clients' sleep onset latency, wake after sleep onset, total sleep time, total time in bed, and sleep efficiency reported at baseline; two copies of the form are prepared; the interventionist keeps one and gives one to the client for review during the session

iii. Group session log for interventionist to take clients' attendance at the session

iv. Pens for clients to take notes as needed and to write down information discussed during the session

(2) Session 2:

   (a) Environment: Sessions should take place in the same room, for consistency.

   (b) Objects:

      i. Form graphing clients' sleep onset latency, wake after sleep onset, total sleep time, total time in bed, and sleep efficiency reported at both baseline and the first week of treatment; two copies of the form are provided to the interventionist who will keep one and give one to the clients for review during the session

      ii. Group session log for interventionist to take client attendance at the session

8.2.3 Section 3: procedure

The third section of the intervention manual contains a description of the procedure to be followed when delivering the intervention. The description details the steps to be undertaken in order to carry out the components and activities of which the intervention is comprised, in the selected mode of delivery, and it provides scripts for the information to be relayed to clients. The detailed description of the procedure clarifies to interventionists what they are exactly to do, how, where, and when, thereby facilitating consistency in the implementation of standardized or tailored interventions across clients and settings.

The steps of the procedure are presented in a logical sequence. The sequence is specified at two levels. The first level relates to the common sense organization of the intervention session into introduction, body or main part, and conclusion.

The introductory steps entail (1) getting to know each other, where the interventionist introduces herself or himself to clients, stating her or his name and role in the delivery of the intervention, and clients are asked to introduce themselves, stating their first name only to maintain confidentiality in group sessions, to share briefly their experience with the presenting problem, and to express their expectations of the treatment. The first introductory step serves as an "ice-breaker" and fosters the development of a rapport between the interventionist and the client in interventions given on an individual basis, and of a supportive relationship and cohesion among clients in interventions offered in a group format; and (2) providing an overview of the intervention, explaining its goals and components as well as the responsibilities, if any, expected of the clients and/or activities in which they are expected to engage. This second introductory step helps clients understand the rationale and the general nature of the intervention, as well as what is expected of them. Clarification of expectations at the beginning of the intervention implementation reduces the likelihood of misinterpretation of what the intervention is set to achieve, and consequently of a sense of disappointment and dissatisfaction with treatment which lead to nonadherence to treatment.

The body or main part of the intervention session consists of the specific steps that represent the application of the components and activities constituting the intervention in the selected mode. The steps undertaken in the main part are discussed later in this section.

The concluding steps relate to termination of the intervention session. For simple intervention given in one session, this involves informing clients of the completion of the intervention session, disconnecting or removing and cleaning any equipment used during the session (e.g., CD player, earphones), inquiring about any question or concern clients may have about the intervention, and highlighting the activities clients are expected to continue carrying out, if any, in their day-to-day life. For complex interventions given in more than one session, additional concluding steps include (1) recapping the main points discussed during the session, (2) assigning homework for clients to do in the time interval between sessions (e.g., setting goals, applying relaxation techniques in different situations, monitoring their sleep), and (3) reminding them of the logistics of the next session (i.e., date, time, location).

The second level at which the procedure is specified relates to the components and activities to be performed within the main part of a session and across sessions of the intervention. The intervention theory points to such sequence, particularly if some components and activities are considered foundational or the building blocks for delivering other components and activities. In the example of the simple intervention, listening to music to alleviate anxiety, the individual client has to be seated comfortably in a recliner, in a room with comfortable temperature and dim light, before listening to the selected music. In the example of the complex intervention, stimulus control therapy, it is essential to first provide sleep education with an emphasis on factors that control sleep (i.e., sleep drive and biologic rhythms) because some of the stimulus control instructions are based on these factors. Specifically, the instruction to avoid napping, if possible, contributes to building the sleep drive, and the instruction to wake up at the same time every day contributes to the development of a consistent sleep rhythm.

Once the sequence of the steps, within and across intervention sessions, is delineated, each step is specified in a statement that identifies who (interventionist, client) is to do what (action) and in what way, as well as conditions under which the step can be altered, if necessary, and how it is altered in a manner that maintains its congruence with the active ingredients of the intervention. Such alterations are necessary if the needs of individual clients cannot be ignored during the implementation of standardized interventions (Dumas et al., 2001). For instance, although the implementation of the stimulus control therapy is standardized whereby all clients are informed of the same set of instructions and asked to apply them faithfully and consistently, it is important to address concerns expressed by clients sharing the same bed with their spouse or partner. These clients indicate that carrying out the instruction of avoiding any activity in bed (such as watching TV) except sleep and sex, and to get out of bed if they do not fall asleep or get back to sleep within 10-20 minutes, could disturb their bed partner. The description of the procedure has to alert interventionists of this often encountered situation and to suggest strategies to assist clients manage it successfully while enabling them to carry out the instructions that form the active ingredients or specific elements of stimulus control therapy. The suggested strategies may involve problem-solving and cognitive reframing, where clients are encouraged to discuss the nature of the instructions with their spouse or partner, to come up with a mutually agreeable plan for handling the situation, to recognize the long-term benefits of applying the instructions to themselves and to their spouse or partner (e.g., consolidated sleep with minimal interruptions), and to weigh the short-term disturbance against the long-term benefits.

Each step is described in a clear statement of the action to be performed and the qualifiers for the performance of the action, followed by a script clarifying the information to be relayed to clients; conditions and ways to alter the step are then presented. The statement may begin with the verb that best reflects the action to be performed. The qualifiers identify the way in which the action is to be performed. The script is written in simple, nontechnical language that is easy to understand by clients of different educational levels. The scripted sentences are short, presenting one idea or point at a time. The sentences are structured in a way that makes it easy for clients to grasp the content and to follow through; that is, the sentences are prepared in spoken language. For instance, the statement of the first introductory step, getting to know each other, of the stimulus control therapy, reads as:

Step 1: Introduce (action) self as therapist (who)

- State first name
- Identify role as therapist responsible for facilitating the sessions (qualifier)

Script:

- I would like to welcome you to this first session.
- My name is Jane. I am the sleep therapist who will facilitate the sessions and work with you throughout the sessions of this treatment.

Tables 8.1 and 8.2 provide excerpts of the manual for delivering, respectively, the simple intervention, listening to music, and the first and second

Table 8.1   Excerpts of manual for delivering the simple intervention: listening to music

Introduction:
   Introduce yourself.
   Explain the intervention: what it is and what it is expected to do (i.e., goal of the intervention).

Main Part:
   Have the client sit in a comfortable chair.
   Adjust the room temperature, as needed, to the client's comfort.
   Dim the light.
   Assist client in putting earphones.
   Have the client play the music for 20 minutes.
   Leave the room and return within 20 minutes.
   Inquire if client engaged in any activity while listening to music (e.g., closing eyes, engaging in some kind of imagery, reading) and record whether or not the client engaged in and the nature of the activity on the intervention form.

Conclusion:
   Assist client in taking off earphones.
   Remind client to listen to music as instructed.

sessions of the complex intervention, stimulus control therapy, for illustrative purposes. The excerpts were selected to represent the introduction, main part, and conclusion of each session of a standardized intervention.

   The procedure section in the manual of tailored and computer- or Internet-based interventions is comparable to the one described for standardized interventions. For tailored interventions, the description of the steps should also delineate the specific actions to be done to assess the characteristics selected for tailoring, to determine the clients' level on the characteristics, and to select the intervention strategies that are consistent with the client's level on the characteristics. The following is a generic account of the steps to be specified for the three main activities constituting tailored interventions:

Activity 1: Assess characteristics selected for tailoring

- Inform participating clients that they have to complete a questionnaire about some characteristics, which is necessary to guide the delivery of the treatment.
- Remind clients that there are no right or wrong answers to the questions and that the interest is in learning about their perspective or opinion.
- Explain that clients take time (i.e., no rush) to complete the questionnaire, and ask for clarification; interventionist can respond, as needed.
- Administer the questionnaire in the selected method.
- Get the completed questionnaire.

Table 8.2 Excerpts of manual for delivering the complex intervention: stimulus control therapy

Session 1

Introduction:

Introduce the intervention, in a standard way, by reading slowly the following script:

The treatment you will receive is a behavioral treatment for insomnia or sleep problem. This means that it does not involve medications or pills. The behavioral treatment for insomnia focuses on learning new ways to approach your sleep. This means you will learn new behaviors.

You must practice the new behaviors you learn so that you benefit from the treatment.

By using this treatment, you will develop skills to manage your insomnia, get your sleep under your control, and be able to cope/deal with any sleep problem that may come up after you finish this treatment.

The behavioral treatment you will receive consists of three behavior-therapy approaches. These are education about sleep, sleep monitoring, and stimulus control instructions.

Education about sleep provides information about sleep and guidelines about things you can do to develop good sleeping habits.

Sleep monitoring is done to help you track your sleep. You will do this by completing the sleep diaries.

Stimulus-control instructions are a set of behaviors or actions that you will have to do. The goal is for you to reassociate the bed and bedroom with sleepiness rather than wakefulness. This means that with this treatment, you learn to associate the bed and the bedroom with sleep, sleepiness, and falling asleep easily so your sleep becomes more consolidated and less broken up.

There are two sessions to this treatment. In addition to this one, you will come to the second session that is scheduled in 2 weeks. The date and time for the second session are written in the intervention session schedule available in the folder I just handed out.

Ask if clients have any questions and address them as needed.

Main Part:

Inform clients of the next topic of presentation: sleep hygiene, using the following script as a guide:

Now that we have discussed what is insomnia, how it starts, and how it keeps going; we will now discuss what can persons with insomnia do to sleep better.

In general, persons with insomnia have to get rid of habits that hurt sleep and develop habits that help sleep.

I will present recommendations that help you be prepared to make the most of your night's sleep.

Explain where clients can find information about these recommendations and what clients are expected to do with these recommendations, using the following script as a guide:

You will find information on these recommendations in the booklet available in your folder.

I would like you to read the booklet when you go home. Then see which of these recommendations are appropriate to you, and start applying the appropriate recommendations tonight.

Table 8.2 (*Continued*)

Review each recommendation by explaining what it is about and how it contributes
   to good sleep, using the following script as a guide:
   Let us review the recommendations. I will explain what each one is about and you
      can follow through in the booklet.
   The first recommendation is: develop a regular schedule of daytime activity or
      exercise.
   Activity or exercise may help improve the quality of your sleep.
   Select the type of activity or exercise that you like/enjoy doing, such as walking,
      gardening, or swimming.
   Do the activity or exercise on a regular basis.
   It is preferable to schedule the activity during the day, late afternoon, or early
      evening but not immediately before bedtime. This is because activity or
      exercise stimulates the body and makes falling asleep soon afterward
      difficult.
After reviewing all recommendations and responding to clients' questions, inform
   clients of the next topic of presentation: stimulus control instructions, using the
   following script as a guide:
   Now, we will discuss the stimulus control instructions.
   There are six instructions.
Explain where clients can find information about the instructions, using the
   following script as a guide:
   You have a list of these six instructions in your folder.
   You may want to pull this list out and follow through while I explain what each
      instruction is about.
Discuss each instruction, using the following script as a guide:
   I am going to explain each of the six instructions, but I have to emphasize that all
      are important.
   The first instruction states: go to bed only when you are sleepy.
   It is often the case that persons with insomnia start thinking about bedtime right
      after dinner. They go to bed too early just to be sure they fall asleep at the
      desired time. However, since they are not sleepy, they are awake in bed. They
      start to do things they hope will bring on sleep, like reading, watching TV or just
      resting. These things seem logical solutions to the sleep problem. But they are
      counterproductive and contrary to what persons with insomnia need to
      improve sleep.
   So, persons with insomnia, like you, spend a lot of time in bed awake. This gets
      you to associate the bed and bedroom with wakefulness or being awake, rather
      than signals for sleepiness.
   It does not pay to go to bed when you are not sleepy. Therefore, you need to stay
      up until you are sleepy and then go to bed.
   It is helpful that you start to be aware of when you actually feel like you are
      getting sleepy. You can start to develop a sense of what sleepiness feels like
      and use that as a signal to go to bed rather than the clock time.
   There are signals that tell you that you are sleepy, such as yawning, heavy
      eyelids, and rubbing your eyes.
   You need to pay attention to these signals and if you feel them, then this means
      you are sleepy. It is only at the time that you feel sleepy that you go to bed
      with the intent to sleep.

Table 8.2   (*Continued*)

Have clients identify signals or cues for sleepiness; ask each client to think about the signals they feel when sleepy and state them, using the following script as a guide:

Now, let us see how each one of you know that you are sleepy.

I would like you to think of the time you feel sleepy; what signals, of the ones I just listed or other ones you may notice, tells you that you are sleepy?

Once all clients identify their signals for sleepiness, summarize the discussion as follows:

You can see that the signals for sleepiness differ from one person to the other.

So, you need to monitor yourself, starting tonight, to learn more your personal signals for sleepiness.

Remember that when you feel these signals, you know that you are sleepy. You go to bed only when you feel sleepy.

Conclusion:

Assign homework as follows:

I am going to ask you, starting tonight to: (1) read the information in the booklet and start following the recommendations that are applicable to you; (2) follow the six stimulus instructions we discussed; and (3) continue to complete the sleep diaries every day. The diary is important to monitor your sleep.

Session 2

Introduction:

Start discussion in implementation of the six stimulus control instructions, using the following script as a guide:

Let us discuss how the last 2 weeks went.

Overall, were you able to carry out the six stimulus control instructions? How tough was it?

Have clients comment about their overall experience implementing the instructions; ask clients to share their experience, one at a time, whether "good" or "bad."

Once all clients give their comments, remind them:

I have to remind you that you are learning new habits and you are performing new behaviors.

These behaviors must be practiced consistently over the treatment period to work and to become routine.

Main part:

Engage clients in a discussion of each stimulus control instruction, with a focus on getting clients to think about their behaviors and to link their performance of the behaviors with the quality and quantity of their sleep, using the following script as a guide:

Now, let us see how you did on each instruction.

How about the first instruction: Go to bed only when you are sleepy?

Use the following questions as prompts for discussion:

Were you able to follow this instruction?

Were you able to know that you are sleepy? That is, did you pay attention to how you feel when you get sleepy?

Tell me how you feel when you get sleepy.

Have clients state the signals for sleepiness they noticed.

Table 8.2 (*Continued*)

Continue exploration of the extent to which clients adhered to the first
introduction, using the following as prompts:
How soon did you go to bed when you felt sleepy? How long did it take you to fall
asleep?
What prevented you from applying this instruction? What can you do about it?

Conclusion:
Remind clients that:
This is the last session of the treatment.
They have to (1) follow the six stimulus control instructions, for the treatment to
work, (2) monitor their sleep, and (3) continue doing the things or behaviors
that helped having a good night sleep and to eliminate those that led to poor
night sleep.

Activity 2: Determine clients' level on the characteristics

- Review the clients' responses to items assessing each characteristic.
- Assign appropriate score to each response, following the rules preset
  for the items.
- Compute the total score for the multi-item scale assessing each characteristic, following the preset rule.
- Document the total scores for all selected characteristics on the respective forms.
- Interpret the clients' total scores on the selected characteristics, by
  comparing the score for each characteristic to normative values or cutoff values preset for the scale measuring the respective characteristics;
  this will determine the clients' level on the characteristics selected for
  tailoring.

*Activity 3: Select the intervention strategies responsive to clients'
characteristics*

- Have the algorithm guiding the tailoring process available.
- Follow the instructions, as specified in the algorithm, to identify the
  strategies to provide to clients.
- Inform clients of the selected strategies.
- Provide the selected strategies as described.

For computer- or Internet-based interventions, the manual provides the
scripts of the information to be relayed to clients and the exercises or homework clients are expected to do. The scripts are presented in a logical sequence.
The scripted information is embedded in the computer program accessed by
clients. The recommendation of preparing the information in simple language,
short sentences presenting one idea at a time, is highly relevant for this format of intervention delivery. Prompts can be incorporated in interactive programs to highlight the key messages, thereby attracting clients' attention and

promoting retention of the information. Exercises can be designed to facilitate the application and retention of the knowledge gained. With advances in technology, videos of healthcare professionals presenting relevant information or laypersons sharing their experiences can be uploaded and reviewed by clients.

In summary, the content of the intervention manual gives an overview of the intervention and specific directions for implementing the intervention. The directions indicate the resources required, the sequence and nature of the steps to be undertaken, and the scripted information to be relayed to clients, when delivering the intervention.

8.3   Use of the intervention manual

The intervention manual is the means for operationalizing the intervention. It informs interventionists or healthcare professionals contemplating the implementation of the intervention, in the context of research or day-to-day practice, of what the intervention is about; what is needed to deliver it; what exactly is to be done, how, where, and when; and ways to modify some of the intervention activities to address nonignorable needs of client subgroups. A cookbook, rigid way of delivering the intervention that ignores the needs of client subgroups is not well received by healthcare professionals and clients. Healthcare professionals are socialized to attend to individual clients' needs and may not feel comfortable with standardization of treatment delivery (Leventhal & Friedman, 2004). Clients dislike nonattendance to their individual needs, which also interferes with the development of a trusting relationship with interventionists (Dumas et al., 2001); this, in turn, may be associated with client dissatisfaction with and nonadherence to treatment, and subsequent attrition (i.e., drop out of treatment) and achievement of poor outcomes. Therefore, it is useful to hint to circumstances where client subgroups have particular needs and to suggest ways to modify the intervention activities to address the needs while still implementing the intervention's active ingredients. The importance of developing a manual for simple or complex interventions relates to the details it provides for carefully implementing the intervention with integrity, that is, as originally planned. Integrity or fidelity of treatment implementation is critical for achieving in the intended outcomes for clients taking part in a research study or seen in practice.

The intervention manual contributes significantly to fidelity of treatment implementation. First, it guides the training of interventionists. It points to the skills that interventionists have to acquire to properly deliver the intervention. It assists in organizing the (1) content of the training, beginning with an overview of the intervention, moving to the resources required for giving it, and ending up with the step-by-step procedure to be followed when implementing it, (2) hands-on demonstration of the procedure, and (3) presentation of case studies representing a range of client subgroups with specific needs requiring alterations in intervention activities to address them. It offers the ground for developing theoretical and practical tests to examine the interventionists' posttraining acquisition of the cognitive, behavioral, and communication skills needed for intervention delivery. Second, the intervention manual serves as a reference to interventionists involved in the implementation of the intervention. It reminds interventionists of the resources required for carrying out the intervention activities in the selected mode, at each planned session, and prompts them to obtain the resources and ensure their proper functioning prior to intervention delivery. It informs interventionists of the nature and sequence of the activities to be carried out. Thus, interventionists can review the step-by-step procedure in preparation for delivering the intervention. Further, they refer to the manual and follow through with the steps as detailed in the manual when actually providing treatment. This maintains fidelity of the implementation of the intervention. Third, the intervention manual forms the basis for monitoring the implementation of the intervention. In practice, such monitoring is part of evaluating the performance of healthcare professionals or of quality improvement initiative, whereas in research, such monitoring is necessary to determine consistency in the delivery of the intervention across all participating clients and identify circumstances and reasons for deviations in its delivery. Examination of these deviations provides necessary feedback for refining the step-by-step procedure to be followed in implementing the intervention; for adapting some activities or steps to be responsive and consistent with the characteristics and needs of particular clients and settings; and for assisting interventionists in improving their skills required for delivering the intervention. Consistency in implementing the intervention across clients is essential for minimizing type III error, increasing statistical power for detecting significant intervention effects, and maintaining validity of conclusions reached in a research study. The intervention manual describes the step-by-step procedure to be followed from which criteria are generated for evaluating interventionists' performance and for monitoring consistency of intervention implementation.

The development of the intervention manual is demanding. It requires attention to details surrounding implementation of the intervention, clear articulation of the steps to be done, and detailed description of alternative ways for carrying out specific intervention activities. Accordingly, the preparation of the manual is time consuming, involving careful thinking and efforts to determine the logical sequence for carrying out the intervention components and activities, the appropriateness of the steps in operationalizing the active ingredients and the nonspecific elements in reflecting the selected mode for delivering the intervention, and the feasibility of carrying out the steps in the selected setting. However, the efforts and time spent in the development of the manual are worthwhile relative to the benefits gained in using the manual, whether in research or in practice.

Chapter 9

Selecting, Training, and Addressing the Influence of Interventionists

In most interventions, the interventionist is the medium through which the active ingredients are provided to clients. In educational interventions, the interventionist relays the information on the presenting problem and self-management strategies to clients. In cognitive-behavioral interventions, the interventionist facilitates discussion of the problem, intervention activities or treatment recommendations to manage it, and ways to address factors that interfere with the implementation of the recommended activities; demonstrates the performance of pertinent skills; and assists in monitoring and offers feedback on skill performance. In physical interventions, the interventionist gives instructions on the application of the skills or treatment recommendations, and provides instrumental support as needed. Even in the delivery of pharmacological interventions, the interventionist is involved not only in the administration of the medication, but also in providing information on its effects, dose, and adverse reactions, and in discussing issues of adherence. Whether these interventions are implemented in an individual or group, face-to-face, telephone, or electronic (e.g., chat room) format, they involve interactions between interventionists and clients.

Although interventionists are the central figure in the implementation of interventions, their contribution to intervention delivery and outcome achievement has often been ignored. However, clinical observation and emerging empirical evidence suggest that healthcare professionals providing care in the natural setting of day-to-day practice and interventionists giving the intervention in the experimental setting vary in their effectiveness in producing beneficial client outcomes. Careful selection, intensive training, and continuous supervision of interventionists are the strategies proposed to maintain proper implementation of the intervention and adequate performance of interventionists while minimizing their influence on client outcomes.

Design, Evaluation, and Translation of Nursing Interventions, First Edition.
Souraya Sidani and Carrie Jo Braden.
© 2011 John Wiley & Sons, Inc. Published 2011 by John Wiley & Sons, Inc.

In this chapter, the traditional perspective on interventionists' influence is summarized and the empirical evidence demonstrating the interventionists' effects is synthesized to provide the context for the emphasis on addressing this potential source of variance in the outcomes expected of the intervention. Characteristics to consider for selecting interventionists are presented. The type of training interventionists should receive prior to entrusting them treatment delivery is described. Methodological features for studies aimed at investigating interventionist effects are highlighted.

9.1   Traditional perspective on interventionist influence

As mentioned previously, the interventionist is the medium through which most, if not all, interventions are provided to clients within the context of research and the context of day-to-day practice. Interventionists represent the mode of intervention delivery, whereby the interactions between the interventionists and the clients are the means for applying the active ingredients of the intervention. As such, the interventionist–client interactions have been traditionally, and still are, considered nonspecific elements that accompany the implementation of the intervention (Okiishi et al., 2003). Nonspecific or common elements are not unique features that characterize particular intervention; rather, they facilitate the delivery of the interventions' active ingredients. Accordingly, they are hypothesized to be inert and to not contribute to the expected improvement in the outcomes. The active ingredients are posited to be responsible for producing the expected improvement in the outcomes.

The traditional perspective on the inert nature of interventionist–client interactions forms the basis of the assumption of interventionist uniformity (Kim et al., 2006). The assumption implies that interventionists are equivalent and play a relatively unimportant role in the achievement of outcomes. This means that interventionists are comparable, and hence intersubstitutable. Thus, interventionists can be trained in the implementation of the intervention, deliver the intervention, and induce the expected changes in the outcomes, regardless of their personal and professional qualities. Consequently, the influence of interventionists on outcome achievement has been ignored.

The traditional perspective on interventionist influence prevails in intervention research and in clinical practice. The interventionist effects are rarely investigated. The majority of reports on studies evaluating the effects of interventions may describe the characteristics of the interventionists selected and involved in the intervention delivery, and indicate that interventionists received training prior to and were monitored during implementation of the intervention; but the reports do not usually point to any observation of differences in the performance of interventionists and/or in the outcomes of participants assigned to different interventionists. In addition, few studies were conducted to determine the effects of interventionists on client outcomes.

Similarly, in the clinical practice setting, it is often assumed that healthcare professionals have gained the same knowledge and acquired the same skills (Marteau & Johnston, 1990) as inferred from successfully passing the licensing examination. As such, they are considered competent in providing care of comparable quality, which is expected to yield improvement in clients' condition. However, emerging empirical evidence and clinical observation suggest otherwise: interventionists do influence outcomes.

9.2   Interventionist influence: the evidence

The assumption of interventionist uniformity may be questioned on the ground that interventionists are, after all, human beings. As human beings, interventionists are unique in that they have individual characteristics. They differ in their socio-demographic profile and in their professional qualities. These differences translate into differences in knowledge, beliefs, and values, which inform their approach to specific situations as well as their behaviors and interactions with clients. Differences in interventionist-client interactions during implementation of the intervention, although considered nonspecific or common elements, appear to contribute significantly to outcome achievement in the contexts of clinical practice and research.

Clinical practice is replete with examples illustrating differences among healthcare professionals. The differences are in various characteristics such as levels of knowledge and competence, behaviors, interactions with colleagues and with clients, and ability to develop a rapport or trusting relationships with clients. Interactions and relationships often are factors that clients consider when rating their satisfaction with care. Healthcare professionals' interactions in which they listen to clients, respect clients' beliefs and values, inform clients of their condition and treatment alternatives, involve clients in treatment decisions, and collaborate with clients on finding the most suitable strategies to carry out treatment recommendations and to overcome barriers, enhance the formation of a trusting relationship. Such interactions and relationships meet clients' expectations in terms of the technical and relational aspects of care, translating into satisfaction with the care received. In addition, through these positive interactions with healthcare professionals, clients develop an appreciation of the value of treatment, and motivation to carry out and adhere to treatment, which, in turn, contribute to achievement of the desired client outcomes (Fuertes et al., 2007; Travaodo et al., 2005). Results of several descriptive studies support the centrality of the healthcare professional-client interactions in improving satisfaction with, adherence to, and outcome of healthcare in the context of day-to-day practice (e.g., DiMatteoa et al., 1993; Van Dam et al., 2003).

Accumulating empirical evidence, primarily in the field of psychotherapy, indicates that interventionists (also referred to as therapists) vary in their effectiveness in producing beneficial client outcomes. Interventionists' influence has been investigated on two indicators of effectiveness, client attrition (i.e., drop out of treatment) and outcomes of treatment (Najavits & Weiss, 1994), in two types of setting: (1) experimental research and (2) natural/day-to-day practice.

In the experimental setting, the results of studies that examined differences in client attrition rates across interventionists were inconsistent. Kleinman et al. (1990) found therapist assignment to predict attrition in substance abusers, whereas Elkin et al. (2006) reported no significant differences in attrition for clients with major depression assigned to different therapists. Inconsistent findings can be explained by differences in the target populations, the nature of treatments, and the statistical tests used to examine interventionist influence. Hierarchical linear models (HLM) have been recently applied to examine differences in client outcomes across therapists while accounting for the nesting of clients within interventionists (Raudenbush & Bryk, 2002). Several studies and one systematic review explored the interventionist effects on client outcomes. The studies were often designed to evaluate the effectiveness of two or more interventions in managing the same presenting problem, such as cognitive behavioral treatment and interpersonal therapy for major depression. The interventions were delivered by a number of therapists ranging from 5 to 54; the therapists received training prior to implementation of the intervention, and for the most part, were requested to follow the treatment manual. Overall, the results showed that therapists accounted for up to 13.5% of the variance in changes in client outcomes observed following treatment (e.g., Elkin et al., 2006; Huppert et al., 2001; Kim et al., 2006; Luborsky et al., 1997; Project MATCH Research Group, 1998). These results are consistent with those of a previously conducted systematic review (Crits-Christoph & Mintz, 1991). It should be noted that in most studies, the amount of outcome variance accounted for by therapists, although not statistically significant, is larger than the amount of outcome variance explained by treatments that clients received; the latter ranged between 0% and 2% (Wampold & Brown, 2005).

In the natural setting of day-to-day practice, investigation of interventionist influence focused on client outcomes. Four studies were conducted in inpatient units or outpatient clinics offering psychotherapy to clients ($n > 1000$ in each study) presenting with various problems. The most common problems were depression, anxiety, and adjustment disorders. Clients were assigned to the care of therapists ($n > 50$ per study) based on availability and area of expertise, which resulted in differences in caseloads across therapists; that is, some therapists had a larger number of clients with high levels of severity of the presenting problem than others, as anticipated in the real world setting. The findings were consistent in showing significant differences in client outcomes among therapists, explaining about 8% of the overall variance in outcomes (Dinger et al., 2008; Lutz et al., 2007; Okiishi et al, 2003; Wampold & Brown, 2005). Lutz et al. and Wampold and Brown recognized that variability in therapists' caseload could confound the observed therapists' effects on outcomes. Wampold and Brown controlled for therapist caseload and found that the variance in client outcomes attributed to differences in therapists decreased to 5.5% (from 8%) after controlling for severity of the problem with which clients presented. This amount of outcome variance, even though reduced, is still larger than the amount of outcome variance (0-2%) explained by the treatments that clients received. This pattern of findings supports therapist effects on outcomes for clients participating in experimental research and for clients in practice. Overall, therapist effects are estimated to be of a small-to-moderate magnitude (Kim et al., 2006).

Some researchers attempted to gain an understanding of the observed interventionists' influence on client outcomes by examining the extent to which interventionists' characteristics were related to client outcomes. Two general categories of characteristics were identified as potentially related to interventionists' effectiveness: (1) preexisting qualities and (2) behaviors exhibited during implementation of interventions (Najavits & Weiss, 1994). Interventionists' preexisting qualities entailed personal profile such as age and sex, and professional attributes such as highest degree obtained, competence, years of experience, and treatment orientation. These were found to have nonsignificant associations with client outcomes (Dinger et al., 2008; Okiishi et al., 2003; Wampold & Brown, 2005), except for years of experience. In their systematic review, Crits-Christoph and Mintz (1991) reported differences in the outcomes for therapists with varying levels of experience. Less experienced therapists, compared to highly experienced ones, showed greater variability in the outcomes among clients assigned to their care. Interventionists' behaviors during intervention delivery were described in terms of "interpersonal functioning" (Najavits & Weiss, 1994) or development of working alliance and emotional bond (Fuertes et al., 2007). Interventionist-client alliance is defined as helping, purposive work in which the interventionist and the client agree on the goals of treatment and collaborate on the activities or tasks to be performed to attain the preset goals within the context of a trusting relationship (Baldwin et al., 2007; Fuertes et al., 2007; Joyce et al., 2003). Results of several studies were consistent in indicating that (1) clients' perception of the working alliance differed across therapists, (2) the relationship between alliance and client outcomes was larger in magnitude than the observed direct influence of interventionists on outcomes operationalized in terms of differences in outcomes for clients assigned to different therapists (Dinger et al., 2008), (3) clients' perception of a positive, helpful working alliance was associated with enhanced adherence to and satisfaction with treatment (Fuertes et al., 2007), and (4) clients' perception of a helpful alliance was positively related with achievement of beneficial outcomes (Dinger et al., 2008; Joyce et al., 2003). The alliance-outcome relationship was of a moderate magnitude, with an average effect size of .45 (Martin et al., 2000).

In conclusion, clinical observation and empirical evidence converge in supporting the effects of therapists, specifically their interactions and working relationship or alliance with clients, on improvement in outcomes expected of interventions. It appears that interventionists' variability is more influential than the active ingredients of interventions in accounting for the benefits of treatment (Messer & Wampold, 2002).

The direct (indicated with differences in outcomes across therapists) and indirect (mediated by working alliance) effects of interventionists on client outcomes may confound the effects of interventions on client outcomes (Elkin et al., 2006). Therefore, it is essential to minimize the potential influence of interventionists in studies aimed at determining the effects of interventions and/or to disentangle the effects of interventionists from those of treatments, if the goal is to demonstrate the causal relationship between the active ingredients of the intervention and the intended outcomes. Four strategies are applied to attenuate interventionists' influence: (1) careful selection of interventionists, (2) adequate training of interventionists, (3) standardization of the intervention, and (4) monitoring fidelity of intervention implementation by interventionists (Najavits & Weiss, 1994; Staines et al., 2006). These strategies are consistent with findings of Crits-Christoph and Mintz's (1991) systematic review indicating that the type of psychotherapy and use of a manual were related to the observed therapist variability. Specifically, structured interventions such as behavioral therapy, and use of a manual to guide delivery of treatment were associated with less therapist variability in client outcomes. Standardization of the intervention, operationalized in the development of a treatment manual that interventionists are requested to adhere to, was discussed in the previous chapters. Monitoring fidelity is addressed in Chapter 10. Selection and training of interventionists are described next, followed by a presentation of issues to consider in planning studies designed to disentangle interventionist from treatment effects.

9.3 Selection of interventionists

Although careful selection of interventionists is recommended as a means to minimize their potential influence, no guidelines are available that specify the attributes to consider when choosing interventionists. The following is a list of preexisting characteristics that could be taken into account:

(1) Socio-demographic characteristics, including sex and age. Congruence between interventionist and client on these characteristics may facilitate the implementation of interventions addressing sensitive topics.

(2) Competence, operationalized in terms of formal training, licensing, and experience. Formal training and licensing are required by regulatory bodies to practice and deliver some types of interventions. Competence is necessary for high quality and safe practice.

(3) General personality style (e.g., introvert or extrovert, humorous or serious) or relational style (e.g., use of support, willingness to collaborate with others). Personality and relational styles affect the nature of the interventionist's interactions with clients during treatment sessions and the development of working alliance, which contributes to motivation to initiate and engage in, satisfaction with, and adherence to treatment.

(4) Knowledge of the theoretical orientation underlying the intervention under evaluation and skills in applying the intervention's components and activities. These support training and the correct implementation of the intervention active ingredients. Dumas et al. (2001) highlighted that interventionists who do not have an understanding and appreciation of the intervention may not perform adequately and hence introduce error in treatment implementation, thereby reducing the chance of detecting significant intervention effects.

In addition, Najavits and Weiss (1994) suggested the following qualities, exhibited during treatment sessions for consideration: empathy, supportiveness, warmth, affirmation and understanding, helping and protecting, and support of client autonomy. These qualities are foundational for developing a helpful working alliance, through which the intervention active ingredients are provided.

Ascertainment of interventionists' characteristics is an ongoing process. It begins with the recruitment of interventionists and with an initial formal interview, and continues with monitoring of interventionists' implementation of the intervention. Different venues can be used to recruit interventionists including advertisement for the position in local newspapers, posting flyers in academic institutions or affiliated healthcare organizations, or word-of-mouth. Regardless of the venue used, the recruitment information should specify the main preexisting characteristics that interventionists should have in order to deliver the intervention, as required by regulatory bodies. These entail the indicators of competence that is, formal training, licensing, and experience. For instance, recruitment of interventionists for the study that evaluated the effectiveness of cognitive–behavioral interventions for the management of insomnia specified the following requirements: a Master's degree in nursing, psychology, or other health-related discipline, and training in cognitive–behavioral therapy. Persons who have these preexisting characteristics are invited to an initial formal interview, and are requested to submit their curriculum vitae (CV) or resume and letters of references. The formal interview is scheduled prior to contracting interventionists and aims at assessing the remaining preexisting characteristics selected for consideration. A preset list of open- and close-ended questions is asked of all applicants. The questions cover indicators of the remaining preexisting characteristics while allowing applicants to elaborate on points of interest, as necessary. Examples of open-ended questions to explore knowledge related to cognitive behavioral treatment for insomnia are: Have you had any training in cognitive–behavioral therapy in general and does it relate to insomnia? What are the basic features of this therapy? How effective do you think it is? Close-ended questions may be developed specifically to assess particular qualities and may consist of short instruments measuring relevant characteristics. The six-item measure of therapeutic alliance developed by Joyce et al. (2003), illustrates short instruments that can be administered to applicants during the interview to assess their relational style. Applicants' responses to open- and close-ended questions are clearly documented. In addition, the interviewer may observe the applicants' demeanor, communication style, interactions, and behaviors during the interview process. Applicants' responses to questions and interviewer's observations are then compared to the applicants' CV and letters of references, seeking convergence of information pertaining to the degree to which applicants have the preexisting characteristics of interest. For example, the CV may confirm educational background, licensure, training, and experience, whereas letters of support may point to the interpersonal or relational style of the applicants.

Once all interviews with all applicants are completed, the information gathered on the applicants is compared and contrasted for the purpose of identifying those who have the preexisting characteristics. A ranking system may be designed and followed to choose applicants demonstrating high levels on the attributes of interest. It may be useful to select a number of applicants that exceeds (e.g., by 1 or 2) the number of interventionists required to deliver the interventions to all clients participating in a research study or seen in practice. The selected applicants are trained in the implementation of the intervention as discussed in the next section. Securing a large number of carefully selected and trained interventionists is essential to offset possible interventionists' (1) attrition, where some may withdraw for various reasons such as moving out of town to pursue further education, (2) schedule conflict, where some may not be able to facilitate treatment sessions offered in the evening at clients' convenience, and others may need to take time off (e.g., vacation, maternity leave), and (3) inadequate performance, where some may consistently fail to adhere to the intervention protocol or to develop an acceptable level of working alliance with clients.

Monitoring interventionists' implementation of the intervention is done on a continuous basis. The purpose is to determine the interventionists' technical performance and relational style. Technical performance relates to the evaluation of the interventionists' skills in applying the intervention activities and adherence to the intervention manual. This evaluation is part of examining fidelity of intervention implementation and will be discussed in more details in Chapter 10. Relational style is operationalized by the qualities that interventionists exhibit during implementation of the intervention. These entail behaviors and interactions reflecting respect, understanding, willingness to help, and provision of support to clients, while carrying out the active ingredients. Information on the interventionists' relational style is obtained from two sources, using different methods, as part of or independent of fidelity check. First, a research staff member (e.g., investigator, project coordinator) is given the responsibility of observing interventionists' relational style, and requested to attend selected intervention sessions. The selection of these sessions varies with the format for delivering the intervention. For instance, when interventions are given on a single individual basis, over the telephone, then the sessions are randomly selected for monitoring. In contrast, when interventions are offered in a group format, in multiple sessions, then the observer attends all sessions to avoid disruption to the group dynamics and to capture the interventionists' relational style when providing different components or activities of the interventions. Observation of the interventionists' relational style can be semistructured or structured. In semistructured observations, the research staff is not given specific instructions on conducting the observation; however, the staff member is told of the general qualities to assess and is requested to write down any piece of information he or she considers as reflective of the qualities. In structured observations, a list is prepared detailing the specific indicators of each quality of interest and the research staff is asked to indicate the occurrence or the level at which the indicators were manifested during implementation of the intervention. The second source for gathering information on interventionists' relational style involves the clients. Clients are asked to provide informal or formal comments. Informally, clients may relay their evaluation of the interventionists, whether favorable or unfavorable, to other research staff members (e.g., those responsible for data collection) verbally or in writing. For example, in the study for evaluating the cognitive-behavioral intervention for managing insomnia, data collectors were instructed to call participants to remind them to complete the daily sleep diary during the 6 weeks of treatment. During calls initiated by the data collectors in the fifth week, some participants receiving the treatment from a particular interventionist complained that the interventionist would schedule the telephone call (to deliver the individual intervention sessions in the last 2 weeks of treatment) but be late in calling, showing disrespect to participants. Formally, clients may be asked to complete questionnaires assessing their perception of the working alliance and/or their satisfaction with the intervention; the latter often contains a subscale inquiring about the interventionists' qualities, behaviors, and/or interactions (e.g., knowledge of the treatment, helpfulness in carrying out the treatment activities). Analysis of the information gathered from the two sources depicts the relational style of interventionists, which can guide further actions such as giving feedback to interventionists on areas for improvement, with the goal of maintaining quality performance and/or positive working alliance.

As stated previously in this chapter, interventionists represent the medium through which interventions are implemented. The quality of the medium is critical for an appropriate delivery of the intervention active ingredients and for accurate conclusions about their effects on the intended outcomes (Simmons & Elias, 1994).

9.4 Training of interventionists

Training of interventionists is another strategy for minimizing their potential influence on outcomes. Initial training is done prior to entrusting the selected interventionists' implementation of the treatment; it is essential for an adequate preparation of interventionists in the competencies required for a successful delivery of the intervention (Borrelli et al., 2005). Ongoing training is offered at regular intervals throughout the research study time frame; it is important for maintaining or reinforcing the acquired competencies and preventing any slippage in performance (Johnson & Remien, 2003). Both types of training are required for a proper implementation of the intervention, which is necessary to accurately carry out its active ingredients; this, in turn, triggers the mechanisms underlying the intervention effects on the outcomes.

Through initial training, interventionists should acquire the cognitive and behavioral or dexterous skills that enable them to perform the intervention activities in the specified format and at the prescribed dose in order to ensure accurate implementation of the intervention active ingredients. Initial training should be comprehensive and intensive, providing a balance between didactic and experiential learning if it is to adequately prepare interventionists. The didactic part of training revolves around the theory underlying the intervention (Johnson & Remien, 2003), which provides the rationale for the intervention, an overview of what the intervention is about and what it is set to achieve and how. The intervention theory also helps interventionists appreciate the value of the intervention and understand the activities to be performed. The topics to be discussed include the following:

(1) The nature of the presenting problem addressed by the intervention, that is, what it is, how it is manifested, what are its determinants with a particular focus on those targeted by the intervention, and what are its consequences. A condensed presentation of the theory of the problem and of empirical and/or experiential accounts of the problem as it is experienced by clients is useful in putting the intervention in context and in anticipating and understanding some clients' perceptions of the problem and reactions or responses to specific intervention activities. For instance, clarifying that clients with insomnia often present for treatment after having had the problem for a long time, during which they may have developed particular sleep habits that are counterintuitive (e.g., spending too much time in bed), alert interventionists to the possibility that some clients may not perceive restricting time in bed (which is an active ingredient of sleep restriction therapy) favorably. Thus, they may question the soundness and utility of this intervention activity and find it difficult to adhere to it.

(2) The nature of the intervention, that is, its name, goal, and active ingredients, as specified in the intervention theory. The discussion focuses on the conceptual underpinnings of the intervention, providing an explanation of how the intervention addresses the problem, what it is set to achieve, and what is absolutely necessary to implement in order to reach the goal. This information serves to promote an appreciation of the significance of the intervention, and an understanding of its rationale. Interventionists who realize the importance of the intervention may be able to convince clients of its value in addressing the presenting problem, particularly if they develop a helpful working alliance. Fuertes et al. (2007) reported that clients who understand treatment and agree to it, and trust their healthcare provider are likely to "buy into" treatment, see it as worthy, and follow through it.

(3) The operationalization of the intervention in terms of its components, activities, mode of delivery, and dose. The congruence between these operational elements and the active ingredients of the intervention is highlighted, pointing to the importance of carrying out the intervention as designed in order to accurately implement its active ingredients which are responsible for producing the intended outcomes. This helps interventionists recognize the importance of implementing the intervention with fidelity and of relaying to clients the need to adhere to the intervention activities or recommendations if they are to benefit from it.

(4) The outcomes expected of the intervention and the time frame during which changes in different outcomes may take place. This information further contributes to interventionists' valuing the intervention and relaying realistic expectations of treatment to clients.

Discussion of the topics related to the intervention theory relies on effective communication skills of the presenter (Dumas et al., 2001) who often is the researcher or his/her delegate. The presenter relays the information in simple terms, clearly, and in a logical sequence; elaborate on key points, giving examples for illustration; asks questions to elicit interventionists' understanding of the content and makes clarification as needed. The verbal presentation is facilitated with necessary audio-visual materials, such as slides highlighting key points of discussion.

In addition to the discussion of the intervention theory, the didactic part of initial training involves a review of the intervention manual. The review is systematic and thorough, led by the presenter (i.e., researcher or delegate). The presenter proceeds by reading each section of the manual, clarifying the intervention activity to be performed as described in the section, reiterating its rationale and way of carrying it out as well as the resources (materials and equipment) for doing it; explaining possible variations in performing the activity to address needs of clients with particular needs or situations while maintaining fidelity in implementing the intervention's active ingredients; discussing issues that may be encountered (e.g., negative comments expressed by clients) and strategies to manage them successfully; giving examples to illustrate the points of discussion; and reiterating the main points to reinforce learning. The presenter reads off a copy of the manual and requests interventionists to follow through with their own copy of the manual.

The experiential part of initial training follows the didactic presentation. The experiential part focuses on skill performance. It provides interventionists opportunities to observe and practice the cognitive and behavioral or dexterous skills needed to carry out the intervention activities. Various educational techniques can be used, including but not limited to case studies or vignettes, role playing or modeling, and review of archived audiotapes or videotapes of actual intervention sessions (Dumas et al., 2001). Case studies or vignettes consist of presenting information about particular hypothetical or actual clients describing their (1) condition or problem and requesting interventionists to analyze the information and delineate the course of treatment, guided by the intervention theory and protocol, or (2) reaction or response to treatment and requesting interventionists to devise and apply relevant strategies to address positive and negative ones. Case studies can be completed on an individual or group basis, and are followed with discussion of the interventionists' answers and rationale for their answers, and provision of feedback as necessary. Role playing or modeling involves having the presenter demonstrate the performance of specific skills, then the interventionists take turn in applying the same skills. The presenter and/or interventionists give comments to reinforce correct and/or to rectify incorrect performance. If available, audiotapes or videotapes of previously offered intervention sessions are played, or the transcripts of taped sessions are reviewed to illustrate the implementation of the intervention. This is followed by a group discussion, facilitated by the presenter, to highlight accurate skill performance; suggest ways to improve skill performance to maintain fidelity of implementation; identify deviations in carrying out specific activities, rationale for the deviations, and the impact on fidelity; and review the appropriateness of strategies used to address emerging issues. Additional experiential learning can be planned as part of an internal pilot study (detailed in Chapter 12), where interventionists in training assume the responsibility of delivering the intervention to a small number of participants under close supervision of the researcher.

It is wise to assess the interventionists' competence in delivering the intervention following training and prior to assuming the responsibility of providing it to clients, as suggested by Dumas et al. (2001) and Bellg et al. (2004). Assessment of competence is accomplished by administering a test to the interventionists who completed initial training. The test contains questions and relevant vignettes. The questions are geared to measure interventionists' understanding of the theory underlying the intervention and of the nature and rationale for carrying out specific activities that operationalize the active ingredients. Short vignettes and associated items are generated to assess interventionists' skills at implementing various aspects of the intervention accurately and with fidelity, and at handling issues that may arise during intervention delivery. The interventionists' responses to the test determine their level of competence and guide further actions, such as offering additional training for remediation of weak performance.

Ongoing training has been recommended to maintain an adequate competence level for all interventionists involved in the implementation of the intervention over time. Ongoing training can take the form of in-service, booster sessions (Bellg et al., 2004; Johnson & Remien, 2003). The sessions are organized into two parts. The first part consists of a review of the intervention theory and activities, and the second entails discussion of particular cases or subgroup of clients who present with specific needs, strategies that interventionists use to address these needs, appropriateness of these strategies in addressing the needs while maintaining fidelity of the intervention active ingredients, and effectiveness of these strategies in meeting clients' needs; and issues encountered during the delivery of the intervention, factors contributing to the issues, strategies used to manage the issues, and utility or helpfulness of the strategies in managing the issues and preventing their re-currence. The in-service booster sessions are held on a regular basis.

Careful selection and initial and ongoing training of interventionists are means to minimize the interventionists' effects on client outcomes. They may not completely eliminate these effects. Therefore, researchers may want to investigate the extent to which client outcomes differed among interventionists in studies designed to evaluate the interventions' effects. The methodological features of such studies are presented next.

9.5 Methodological features of studies aimed at investigating interventionist effects

Researchers planning to examine the interventionist effects, in addition to the intervention effects, should consider the following methodological features when designing the evaluation studies:

(1) The number of interventionists has to be large enough (at least 30) in order to obtain meaningful estimates of interventionist effects. Each interventionist is to provide treatment to a reasonable number of clients (at least 10). The number of clients is balanced across interventionists. Also, assignment of clients to interventionists is done in a way that minimizes potential selection bias, so that the baseline characteristics (such as level of severity of the problem) of clients assigned to different interventionists are comparable. Differences in the number and characteristics of clients across interventionists may confound interventionist effects (Lutz et al., 2007; Wampold & Brown, 2005).

(2) A crossed design is most appropriate to dismantle the interventionist from the intervention effects. In this design, each interventionist is asked to deliver each intervention offered within the context of the study (Staines et al., 2006). The interventions include two distinct treatments (e.g., inter-personal therapy and cognitive–behavioral treatment) or an active inter-vention and a placebo (which has the same structure as the intervention but not the active ingredients characterizing the intervention under eval-uation). The crossed design prevents the confounding of interventionists with treatments and permits the examination of the interventionist-by-treatment interaction effect. Confounding occurs when the same inter-ventionist provides the same intervention. In this situation, the observed outcomes may be attributable to the characteristics of the interventionist rather than the intervention active ingredients or vice versa. By hav-ing different interventionists deliver different treatments, variability in interventionists and in treatments is generated; each source of variabil-ity induces its unique influence on client outcomes, thereby allowing to detect the interventionist influence separately/independently from the treatment effects. Use of the crossed design requires the selection of in-terventionists who are willing to learn, acquire competency in, and deliver

interventions with which they may not be familiar or that differ from their theoretical orientation.

(3) Collection of data on the preexisting characteristics of interventionists and on the qualities that interventionists exhibit during implementation of the intervention. These variables could explain the observed interventionist effects.

(4) Tracking which clients received which treatment from which interventionist, and documenting these data, which are required for conducting the planned analysis.

(5) Application of HLM to analyze the data. HLM is a statistical technique that accounts for the nesting of clients within interventionists and interventions when estimating the effects of interventionist and of treatment on client outcomes assessed following implementation of the intervention or on changes in client outcomes over time. It is recommended to consider the interventionists as a random factor and the treatment as a fixed factor in the data analysis. Representing interventionists as a random factor has the advantage of generalizability or applicability of the observed effects to other interventionists with characteristics similar to the qualities of interventionists who were involved in intervention implementation (Lutz et al., 2007).

These methodological features are not always practical and feasible. The number of interventionists needed to examine their influence on client outcomes may exceed the financial resources available for a study, and/or the human resources that are locally accessible. Similarly, the required client sample size is large. Few competent interventionists may agree to the implementation of different treatments, and those who do agree may not be representatives of the respective population. Investigating interventionist influence is best done in large multicenter experimental studies, or in large cohort studies conducted in the natural, real world, practice setting.

Chapter 10

Intervention Fidelity

Whether simple or complex, interventions must be implemented with fidelity to be successful in producing the outcomes in the contexts of research and day-to-day practice. This implies that interventions are delivered as originally designed, ensuring that their active ingredients are carried out in the selected mode and dose, which is essential for triggering or initiating the mechanisms responsible for producing the desired changes in outcomes. The development of an intervention manual that meticulously operationalizes the intervention and details the step-by-step procedures for delivering the intervention, the careful selection of competent interventionists with ability and skills to maintain a helpful working alliance with clients, and the intense training of interventionists in the skills required to provide the intervention and requesting them to follow and adhere to the intervention protocol are strategies that enhance fidelity of treatment implementation; however, they do not guarantee it (Forgatch et al., 2005).

Actual implementation of the intervention may still fall short of the original plan, resulting in deviations in what was delivered from what was designed and in variations in what was provided to different clients. With these deviations and variations, active ingredients that characterize the intervention under evaluation may be omitted and/or given in a less than optimal dose, potentially resulting in nonsignificant effects on outcomes. Monitoring fidelity of intervention implementation is critical for identifying variability in treatment delivery and for examining the impact of such variability in the intervention on outcome achievement. In this chapter, the focus is on the conceptualization, operationalization, and assessment of intervention fidelity. The definition of fidelity and methods for monitoring fidelity are reviewed. The importance of fidelity is discussed from a research and a clinical perspective.

10.1 Definition of fidelity

Traditionally, fidelity of intervention implementation has received limited attention in intervention evaluation research. This was based on the

Design, Evaluation, and Translation of Nursing Interventions, First Edition.
Souraya Sidani and Carrie Jo Braden.
© 2011 John Wiley & Sons, Inc. Published 2011 by John Wiley & Sons, Inc.

assumption that well-trained interventionists strictly follow the treatment manual, which ensures standardization and consistency of intervention delivery across clients. The assumption proved to be untenable in light of observations in clinical practice and in research, of variability in the way different interventionists provide treatment (as presented in Chapter 9), and in the intervention components and dose given to clients. Differences in the implementation of interventions have been found to affect their effectiveness in producing the intended changes in outcomes (Lipsey & Wilson, 2001).

Fidelity of intervention implementation emerged as a concern in intervention research in various fields of study, most notably psychotherapy, program evaluation, and recently behavioral medicine. Differences in theoretical and methodological orientation across fields of study may have contributed to differences in the conceptualization and operationalization of fidelity. Accordingly, different terms have been used to refer to intervention fidelity, and the definition and respective elements indicative of intervention fidelity varied. The terms such as integrity (appearing primarily in the program evaluation literature), adherence to treatment protocol (mentioned in the psychotherapy literature), and fidelity (reported in psychotherapy and behavioral medicine) have been used, sometimes interchangeably, to refer to the extent to which the implementation of an intervention is consistent with the original intervention design. The term fidelity is used throughout this book as it is the most widely employed in current writings. Earlier work on intervention fidelity focused on issues related to treatment delivery, as executed by interventionists, whereas recent conceptualization has extended fidelity to the implementation of the intervention by clients. This change in perspective further contributed to differences in the definition and operationalization of fidelity, as reported in Table 10.1.

Embedded in the definitions and operationalizations presented in Table 10.1 is a comprehensive conceptualization of intervention fidelity that posits two levels of fidelity: (1) theoretical, which has to do with the design of the intervention, and (2) operational, which has to do with the implementation of the intervention.

At the theoretical level, fidelity refers to the consistency between the components and activities of which the intervention is comprised and the active ingredients that characterize the intervention as specified in the intervention theory. In other words, the intervention activities accurately represent and are in alignment with the active ingredients, as alluded to in the definitions of fidelity reported by Dumas et al. (2001), Pearson et al. (2005), Carroll et al. (2007), and Keller et al. (2009), and the element of design suggested by Bellg et al. (2004) and Borrelli et al. (2005). Fidelity at the theoretical level is maintained through the systematic process for developing interventions described in the previous chapters. The process begins by specifying the active ingredients of the intervention that are hypothesized to bring about the intended changes in the outcomes. Pertinent components and activities are selected to operationalize the active ingredients. The components and activities are then translated into a series of specific actions that interventionists perform in a

Table 10.1 Definitions and operationalization of intervention fidelity

Source	Definition	Operationalization
Bellg et al. (2004), Borrelli et al. (2005), Resnick et al. (2005)	Methodological strategies used to monitor and enhance the reliability and validity of interventions	Design Training of interventionists Delivery of intervention Receipt of treatment Enactment of treatment skills
Brandt et al. (2004)	Degree to which an intervention is actually delivered as planned	
Carroll et al. (2007)	Degree to which programs are implemented as intended by the program developer	Adherence to intervention Exposure or dose Quality of delivery Client responsiveness Differentiation of intervention Facilitation strategies
Dumas et al. (2001)	Demonstration that an experimental manipulation is conducted as planned, i.e., all components of the intervention are delivered in a comparable manner to all clients and true to theory	Content: Delivery of intervention specified in treatment protocol Process: Manner in which content is supposed to be delivered
Forgatch et al. (2005)		Adherence to intervention's core content Competence in intervention's execution
Hart (2009)	Use of quantitative or qualitative criteria to ensure that the intervention has been implemented as designed	Treatment receipt Treatment enactment
Keller et al. (2009)	Consistency with the components of the intervention theory	
Leventhal and Friedman (2004)	Meeting or exceeding a high standard of success in implementation of change/practice	
Mowbray et al. (2003)	Proportion of program components that were implemented Adherence to actual intervention delivery to the protocol originally developed	Adequacy of implementation of a program model Conformity with prescribed elements and absence of proscribed elements

(Continued)

Table 10.1 (*Continued*)

Source	Definition	Operationalization
Oxman et al. (2006)	Degree to which a treatment is delivered within its established parameters	Implementation of intervention activities
Pearson et al. (2005)	Alignment of activities with elements of intervention	Implementation of intervention activities
Judge Santacrocce et al. (2004)	Adherent and competent delivery of intervention as set forth in the research plan	Adherence Competence
Saunders et al. (2005)	Quality of program implementation	
Stein et al. (2007)	Reliable and competent delivery of the experimental intervention by interventionists	Adherence to treatment protocol Competence in treatment delivery

logical sequence to carry out the interventions. These actions are detailed in the intervention manual. Accordingly, fidelity at the theoretical level is indicated by the correspondence among the active ingredients, components, and activities identified in the intervention theory as distinguishing the intervention and the actions to be undertaken as delineated in the intervention manual.

At the operational level, fidelity refers to the degree to which the intervention is implemented as planned. Implementation of most interventions, in particular those targeting health behaviors, is the responsibility of the interventionists and the clients. Interventionists are ascribed the function of delivering the intervention, that is, carrying out the actions specified in the manual, whereas clients exposed to the intervention are expected to enact the recommended practices or the treatment recommendations. The actions of both interventionists and clients are necessary for a successful attainment of the intervention goals and achievement of the intended changes in the outcomes. Accordingly, fidelity at the operational level is reflected in the implementation of the intervention by interventionists and clients.

Interventionists' implementation of the intervention has to be of high quality in terms of content and process (Dumas et al., 2001) to promote valid, reliable, and competent delivery of the intervention's active ingredients. Fidelity of content delivery is concerned with the provision of the intervention components and activities in a manner that accurately reflects the active ingredients and that is consistent across clients. It is enhanced by having an intervention manual that clearly specifies the nature and method for carrying out the intervention activities at the prescribed dose; training interventionists and assessing their conceptual knowledge of and behavioral/dexterous skills required for delivering the intervention; and requesting interventionists to follow the treatment protocol, as specified in the manual, when implementing the intervention. Fidelity of content delivery is manifested by the interventionists' adherence to or conformity with the treatment protocol (Forgatch et al., 2005; Judge Santacrocce et al., 2004). They (1) perform the prescribed activities or behaviors operationalizing the active ingredients and refrain from engaging in proscribed activities or behaviors used in alternative treatments (Stein et al., 2007), which is necessary for maintaining validity of treatment implementation, and (2) carry out these behaviors in the same way when giving the intervention to different clients, which is crucial for reliability of intervention delivery. Process fidelity focuses on the manner in which the intervention content is supposed to be given (Dumas et al., 2001). It relates to the interventionists' skillfulness at providing the intervention (Stein et al., 2007), encompassing the qualities they exhibit (as described in the previous chapter) such as communication and development of a helpful working alliance (Judge Santacrocce et al., 2004). Process fidelity is enhanced with careful selection of interventionists, and is indicated by competent implementation of the intervention that actively engages clients in understanding, valuing, and enacting treatment recommendations.

Clients' implementation of the intervention, traditionally discussed under the rubric of client adherence to treatment (Leventhal & Friedman, 2004), is equally important for its success in producing beneficial outcomes. Clients' adherence to the intervention broadly refers to the extent to which clients are exposed to and engage in the intervention, and apply the treatment recommendations for the management of the presenting problem. This functional definition implies three indicators of adherence. The first is exposure to treatment; it reflects the extent of contact with the intervention content and is often represented with the intervention dose that clients receive, such as the number of treatment sessions attended and the amount of written materials read and the frequency of reading. The second indicator of adherence is level of engagement in treatment, which denotes clients' active involvement in the intervention activities (Carroll et al., 2007). Clients' involvement is facilitated by the interventionists during the intervention sessions and aimed at improving clients' understanding and adequate performance of the treatment recommendations. The type of activities to enhance clients' engagement in treatment varies with the nature of the intervention exemplified by participation in group discussion, completing homework, and setting goals. The third indicator of adherence is enactment of intervention, which is defined as the degree to which clients actually apply the treatment recommendations in their everyday life (Bellg et al., 2004; Borrelli et al., 2005; Hart, 2009) during and following attendance at the intervention sessions. Figure 10.1 illustrates the conceptualization of intervention fidelity described above.

10.2   Methods for monitoring fidelity

Fidelity at the theoretical and operational levels is critical for a valid, reliable, and competent implementation of interventions. Both types of fidelity are to

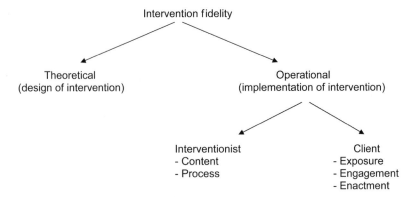

Figure 10.1 Conceptualization of intervention fidelity.

be assessed in research and clinical practice contexts to minimize deviations in treatment delivery and to determine the nature of variability in intervention delivery and its impact on outcomes. Whereas different methods have been proposed and used to collect data on fidelity at the operational level, none has been suggested for fidelity at the theoretical level. Section 10.2.1 presents strategies devised to examine fidelity at the theoretical level and a review of methods for assessing fidelity at the operational level.

10.2.1 Theoretical fidelity

Assessment of theoretical fidelity involves thorough examination of the alignment among the intervention's active ingredients, components, and activities as specified in the intervention theory, and the actions to be performed during treatment implementation as delineated in the intervention manual. Assessment of theoretical fidelity is usually done in the early stages of intervention development. Two strategies can be applied to conduct this assessment: (1) generation of a matrix and (2) content validation.

10.2.1.1 Generation of a matrix
The matrix identifies (1) the active ingredients of the intervention hypothesized to bring about the intended changes in the outcomes, (2) the components and activities that operationalize the active ingredients, and (3) the series of actions to be performed to carry out the components and activities, including the specific ones that represent the unique features of the intervention, and the nonspecific ones that facilitate the delivery of the intervention. Table 10.2 illustrates the matrix for one ingredient of the stimulus control therapy introduced in the previous chapters. The matrix shows the linkages among the theoretical and operational elements of the intervention. A thorough review of the content provided in the matrix determines the extent of correspondence of the intervention active ingredients, components, activities, and actions. The matrix is used by the intervention developer or the experts given the responsibility of assessing theoretical fidelity. The intervention developer generates

Table 10.2   Matrix for examining theoretical fidelity of one ingredient of stimulus control therapy

Active ingredient	Component	Activities	Actions
Associate bed and bedroom with sleepiness	Stimulus control instructions		
	Instruction 1: Go to bed only when sleepy	*Specific:*	*Specific:*
		Discuss Instruction 1	State Instruction 1 and point to written material where it is listed
			Explain rationale for the instruction
			Assist in identifying cues for sleepiness:
			Mention commonly reported cues
			Ask each participant to reflect on their experience and recognize relevant cues
			Reinforce the instruction by restating it
		Nonspecific:	*Nonspecific:*
		Assign homework	Describe homework:
			Have participants monitor cues for sleepiness
			Have participants follow Instruction 1 every night
	Instruction 2: Use bed only for sleep	*Specific:*	*Specific:*
		Discuss Instruction 2	State Instruction 2 and point to written material where it is listed
		Explore difficulties/ barriers to carrying out Instruction 2	Explain rationale for the instruction
			Explore current practices and strategies to change and follow Instruction 2

(Continued)

Table 10.2 (*Continued*)

Active ingredient	Component	Activities	Actions
			Engage in problem-solving as needed (e.g., issues with bed partner)
		Nonspecific: Facilitate group discussion Assign homework	*Nonspecific:* Involve group in providing instrumental support during problem-solving Describe homework: Have participants follow instruction 2 every night

the matrix in the process of developing the intervention and preparing the intervention manual; it serves as an "internal check" on the alignment of the intervention elements and the content of the intervention manual. Experts may be consulted on the conceptualization and operationalization of the intervention, and requested to assess theoretical fidelity. The consultation can proceed in two ways. First, experts are provided with written information about the intervention including presentation of the intervention theory that specifies the active ingredients, components, and activities, and a copy of the intervention manual. They are asked to examine the correspondence among these elements by generating the matrix to facilitate their analysis. Second, experts are invited to validate the content of the intervention by reviewing the matrix generated by the intervention developer, as described next.

10.2.1.2 Content validation

Content validation is a strategy to assess theoretical fidelity. This strategy draws on the method for determining content validity of measures described by Lynn (1986) and Armstrong et al. (2005). It involves having experts validate the correspondence among intervention active ingredients, components, activities, and actions. Experts are selected to represent academics and clinicians who have been involved in the development, implementation, and/or evaluation of interventions similar to the one of interest. Similarity is inferred from the general type and approach of interventions. For instance, to determine the theoretical fidelity of a behavioral intervention designed to promote self-efficacy in diabetes self-management, experts are academics and clinicians who have designed and delivered interventions that focus on self-efficacy and/or that applied a behavioral approach to induce changes in health-related practices. The number of experts to take part in content validation varies with availability, and could range from a minimum of three to a maximum of ten, as recommended by Lynn (1986) and Polit and Beck (2006). Experts are given the matrix generated to identify the conceptual elements of the intervention (active ingredients, components, activities) and to delineate its operational-ization (specific and nonspecific actions). They are requested to (1) review the active ingredients, components, and activities of the intervention as de-scribed in the matrix and derived from the intervention theory; (2) comment on the consistency and comprehensiveness of the components in capturing all active ingredients; (3) comment on the appropriateness of the activities in operationalizing the components; (4) comment on the accuracy and relevance of specific and nonspecific actions in carrying out the intervention activities; (5) determine any omission of important components, activities, and actions; and (6) suggest ways to revise the intervention elements in order to improve correspondence among them. The experts' qualitative comments can be sup-plemented with overall quantitative ratings of the extent to which the active ingredients, components, activities, and actions are aligned. Experts' feed-back guides the refinement of the intervention design to enhance theoretical validity.

The two strategies (i.e., "Generation of a matrix" and "Content validation") have not been applied to examine theoretical fidelity. However, they parallel techniques that have been used to develop valid instruments measuring con-cepts that represent independent and dependent variables of interest. The techniques include: clarification of the theoretical definition of the concept to be measured that identifies its critical attributes; operationalization of each attribute into relevant empirical indicators; and generation of items to as-sess the empirical indicators. The measure is subjected to content validation as a means for determining its accuracy in capturing the concept of inter-est. Considering the intervention as the independent variable in a research study demands careful attention to its conceptualization and operationaliza-tion. The same process for developing instruments is followed in the process of designing interventions and assessing theoretical fidelity. The matrix fa-cilitates the identification of the intervention's active ingredients (same as critical attributes), components and activities (same as empirical indicators), and actions (same as items). The matrix is reviewed by experts to determine alignment among the intervention elements, particularly the accuracy of the actions in reflecting the active ingredients. Such correspondence provides evidence of construct validity of the intervention implementation.

10.2.2 Operational fidelity

Assessment of operational fidelity entails examination of the interventionists' performance when implementing the treatment and of the clients' exposure, engagement, and adherence to the recommended practices. Different sources and methods have been proposed and used to assess these indicators of operational fidelity.

10.2.2.1 Interventionist
Examination of interventionists' performance when implementing the treat-ment has been discussed in terms of process evaluation. Interventionists'

performance is evaluated in terms of content fidelity and process fidelity; in addition, factors that could influence implementation of the intervention are explored. Data on content and process fidelity are gathered from different sources: research staff's observation of intervention delivery, interventionists' self-report, and clients' report, using quantitative or qualitative methods. Data on factors that could influence treatment implementation are collected from interventionists and through research staff field notes, relying primarily on qualitative methods.

Observation of intervention delivery

Observation of interventionists during actual delivery of the intervention to clients is done to assess content fidelity, that is, the extent to which interventionists conform to the intervention protocol, and process fidelity, that is, the interventionists' competence or skillfulness in providing the intervention. The observation can be direct or indirect.

In direct observation, the research staff members responsible for assessment of fidelity are physically present during the implementation of the intervention. They attend the sessions with individuals or group of clients; however, they do not participate in any intervention-related activities (i.e., they assume the nonparticipant observer role). While research staff's presence is useful in capturing nuances of what is actually taking place including demonstration of skills or practices and the nonverbal responsiveness of interventionists and clients, it may be logistically difficult and potentially inappropriate. For instance, it may be overwhelming for staff members to simultaneously follow through the intervention content covered, note the interventionists' competence or skills at providing the intervention, and recording their observations. Two well-trained observers are needed to overcome this difficulty and to reduce potential observer bias (Melder et al., 2006). Further, the mere presence of research staff at the intervention sessions may not be well received by clients, which interferes with their engagement in treatment; also, it may potentially lead to social desirability where clients and interventionists behave in socially expected and appropriate manner, thereby introducing bias.

Indirect observation is one strategy for enhancing complete and accurate assessment of interventionists' performance. It consists of reviewing video-recording or audio-recording of the intervention sessions to examine content and process fidelity. Both types of recording require clients' written consent. Videotaping, if done by a staff member who would manipulate the video recorder as necessary to capture the interventionists' and the clients' verbal and nonverbal expressions, has the potential of yielding a sense of uneasiness or discomfort, social desirability, and bias. It also is expensive. However, review of the video-recording is done at the required pace, which allows for comprehensive and detailed examination of fidelity, as well as clients' expressions of responsiveness to treatment. Alternatively, video-recordings done without the presence of a staff member would capture voices of interventionists and clients while remitting images focused on only one aspect of the setting in which the intervention is delivered; thus, nonverbal behaviors of participants in the session may not be recorded. Audiotapes of the intervention sessions are frequently proposed (Borrelli et al., 2005; Dumas et al., 2001; Resnick et al., 2005; Waltz et al., 1993) and used (e.g., Bruckenthal & Broderick, 2007) to assess content and process fidelity. Audio-recording equipment may be less expensive, cumbersome to operate, and intrusive than video-recording when used in-session. Recent models of tape recorders have the ability to clearly record voices of different individuals participating in group sessions and telephone sessions. The drawback of audio-recording is inability to observe demonstration of skills or practices as well as interventionists' and clients' nonverbal expressions, thereby limiting assessment of process fidelity if such behaviors are important in operationalizing interventionists' competence.

Direct observation is done in an unstructured or structured format. In the unstructured format, research staff members are asked to record the content covered and the interventionists' behaviors they observe during the delivery of intervention sessions. Research staff members are not provided with a guide to direct their observations; rather they document information as the session proceeds. The unstructured format is useful in that it yields rich data on the implementation of complex, tailored, or ill-defined interventions, and it gathers data on the interventionists' (1) coverage of content and/or use of strategies which deviate from those featuring the intervention under investigation, (2) alteration of some aspects of the intervention to accommodate or be responsive to the needs of client subgroups, and (3) way of dealing with client- and/or setting-related factors that interfere with the implementation of the intervention. The qualitative data obtained from unstructured observations are content analyzed to identify the content covered in the sessions and strategies or skills the interventionists' used to deliver the content. The emerging themes or categories (1) are compared to active ingredients, components, and activities of which well-defined interventions are comprised, (2) provide the evidence to support the delineation of the elements characterizing complex, tailored, or ill-defined interventions, or (3) guide the refinement of interventions' design and of interventionists' training.

In the structured format of direct observation, research staff members are given a checklist to guide their observation and documentation of intervention implementation. The checklist is meticulously developed to enhance its validity in assessing content and process fidelity. Stein et al. (2007) described and illustrated the steps of the procedure for generating the checklist. The procedure is founded on the content of the matrix that delineates the intervention-active ingredients, and respective components, activities, and specific and nonspecific actions to be performed during treatment implementation.

As mentioned by Stein et al. (2007), McGrew et al. (1994), Oxman et al. (2006), and Waltz et al. (1993), the first step focuses on the identification of the critical elements of the intervention. These include (1) the active ingredients (or unique features) as referred to by Stein et al. that characterize the intervention and are hypothesized to produce the intended changes in the outcomes; these active ingredients form the basis for assessing content validity; and (2) the nonspecific or common factors that facilitate the provision of the active ingredients such as application of instructional strategies that are also used in other interventions (e.g., homework, setting goals) and interventionists' qualities (e.g., communication skills and development of working alliance); these nonspecific factors guide examination of process fidelity. The second step in the generation of the checklist is the specification of the active ingredients and nonspecific factors in observable behaviors (Stein et al., 2007), exhibited by interventionists during treatment implementation; these correspond to the activities listed in the matrix (Table 10.2) relative to each intervention component. These behaviors or activities constitute the content of the checklist, which provides a rather macro-level information of the behaviors/activities to observe. If the interest is in micro-level behavioral information to closely monitor interventionists' conformity with the treatment protocol, then the actions listed in the matrix (Table 10.2) and derived from the intervention manual are used in the next step. The selection of the intervention actions, instead of activities, gives a comprehensive and detailed picture of what was actually implemented; however, it increases the number of items in the checklist and subsequently the efforts expended on the observation.

The third step in the development of the checklist consists of generating the items by translating the behaviors, activities, or actions into statements that clearly depict what is to be observed. Each statement details one behavior or activity in terms of its nature and specific indicators; examples are provided for illustration if necessary, to enhance understanding and recognition of the behavior or activity when exhibited. The items are organized by intervention components (where the set of items assessing a particular component form a subscale of the checklist) or by sequence of occurrence within each intervention session (as specified in the intervention manual). The former organization is conceptually meaningful and the latter organization makes it easier to complete the checklist during direct observation. The fourth step in the development of the checklist involves the selection of a scale (or response options) to rate the interventionists' performance in terms of context and process fidelity. The most commonly used rating scale is the occurrence of the specified behaviors or activities: observers indicate whether the behavior did or did not take place or the activity was or was not performed (Melder et al., 2006; Oxman et al., 2006; Waltz et al., 1993). Other multioption scales can be used to rate the quality of interventionists' performance, particularly as it relates to some of their qualities such as communication skills (with a scale ranging from "poor" to "excellent").

In addition to these steps for generating the checklist of interventionists' behaviors to observe, a manual is developed to inform observers on how to use the checklist (Hart, 2009) and to guide observers' training. The manual (1) introduces the intervention in terms of its goals, active ingredients, components, activities, and dose, which is summarized in the matrix; (2) clarifies the nature of the interventionists' unique behaviors (reflecting the active ingredients) and common behaviors or activities (reflecting the nonspecific factors) and illustrates them with examples; (3) explains how to conduct the observation and code the behaviors or activities, such as in time or event segments (Stein et al., 2007); and (4) specifies the procedure for computing total scores that quantify the level of content and process fidelity. Whether the codes are for time or event segments, the observation is usually done for the whole session and for all sessions planned to implement the intervention with an individual client or a group of clients. This is essential to comprehensively assess interventionists' performance, particularly when the content of the sessions is cumulative, demanding engagement in different sets of nonspecific behaviors or activities and exhibition of different qualities in different sessions. Although the ideal is to conduct the direct observation on all interventionists providing all sessions to all clients, this may not be feasible. Therefore, the direct observation can be done on each interventionist for 10% to 20% of their clients or sessions they deliver. Total scores are calculated separately to quantify content fidelity and process fidelity within and across session. For content fidelity, the total scores are computed for each subscale of the checklist that represents a component of the intervention and for the overall scale. Two mathematical functions are used in this endeavor, when each item score indicates the occurrence (scored as 1) or nonoccurrence (scored as 0) of the behavior. One function is to sum the items' scores and the other is to calculate the proportion of the behaviors or activities observed to have been performed out of those listed. Higher scores suggest higher levels of content fidelity. For process fidelity, the total scores are based on the items assessing nonspecific interventionists' behaviors. Total scores are computed for each type of behavior captured in the checklist, using the same mathematical functions for dichotomously scored items, or by taking the sum or the mean of the respective items scored with a polytomous scale/response format.

Although some authors proposed to assign weights to indicate the relative importance of intervention ingredients (e.g., McGrew et al., 1994) based on feedback of experts (Oxman et al., 2006), such weighting system is no longer recommended. It is cumbersome and performs as well as equal weighting. Furthermore, all ingredients are necessary to trigger the mechanisms underlying the intervention effects.

As mentioned by Stein et al. (2007), the checklist is subjected to testing of its psychometric properties prior to use in examining fidelity of intervention delivery in research or practice setting. The content validity of the checklist is evaluated with selected experts. Interrater reliability is assessed by having at least two research staff members observe and rate the same interventionists. Construct validity is examined by exploring the relationship between the observed level of content and process validity, and the outcomes attained following implementation of the intervention or the changes in outcomes from pre- to postintervention delivery, as reported by Oxman et al. (2006) and Forgatch et al. (2005).

Interventionists' self-report

The interventionist is another valuable source of data on content and process fidelity, specifically in situations when observation of intervention delivery is not appropriate such as interventions addressing sensitive topics and requiring maintenance of clients' privacy and confidentiality. Interventionists are requested to document the intervention activities they provide during the session. The documentation can be unstructured or structured. With the unstructured documentation, interventionists write down the activities they carry out during the treatment session. This method for data collection is time consuming and tainted by recall bias as some interventionist may not remember or forget to document specific activities. The structured documentation consists of having interventionists complete the checklist of specific/unique and nonspecific/common behaviors or activities, indicating performance of these behaviors or activities during the session. Regardless of the method used, interventionists' self-report should be obtained immediately following completion of each intervention session in order to minimize potential recall bias (Melder et al., 2006). In addition, interventionists are asked to rate their competence and level of confidence in implementing various aspects of the intervention, as well as their qualities at different points in time, such as immediately and 3 and 6 months following training. Although interventionists' self-report is valuable, it is likely to be biased, relying on subjective perception (Waltz et al., 1993); therefore, it may not be wise to have interventionists' self-report as the sole source of fidelity data.

Clients' report

Clients who receive the intervention are in a position to report on the occurrence of key activities of which the intervention is comprised, such as discussion of specific topics. Most importantly, they represent a valuable source of information on the interventionists' qualities such as development of working alliance (Waltz et al., 1993) and interpersonal skills (Bruckenthal & Broderick, 2007). Clients' data can be collected using qualitative, quantitative, or mixed methods, upon completion of the intervention. Validated items or instruments are available for measuring interventionists' qualities; most notable is the one developed by Forgatch et al. (2005) to capture various indicators of process fidelity or interventionists' qualities including teaching skills and provision of support, and the one reported by Joyce et al. (2003) to assess helpfulness of working alliance.

Factors influencing intervention implementation

Well-designed interventions may not be implemented as designed because of interference of various factors related to the interventionists, clients, and setting in which it is delivered, as discussed in the previous chapters. Therefore, it is crucial to identify these factors and understand their influence on intervention implementation in order to guide further decisions or actions related for instance to (1) the provision of additional, focused training to improve interventionists' knowledge and skills in delivering some aspects of the intervention; (2) the refinement or extension of the intervention protocol to account for the needs of particular client subgroups; (3) the adjustment of elements in the setting to enhance intervention delivery; and/or (4) the collection of data pertinent to influential factors so that their impact on treatment implementation and outcome achievement is accounted for when analyzing the research study data and interpreting the findings. Examination of barriers and facilitators to implementation is a frequently recommended part of fidelity assessment (Bellg et al., 2004; Spillnane et al., 2007). Pertinent data are obtained through research staff field notes recorded immediately following implementation of the intervention and interviews with interventionists held at regular intervals over the study period. The field notes and interviews focus on difficulties encountered during provision of intervention (Bouffard et al., 2003; Mahoney et al., 2006). Interviews can prompt for more details on the nature of the interfering factors and the condition under which they arise, and explore strategies for addressing them successfully.

It is evident that each source and method of data on content and process fidelity has an inherent bias. Therefore, using a combination, where the bias inherent in a source and/or method is counterbalanced by the bias inherent in another, is an effective strategy to enhance validity of fidelity data. This advantage should be weighted against possible response burden, which is well known to negatively affect the quality (i.e., extent of missingness and carelessness in responses) of the data.

10.2.2.2 Client

The elements of operational fidelity pertaining to clients are exposure, engagement, and adherence to the intervention activities or treatment commendations, with the aim of effectively addressing the presenting problem. Whereas multiple strategies have been used to assess clients' adherence to treatment, few have been proposed to examine exposure and engagement. These are reviewed next.

Exposure

Clients' exposure to the intervention reflects the extent to which they get in contact with the content of the intervention that operationalizes its active ingredients. For interventions delivered by interventionists, in single or multiple, individual or group, face-to-face or telephone sessions, exposure to treatment is logically represented by the number of sessions attended and the length of time spent in the session. As such the indicators of exposure are comparable to those of intervention dose described in the intervention theory. Accordingly, data on exposure are collected by the interventionist or research staff who are requested to complete the session attendance log. The log is used to document attendance of each client at each session, the length of each session, and any additional observation on each client such as if s/he left before the end of session and the time at which s/he left, and if s/he was accompanied by a significant other. For interventions given in a written passive or interactive format, including paper- and computer-based deliveries, clients assume primary responsibility of reviewing the material. The review is done in the presence of the interventionist or research staff, or at a time and place convenient to the clients, on their own. Data on exposure to interventions with paper-based delivery format are obtained through clients' self-report. Upon completion of the intervention, clients are requested to indicate whether they read the written material and the number of times it was reviewed, and to estimate the amount of the material read (e.g., few, most, or all sections of a booklet). The same information is gathered from clients receiving computer-based interventions to quantify exposure; in addition, built-in systems can be designed to track clients' access to the intervention content, the number of times it was accessed, and the sections frequently reviewed.

Engagement

Clients' engagement in treatment refers to their participation in the activities planned as part of the intervention delivery. Examples of such activities include group discussion, goal setting, task or action planning, completing homework, and demonstration of skill performance. Different sources and methods are devised to monitor clients' engagement in the intervention, based on the nature of the specific activity to be monitored and the circumstances in which it is performed. For instance, in-session direct or indirect (through video-recording) observation is most appropriate to assess clients' participation in group discussion and demonstration of skill performance. A checklist is used to document clients' engagement in these activities. A copy of written goals, action plan, and homework is obtained from clients and reviewed for completeness and appropriateness. Clients' self-report on engagement in these activities, using qualitative interviews or quantitative checklist, is an alternative strategy for obtaining data on this indicator of operational fidelity (Bruckenthal & Broderick, 2007).

Adherence

Clients' adherence to treatment involves application of the intervention activities or treatment recommendations in everyday life. Assessment of adherence has been extensively discussed in different fields of study such as behavioral and medical sciences; it is beyond the scope of this book to review this literature. However, three general approaches for investigating clients' adherence to recommended practices that represent the intervention active ingredients, are described.

The first approach relies on clients' self-report. Clients are requested to indicate whether they performed the recommended activities and the circumstances or conditions under which they engaged in them. A checklist of the treatment recommendations, supplemented with global questions on adherence, is used to collect pertinent data. The checklist contains the treatment activities or recommendations clients are expected to perform in their life. Each activity or recommendation is defined in terms of the specific action to perform. The checklist is then administered in the form of the following:

(1) A daily log (Hart, 2009) kept by clients over a specified period of time (such as 1 week). Clients are requested to complete the log prospectively,

indicating whether they engaged in treatment activities or recommendations, the number of times and the time of the day they did so, and to
write any comment related to their performance such as difficulties encountered or the nature and reasons for any alterations in performance.
The log can be completed during the treatment period (which may be
required for the interventionists to monitor clients' performance and provide feedback), and at each planned encounter or data collection occasion
following completion of the intervention.

(2) An instrument completed by clients toward the end of treatment and
at planned follow-up encounters or data collection occasion. Clients are
instructed to report on the performance of the activities as well as on the
frequency with which they did so over a particular time period, such as
the past 2 weeks. The latter form for administering the checklist is less
demanding or burdensome than completing a log of activity performance;
however, it has the potential for introducing recall bias more so than the
log that is completed on a daily basis prospectively.

Global questions on adherence to treatment activities or recommendations
can be used to gain a general sense of clients' implementation of the intervention. The questions inquire about clients' perception of the extent to which they
complied with the treatment and of reasons for noncompliance (Bellg et al.,
2004). They are administered at the planned encounters following treatment
completion. Responses to these questions provide some information on the
extent of adherence and on barriers and facilitators as perceived by clients;
however, they are possibly influenced by recall bias leading to underestimation
or by social desirability yielding overestimation of levels of adherence.

The second approach for assessing clients' adherence to treatment activities or recommendations involves significant others' report (Hart, 2009). Significant others (spouse, family members, friends) are in a position to observe
clients' performance of treatment recommendations (e.g., filling in prescription for medications, smoking), and in some instances, assist clients in the
application of the recommendations (e.g., serving as "buddy" for physical
activity, preparing meals). Accordingly, significant others represent an alternative source of data on clients' adherence to treatment. An adapted version
of the instrument and global questions, described for clients' self-report, is
generated to obtain data on adherence from clients' significant others. The
adaptation consists of (1) restating the instructions and items to point to
the interest in the significant others' perception of the clients' engagement
in treatment recommendations; for example, the global question is restated
as: In your opinion, how compliant has your partner been in following the
treatment recommendation in the past week?; and (2) listing the treatment
activities or recommendations that can be easily noted by significant others
and requesting them to indicate whether or not the client performed them and
the frequency of performance. The information on client adherence provided
by significant others may be limited to what significant others observe during
their interactions with the client. These interactions are determined by the

nature of their relationships and by their living condition. For example, a spouse living with the client interacts with the latter in various conditions and over extended time periods; hence, s/he is able to report on the client's enactment of the treatment recommendations more comprehensively than a friend who meets with the client at social events. Thus, significant others' report can also be biased, similar to the clients' self-report on adherence.

The third approach for assessing clients' adherence to treatment activities or recommendations rests on identifying and collecting data on objective indicators of adherence. Appropriate equipment is used to monitor performance of treatment activities or recommendations amenable to objective assessment. These are illustrated by tracking the number of refilled prescriptions from the pharmacists' database or the number of times the container was opened (detected through a built-in sensor) to monitor adherence to prescribed medications; using pedometers to record the number of steps or the distance walked to monitor adherence to recommended physical activity; and using actigraphs to capture periods of activity and rest to monitor adherence to prescribed time in bed, which represents the active ingredient of sleep restriction therapy.

Although it is advisable to use the three approaches (i.e., Exposure, Engagement, and Adherence) for assessing clients' adherence to treatment recommendations, such practice is not always feasible. Incorporating different approaches or sources and methods for data collection is a means for reducing potential bias and enhancing validity of adherence measurement. However, the selection of an approach is based on the nature of the treatment activities or recommendations to be monitored. The performance of several behaviors may not be readily observed by significant others, if available, nor detected objectively through available technology; therefore, it is most appropriately captured through clients' self-report. In this case, different measures (such as log, instrument, global questions) of adherence can be administered to maintain construct validity (Shadish et al., 2002). The measures should be carefully designed and selected to reduce response burden, which result in low quality of data and incomplete responses. To illustrate this point, assessment of clients' adherence to stimulus control therapy is conducted in the following three ways:

(1) Adding items to the daily sleep diary maintained throughout the treatment period and for 1 week at each follow-up data collection occasion, requesting clients to indicate whether they take a nap, the time the nap started and ended, and the location of the nap (e.g., bed); whether they used the bed for any activity other than sleep; whether they get out of bed when they cannot fall asleep or fall back to sleep within 15–20 minutes; and the time they wake up and get out of bed.
(2) Having clients complete a checklist of strategies to help with their sleep, including those recommended generally in the sleep hygiene (e.g., engage in physical activity during the day; avoid nicotine and caffeine at night) and specifically in the stimulus control instructions (e.g., go to bed only

when sleepy, wake up at the same time every day) components of the intervention. Clients are asked to indicate performance of these strategies within the past week (in concordance with the daily sleep diary time frame) at each occasion of follow-up assessment.

(3) Requesting clients to respond to the global question: How compliant have you been in following the treatment recommendations in the past 2 weeks? The question is asked at each follow-up assessment.

Convergence of responses supports construct validity of adherence measurement.

10.3 Importance of monitoring fidelity of intervention implementation

Whether offered in the context of research or clinical practice, interventions are to be implemented with fidelity in order to reach valid conclusions about effectiveness in addressing clients' presenting problem and promoting general health. Inadequate attention to fidelity has dire consequences for the validity of an intervention evaluation study. Deviations in what was actually delivered from what was originally planned contribute to failure of implementation. These deviations could introduce an unknown or new active ingredient; omit a planned specific ingredient that characterizes the intervention or a nonspecific or common element that facilitates the delivery of the intervention's active ingredients; or add an ingredient that is unique to competing, alternative intervention (serving as reference for comparison), thereby contaminating the intervention of interest (Borrelli et al., 2005). These deviations alter the conceptualization and/or operationalization of the intervention, and present a major threat to construct validity. Thus, it is difficult to know what intervention is actually provided to clients, to accurately interpret the client outcomes observed following treatment delivery, and to understand what exactly contributes to the favorable or unfavorable results. Variations in what was delivered to different clients, although done to be responsive to the characteristics of individuals or subgroups (Leventhal & Friedman, 2004), result in inconsistency in the specific and nonspecific activities, and/or the dose of the intervention to which clients are exposed and/or are expected to enact. Such inconsistency in intervention implementation by the interventionists and/or clients is associated with variability in outcome achievement. The level on the intended outcomes observed following delivery of the intervention differs across clients where some demonstrate the hypothesized changes in the outcomes, others show no changes, and still others experience worsening on these outcomes. This variability in outcomes inflates the error variance, which is a component of the statistical tests used to compare clients who did receive the intervention under evaluation to those who did not, on the outcomes. Increased error variance reduces the statistical power to detect significant intervention effects and the magnitude of the effect size, yielding incorrect conclusions about the effectiveness of the intervention (Bellg et al., 2004; Borrelli et al., 2005; Dumas et al., 2001; Sidani & Braden, 1998). Reaching incorrect conclusions regarding treatment effectiveness when the intervention has not been implemented successfully, with fidelity, has been referred to as type III error (Brandt et al., 2004; Sidani & Braden, 1998).

Monitoring fidelity of intervention implementation is a means for enhancing the validity of conclusions. Documenting the intervention specific and nonspecific activities carried out by interventionists and clients, as well as the dose received, is essential for maintaining internal and external validity in a research study, and for facilitating translation and incorporation of the intervention into practice. Pertinent fidelity data provide information on the intervention elements that were implemented as designed, on the way they were delivered, on modifications made in these elements to accommodate for needs or characteristics of particular subgroups of clients, on barriers and facilitators of implementation, and clients' exposure, engagement, and adherence to treatment, as well as report on factors that affected exposure, engagement, and adherence. These data are extremely informative and useful:

(1) To determine the extent to which the observed changes in the outcomes are attributable to the intervention as designed, rather than other treatment active ingredients or nonspecific elements introduced inadvertently during intervention delivery (Spillnane et al., 2007).

(2) To disentangle the contribution of the intervention's active ingredients and of the nonspecific or common elements, particularly those associated with the interventionists' qualities (Bellg et al., 2004).

(3) To examine the consistency in intervention delivery and the achievement of the hypothesized outcomes at a comparable level post treatment across clients, which increases the confidence in attributing the observed changes in the outcomes to the intervention (internal validity) (Bellg et al., 2004; Borrelli et al., 2005; Bruckenthal & Broderick, 2007; Melder et al., 2006).

(4) To explore specific/unique activities, nonspecific activities, and dose level that have been implemented as designed and contributed to favorable or unfavorable outcomes (Bellg et al., 2004). This information guides specification of intervention elements that are crucial for success and hence should be replicated, as well as refinement of the intervention where ineffective elements are eliminated to enhance efficiency of treatment (Borrelli et al., 2005), and elements of the intervention or its delivery are modified to address needs of particular client subgroups; the nature and ways to implement specific modifications are delineated. Clearly defined ways to adapt the intervention delivery are important for its ease of translation (Melder et al., 2006) and successful uptake and applicability by various interventionists and clients, in different settings (Carroll et al., 2007).

(5) To identify factors that influence intervention implementation. Strategies to address these factors are derived in order to facilitate its delivery, as designed, in a variety of contexts.

In summary, examining fidelity of intervention implementation helps in correct interpretation of research findings. When the results demonstrate significant differences in the outcomes between clients who did and did not receive the intervention under evaluation, fidelity data clarify what contributed to the observed outcomes: the intervention as designed or the influence of other variables. When the results show nonsignificant differences between groups, fidelity data point to possible responsible factors such as ineffective intervention-as-designed or problems with its implementation (Sidani & Braden, 1998). Accurate interpretation of findings prevents rejection of effective interventions and dissemination of ineffective ones (Dumas et al., 2001). Last, fidelity data promotes translation and reproducibility of treatments in the practice setting.

Final thoughts: Interventionists' adherence to the intervention protocol has been recently critiqued on two grounds. First, empirical evidence of the association between adherence to protocol and outcome achievement is mixed, showing that strict adherence may lead to deterioration in the rapport and trusting relationship or working alliance between interventionist and client (Messer & Wampold, 2002), which can negatively affect client's uptake and adherence to treatment and hence attainment of the intended changes in outcomes. Second, experience indicates that clinicians resent standardized delivery of the intervention and strict adherence to its protocol. They believe in the importance of tailoring aspects or elements of the intervention to clients' characteristics and initial response to treatment for successful outcome (Leventhal & Friedman, 2004). Therefore, it is critical to clarify the intervention ingredients responsible for producing beneficial outcomes in the manual used for translating the intervention, and to request clinicians to implement the ingredients with fidelity rather than stress that they strictly adhere to the intervention protocol (Waller, 2009). That is, clinicians are given flexibility in the delivery of the intervention to different clients, as long as they provide the active ingredients faithfully.

Section 4

Evaluation of Interventions

Chapter 11

Overview of Evaluation of Interventions

A clear and comprehensive conceptualization and a meticulously specified operationalization of interventions are prerequisites for intervention evaluation. In general, evaluation entails a systematic process for determining the merit, worth, or value of interventions. The value of interventions is indicated by their effectiveness in producing the intended outcomes. Demonstrating the benefits of interventions is necessary for their appropriate and safe use in managing the clients' presenting problem and enhancing clients' health. Therefore, the aim of evaluation is to determine the causal relationship between the intervention and the immediate and ultimate outcomes. This relationship implies that the changes in the outcomes observed following the implementation of the intervention are the consequences of treatment and are not associated with other factors inherent in the context in which the intervention is delivered. To attain this aim, evaluation is done systematically in sequential phases, beginning with an investigation of feasibility and acceptability of the intervention, moving to an examination of its efficacy in achieving the intended outcomes under ideal conditions, and ending with a determination of its effectiveness in producing beneficial outcomes under conditions of the real world of day-to-day practice. Empirical evidence supporting acceptability and effectiveness is needed for translating and incorporating the intervention in various practice settings. Different research designs are useful to address the objectives set for each phase of intervention evaluation. In this chapter, the criteria for inferring the causal relationship between the intervention and the outcomes are identified. An overview of the phases for evaluating interventions is presented. The chapter concludes with the role of intervention theory in guiding the design of evaluation studies.

11.1 Criteria for inferring causality

Demonstrating the benefits of an intervention involves the provision of empirical evidence that supports the causal relationship between the intervention

---

Design, Evaluation, and Translation of Nursing Interventions, First Edition.
Souraya Sidani and Carrie Jo Braden.
© 2011 John Wiley & Sons, Inc. Published 2011 by John Wiley & Sons, Inc.

and the outcomes. Causality refers to a structural relation that underlies the dependence among phenomena or events, whereby the occurrence of one phenomenon or event is contingent on the occurrence of another. As applied to interventions, causality implies an association between the intervention and the outcomes, whereby changes in the outcomes are attributed solely and uniquely to the intervention.

Traditionally, causality was focused on the simplistic direct connection between the intervention and the outcomes of interest, and rested on the counterfactual claim that if an intervention has occurred, then the effect would have occurred and conversely, if an intervention has not occurred, then the effect would not have occurred (Cook et al., 2010; Stanford Encyclopedia of Philosophy, 2008). Five criteria were considered to infer a causal relationship between the intervention and the outcome, as proposed by Einhorn and Hogarth (1986) and clarified by Sidani and Braden (1998). The criteria included the following:

(1) *Temporal order:* It is typical to think that phenomena or events causally depend on earlier, and not later, ones. It follows that the expected changes in the outcomes should be observed after the implementation of the intervention. If the changes precede treatment delivery, they cannot be logically attributed to the intervention because they occurred irrespective of its implementation. To demonstrate this criterion, the outcomes are measured before and after implementation of the intervention, with the expectation that the hypothesized changes in the outcomes are observed following receipt of treatment.

(2) *Covariation:* This criterion for inferring causality is an adaptation of the counterfactual claim. This claim implies that for the same clients observed under the same conditions, changes in the outcomes occur with the implementation of the intervention, and no changes in the outcomes take place in the absence of the intervention. Evidence supporting the counterfactual claim is derived from having the same clients undergo both treatment and no-treatment at exactly the same time and under exactly the same context to control for factors, other than the intervention, that may influence outcome achievement. Because meeting this requirement is unrealistic and logistically impossible, it has been substituted by the generation of two groups of clients who are comparable in all respect except receipt of treatment (Cook et al., 2010). Therefore, covariation is shown with the observation of the expected changes in the outcome with the presence of the intervention (i.e., among clients who receive treatment) and of no changes in the outcomes in the absence of the intervention (i.e., among clients who do not receive treatment). Covariation is inferred from comparability or equivalence of the two groups of clients on all characteristics and outcomes assessed before the implementation of the intervention, and differences in the outcomes' level between the two groups following treatment delivery or differences in the magnitude of change in the outcomes over the treatment period

(i.e., before and after the implementation of the intervention) between the two groups.

(3) *Contiguity:* This criterion implies that the implementation of the intervention results in the expected outcome changes relatively soon; thus, the time frame between treatment delivery and outcome achievement is rather short. With longer time frames, other factors may take place and mediate the causal relationship between the intervention and outcomes. Observing the hypothesized changes in the outcomes in clients who receive the intervention, immediately following treatment delivery, supports contiguity.

(4) *Congruity:* Congruity means that the amount of the changes in the outcomes is congruent with the nature and strength of the intervention. The outcomes are meaningfully related to the intervention, and the magnitude of the intervention effects is commensurate with its dose, where it is not logical to expect large changes in outcomes as a result of weak treatments.

(5) *Ruling out all other plausible causes of the effects:* This criterion for causality means that the changes in the outcomes observed following treatment delivery are validly attributable to the intervention itself and not to any other factor inherent in the context under investigation. The factors can be substantive or methodological in nature. Substantive factors are related to the characteristics of clients, interventionists, or context. Methodological factors are related to issues encountered in the conduct of the study such as those pertaining to outcome measurement and sample size. Whether substantive or methodological, these factors pose threats to the validity of conclusions regarding intervention effects, because these present alternative explanations of the observed changes in outcomes. Several strategies can be applied to minimize these potential threats and rule them out as possible contributors to the outcomes (Shadish et al., 2002).

With (1) the recognition of multidimensional and multilevel determinants of health in general, of clinical problems with which clients present, and of clients' response to treatment; (2) the design of complex interventions to address the multiple needs of clients; and (3) the acknowledgement of interrelationships among consequences of interventions, recent formulation of causality has been extended to encompass chains of phenomena or events. The formulation represents the interdependence among phenomena or events in that they are posited to influence each other, forming a complex system of causal relationships (Hill, 1965). The application of the notion of multicausality to interventions translated into the propositions that the effects of an intervention on the ultimate outcomes are mediated by changes in a series of phenomena (including reactions and adherence to treatment and immediate outcomes), and are moderated by other phenomena (including characteristics of clients, interventionists, settings). These propositions highlighted the role of theory in explaining the mechanisms underlying the intervention effects

(Lipsey, 1993; Scriven, 2004; Sidani & Braden, 1998) and led to some revisions in the criteria for inferring causality (Cook et al., 2010). The intervention theory (1) identifies the nature of outcomes that are meaningfully related to the intervention, (2) distinguishes immediate and ultimate outcomes expected as a result of treatment, (3) specifies the timing, magnitude, and direction of the anticipated changes in each of the immediate and ultimate outcomes to take place, and (4) points to factors, in particular substantive, that could contribute to outcome achievement and hence should be accounted for in intervention evaluation initiatives in order to enhance the validity of inferences regarding treatment effects. Further, intervention theory guides the design of the intervention evaluation study, the analysis of data, and the interpretation of findings.

The revisions of criteria for inferring causality entailed modification of the evidence required to support some criteria and an emphasis on the importance of other criteria.

(1) *Temporal order or temporality:* This criterion remains unchanged, as it is not quite logical to attribute observed changes in immediate and ultimate outcomes to the intervention if the changes precede the implementation of the intervention. Accordingly, it is necessary to assess the outcomes before and after implementation of the intervention and to examine changes in the level of the outcomes following treatment delivery. Finding changes that are consistent with theoretical expectations is ground for inferring causality.

(2) *Covariation:* The importance in demonstrating causality of having two groups of clients who are comparable on all characteristics and outcomes measured at pretest and of providing the intervention to one group and withholding it from the other is being questioned. The history of health sciences shows that the effectiveness of treatments such as insulin for the management of diabetes, blood transfusion for hemorrhagic shock, and closed reduction for fracture was inferred from empirical evidence derived from series of case studies, rather than comparison between groups of clients who did and did not receive the intervention (Cook et al., 2010; Glasziov et al., 2007). Withholding the intervention may be unethical, particularly when equipoise cannot be maintained and when the target population is in great need for treatment. In addition, creating a comparison group of clients who are denied a potentially useful intervention may be associated with unfavorable clients' reactions that influence the validity of conclusions regarding the intervention effects under some circumstances. Therefore, the evidence supporting covariation can be derived from alternative situations such as repeated observations of the same group of clients under the comparison condition (i.e., withholding the intervention, which usually precedes treatment delivery), and the treatment condition (i.e., implementing the intervention) (Rossi et al., 2004). These alternatives are considered if having a comparison condition is not ethical (e.g., withholding treatment for patients with an infectious disease or a serious

illness) or feasible (e.g., evaluating the impact of public health interventions or health-related policies on community- or society-level outcomes).

(3) *Contiguity and congruity:* These two criteria are reframed within the context of multicausality to account for the mechanisms underlying the effects of the intervention. Contiguity may still be applicable in the case of immediate outcomes, but may not be relevant in the case of ultimate outcomes. Thus, it is theoretically expected that well-designed interventions result in changes in the immediate outcomes within a relatively short time, if not immediately, following their implementation; however, the hypothesized changes in the ultimate outcomes occur within a longer time frame, and once the desired immediate outcomes are achieved. Congruity is emphasized, where the strength of the association between the intervention and the outcomes should be theoretically plausible and follows the hypothesized dose-response relationship. Accordingly, the evidence supporting contiguity and congruity is based on outcome data collected at least once before and repeatedly after the implementation of the intervention. The empirical evidence has to be consistent with the following theoretical expectations:

(a) Large changes in the immediate outcomes are observed immediately following the implementation of the intervention; these changes are maintained or smaller additional changes are reported over time.

(b) Small changes in the ultimate outcomes are observed immediately following the implementation of the intervention, but the amount of change increases, either gradually or sharply, in the hypothesized direction, over time.

(c) The strength of the association between the intervention and the ultimate outcomes is expected to be lower than that of the relationship between the intervention and the immediate outcomes; this expectation is congruent with the notion of mediation advanced by Baron and Kenny (1986), where the immediate outcomes mediate the connection between the intervention and the ultimate outcomes.

(4) *Ruling out other plausible causes of the effects:* The importance of this criterion is greatly emphasized; it is considered the most, if not the only, defensible warrant for causation (Cook et al., 2010) because it demonstrates that the intervention effects on the outcomes are unconfounded with the effects of alternative, plausible biases related to the interference of conceptual or substantive and methodological factors (Glasziov et al., 2007). Two general approaches can be used to rule out plausible causes of the effects. The first entails the application of experimental control over the conditions under which the intervention is implemented. This control consists of eliminating the sources of potential biases so that the observed changes in the outcomes can be validly attributed to the intervention and not to any other factors present under the conditions of intervention delivery. This approach has been traditionally used in intervention research and is well illustrated with the experimental or randomized controlled/clinical trial design. The second approach involves the a priori identification of

factors present under the conditions of treatment delivery and potentially affecting outcome achievement (i.e., serving as potential sources of bias that confound the intervention effects); collection of pertinent data; and examination of the extent to which these factors influenced the outcomes expected of the intervention. The application of this approach requires the availability of intervention theory (Scriven, 2004) and the acceptability of a range of research designs to evaluate the intervention. It is recommended when the concern is in determining the effectiveness of the intervention delivered under the less well-controlled conditions of day-to-day practice.

The reformulation of causality and the reframing of the criteria for inferring causality have implications for the design of intervention evaluation studies. The design is guided by the theory underlying the intervention, and may involve a range of methodologies that are most appropriate to address the study objectives. The study objectives and respective methodologies vary with the phases of intervention evaluation, which are discussed next.

11.2   Phases for intervention evaluation

Despite differences in terminology used to label the phases, there is general agreement within the scientific community on the number of and on the overall aims to be attained within and across phases of intervention evaluation. The four phases are applicable to the evaluation of simple and complex interventions, and parallel the steps of the systematic process for designing, implementing, evaluating, and translating interventions discussed in this book.

11.2.1   Phase 1

The first phase, referred to as modeling phase within the Medical Research Council framework (Campbell et al., 2000; Forbes and While, 2009) aims at developing an optimal intervention. This involves conceptual and empirical work to define and understand the problem to be targeted (Campbell et al., 2007), to select treatment components and activities that are most appropriate to address the problem, to identify components, and activities that are most relevant and acceptable to the target population, and to develop in-depth understanding of how the intervention comprising appropriate and relevant or suitable components works, that is, produces the intended outcomes (Campbell et al., 2000; Walker et al., 1989). The conceptual work consists of critically reviewing theoretical, empirical, and experiential literature, and synthesizing pertinent literature to develop a comprehensive understanding of the problem, of intervention's active ingredients and respective components and activities to address the problem, and of the mechanisms underlying the intervention effects on outcomes. The empirical work entails quantitative and qualitative studies to determine adequacy of the problem conceptualization and appropriateness of the intervention components in addressing the problem, to refine the operationalization of the intervention's components, and to clarify and specify the mechanisms underlying their effects. Details of the strategies to be used in this phase are provided in Section 2 of the book. The refined intervention is subjected to further evaluation.

11.2.2   Phase 2

The second phase focuses on examining the acceptability, feasibility, and preliminary effects of the intervention. Acceptability refers to clients' view of the intervention as appropriate to address the presenting problem, reasonable, suitable, and convenient for application in daily life, and meeting their expectations about treatment (Kazdin, 1980). Feasibility relates to the practicality of treatment delivery, that is, the extent to which the intervention components and activities are implemented smoothly, in the suggested mode of delivery, and at the recommended dose and with ease (Hertzog, 2008). Preliminary effects reflect the extent to which the intervention is successful in producing the hypothesized changes in the immediate and ultimate outcomes. The second phase represents a critical step in the evaluation of interventions. Acceptability of interventions influences their uptake; clients who perceive an intervention as unacceptable will not adopt it, whereas those who rate it favorably will use and adhere to it, and consequently experience the intended changes in outcomes (Eckert & Hintze, 2000). Feasibility of intervention affects the fidelity of its implementation; problems encountered when applying any aspect of the intervention interfere with its delivery-as-designed and potentially detract from its utility in achieving the desired outcomes and subsequently its incorporation in the day-to-day practice setting. Preliminary effects contribute to the assessment of the intervention's value; interventions that do not show any meaningful effects on the outcomes are abandoned.

Pilot exploratory studies are planned to test the intervention's acceptability, feasibility, and preliminary effects. It is important to clarify here that pilot studies are conducted for two different purposes: one relates to the examination of the *intervention*'s acceptability, feasibility, and preliminary effects and other relates to an exploration of the *research methods* and/or *study protocol*'s acceptability and feasibility. These purposes have different implications for the primary focus, the design, and the interpretation and use of the pilot study's findings as discussed next.

11.2.2.1   Examination of intervention's acceptability, feasibility, and preliminary effectiveness

When the primary purpose of the pilot study is to examine intervention's acceptability, feasibility, and preliminary effects, then the research focus is on the intervention itself. Of particular concern are: (1) the clients' and interventionists' view of the intervention; (2) the adequacy of the intervention's operationalization and the fidelity of its implementation by clients and interventionists, and ease of its delivery within the selected context; (3) the clients' experience and satisfaction with the intervention; and (4) the generation of the mechanisms mediating the intervention effects on the anticipated ultimate outcomes. Evaluating these aspects of treatment is necessary for interventions that are newly developed to address the presenting problem, recently adopted to prevent or manage a new problem, and adapted to enhance their relevance to a specific target population. A preexperimental mixed-methods design is appropriate to address the preset purpose for the pilot study.

The pilot study results (1) shed light on issues with the implementation of the intervention related to competence of interventionists, consistency of treatment delivery, clients' exposure, and enactment of treatment (Kovach, 2009); (2) validate and expand understanding of the intervention conceptualization (i.e., clarification of the active ingredients and nonspecific elements of the intervention, and mechanisms underlying its effects) and operationalization (i.e., feasibility of implementing the components and activities in the selected mode and at the specified dose); (3) indicate the range of clients' responses to the intervention (i.e., changes in the immediate and ultimate outcomes); and (4) identify aspects of the intervention and of its implementation that need refinement in order to enhance treatment acceptability, feasibility, and effects.

11.2.2.2 Exploration of research methods and/or study protocols

Where the primary purpose of the pilot study is to explore the acceptability and feasibility of research methods, then the research focus is on the study protocol. Of concern is the extent to which the research steps and activities can be carried out as planned, and are well received by clients. The research steps and relevant questions to be addressed in a pilot study include the following:

(1) *Recruitment:* How adequate and effective are the planned recruitment strategies in reaching the target population? How many persons showed interest in the study over a specified period of time? What are issues or barriers to recruitment?

(2) *Screening:* Of individuals expressing interest in the study, how many agree to undergo screening for eligibility? What difficulties are encountered in the screening process (e.g., clarity of screening measures, adequacy of cutoff scores)? Of those screened, how many individuals meet all prespecified eligibility criteria?

(3) *Enrollment:* Of persons meeting the study eligibility criteria, how many consent to participate and how many decline enrollment? What are reasons for nonenrollment (with a special focus on those related to the characteristics of the intervention and/or study protocol and logistics)?

(4) *Randomization:* How feasible is it to carry out the randomization procedure as planned? How acceptable is randomization to participants, that is, how many express willingness and unwillingness to receive the intervention on the basis of chance? Do participants have a strong preference for a treatment condition? Do they perceive randomization to be unfair and/or

inappropriate as it deprives some individuals of treatment they need? What is the reaction of healthcare professionals at the setting where the study is conducted toward random assignment?

(5) *Data collection methods:* How do clients respond to the planned methods for data collection? For instance, how many agree or refuse to be observed or to complete daily diaries? How convenient are the planned methods to the research staff and participating clients or what issues are encountered? For example, how easy is it to plan for and how many participants attend a focus group session? How many decline attendance because of logistics (like need for child care)?

(6) *Measurement:* Are the measures used to assess the variables of interest comprehensive (i.e., content captures all domains of the concept)? Are the measures appropriate and can be completed by members of the target population, that is, how many participants with which characteristics express difficulty responding to the measures because of unclear instructions and content, irrelevant or inapplicable content, and limited response range? How long does it take participants to complete the measures? What is the quality of the data provided? Are the outcome measures sensitive to change (i.e., able to detect a change in the outcome level from pretest to posttest)? Is the timing of collecting data optimal for capturing the anticipated changes in the outcomes following implementation of the intervention?

(7) *Attrition:* Of consenting participants, how many withdraw from the study? What are reasons for withdrawal? What are appropriate and effective strategies to minimize attrition (e.g., type and amount of incentive)?

(8) *Intervention implementation:* How adequate is the training in preparing interventionists to deliver treatment? How competent are the interventionists in implementing the intervention as designed? What issues do interventionists face during treatment delivery? Of consenting participants, how may get exposed to the intervention, engage in its activities, and enact it in their daily life? What difficulty do participants face in implementing the intervention?

(9) *Resources:* Are the planned human and material resources for conducting the study available and appropriate? Are the resources adequate to complete the study within the proposed time frame?

In summary, the pilot study is conducted to determine the adequacy of the planned study protocol, to identify any methodological problem that may arise during the study implementation and to refine the study methods and procedures as necessary. This information is required to prepare for undertaking a large study aimed at evaluating the intervention effects in Phase 3 (Hertzog, 2008; Kovach, 2009; Lancaster et al., 2004; Thomas Becker, 2008). Accordingly, the design of the pilot study should parallel the design of the large study, whether it is a randomized clinical trial or an alternative trial type. In addition, the research methods and protocol of the pilot study should replicate those planned for the large study. What differs is the sample size, where it is expected to be smaller ($n \leq 30$; Hertzog, 2008) in the pilot study than the large study. Evaluation of the feasibility and acceptability of the research methods is to be performed for any study protocol, whether it is recently planned (i.e., newly designed and innovative protocol) or adapted from previously used ones as may occur with replication studies with the same or different target population.

Lancaster et al. (2004) distinguished between external and internal pilot studies. External pilot studies are "stand alone" studies, conducted independent and prior to the large study. They are planned to address the questions mentioned above, relative to each research step. Answers to these questions provide feedback on the appropriateness, adequacy, and ability to carry out the study protocol and point to challenging areas that may require modification. Necessary modifications in the research methods are incorporated with the aim of improving the implementation of the large study and reducing the potential of any logistic or methodological problem that may threaten the validity of the large study conclusions regarding the effects of the intervention on the outcomes. As such, it appears appropriate to undertake an external pilot study to explore the feasibility and acceptability of new protocols and protocols adapted for use with a new/different target population. Internal pilot studies are done as part of the large study, where the protocol is tested on the first few participants. The aim is to iron out any problem with the implementation of the protocol, in addition to recalculating the sample size as suggested by Lancaster et al. (2004). It is important to caution against relying heavily on the results of pilot studies in guiding future intervention evaluation research. Although these results are only descriptive, providing estimates of measures of central tendency (e.g., mean) and dispersion (e.g., standard deviation), they are based on a small sample. Therefore, the estimated parameters may be biased, yielding under- or overestimation of the population parameters (Hertzog, 2008). Biased estimates may contribute to incorrect conclusions such as abandoning potentially effective interventions.

11.2.3 Phase 3

The third phase for evaluating interventions focuses on determining the efficacy of the intervention. The emphasis is on demonstrating the causal relationship between the intervention and the outcomes. A causal relationship implies that the intervention, and not any other factor, produces the expected changes in the outcomes following the implementation of the intervention. Consequently, the intervention is evaluated under "ideal conditions" (Whittemore & Grey, 2002), which control for factors that potentially influence the achievement of outcomes and present alternative plausible explanations for the observed changes in the outcomes. Of particular concern are factors related to the characteristics of clients who receive the intervention, the characteristics of interventionists delivering treatment, the setting or environment in which the intervention is provided, and the actual implementation of the intervention. The experimental or randomized controlled or clinical trial

(RCT) design has been traditionally considered the most appropriate design to determine the efficacy of the intervention, that is, to demonstrate its causal effects on the outcomes, under the ideal conditions. Its main features are conducive to the establishment of the criteria for causality. These features include manipulation of the intervention implementation, random assignment of participating clients (referred to as participants) to treatment conditions, careful selection of participants, and assessment of outcomes before and after treatment delivery. Manipulation of intervention implementation involves (1) providing it to a group of participants and withholding it from another, which generates a situation (i.e., intervention and no intervention conditions) prerequisite for covariation; (2) controlling the timing of its delivery relative to outcome assessment, which is necessary for maintaining temporality, and (3) implementing the intervention as designed in a standardized and consistent way across all participants, thereby minimizing variability in the content, mode of delivery, and dose of treatment to which participants are exposed. Variability in treatment delivery influences outcome achievement and poses a threat to the validity of the study results (Shadish et al., 2002). Random assignment or randomization consists of allocating eligible participants to the intervention and comparison treatments on the basis of chance. This is believed to enhance the comparability of participants in the two treatment groups on all characteristics and outcomes measured at pretest. This initial group comparability reduces the potential confounding influence of participants' characteristics on the outcomes, which represents an alternative plausible explanation of the changes in outcomes observed following implementation of the intervention. Selection of participants is done on the basis of strictly specified inclusion and exclusion criteria. The inclusion criteria ensure that individuals representative of the target population are selected. The exclusion criteria serve to exclude participants who possess characteristics known to be associated with the outcomes and confounding the effects of the intervention on the outcomes, thereby weakening the validity of conclusions regarding the intervention effectiveness. Assessment of outcomes before and after implementation of the intervention in the intervention and comparison groups provides the evidence for covariation. The evidence should indicate a difference in the outcomes between the two groups, where participants in the intervention group show the expected changes in the outcomes from pretest to posttest and participants in the comparison group report no changes in the outcomes.

Despite these advantages, the experimental or RCT design may not always be feasible (US Government Accountability Office, 2009). This may be the case when the intervention targets the community or an organization and when the likelihood of treatment contamination is high. The target community or organization may have unique characteristics, which makes it difficult to find comparable ones to serve as comparison. In this instance, time series or repeated measure design is a suitable alternative as the same community or organization is observed under the control and intervention conditions. Differences in the outcome levels following implementation of the intervention are indicative of its efficacy. Treatment contamination occurs when participants in the comparison group become aware of and enact the treatment under evaluation. This is likely to happen when clients accessible at one site are randomized to the intervention and comparison groups, but continue to interact with each other. To minimize the potential for contamination, sites with comparable characteristics are selected and randomly allocated to the intervention and comparison group. This design, called quasi-experimental or cluster RCT, is an appropriate alternative to the RCT for evaluating the efficacy of interventions.

Examining the efficacy of interventions, using an RCT design, is crucial for determining its causal effects on the outcomes. However, demonstrating the causal relationship between the intervention and the outcomes under the ideal conditions is not informative as to its potential success in achieving the immediate and ultimate outcomes when it is implemented in the real world of day-to-day practice. Therefore, efficacious interventions are subjected to further testing in Phase 4.

11.2.4 Phase 4

The fourth phase for evaluating interventions focuses on examining the effectiveness of the intervention. The primary concern is on determining the extent to which the intervention produces the expected outcomes when implemented in the real world of practice (Campbell et al., 2000; Whittemore & Grey, 2002). The real world of practice is characterized by variability in clients who receive the intervention, in the interventionists or healthcare professionals who deliver the intervention, the setting or environmental conditions under which the intervention is delivered, and the treatment components, mode of delivery, and dose provided to clients. Therefore, it is important to account for this variability in order to provide the evidence required to translate the intervention and incorporate it in day-to-day practice. To be useful in guiding practice, the evidence should answer the following clinically relevant questions: Which client subgroups, presenting with which personal and clinical characteristics, benefit to what extent from the intervention delivered in what mode and at what dose, and under what conditions? How effective is the intervention in producing beneficial outcomes compared to alternative interventions available and used in practice? To what extent does providing treatment that is responsive to clients' preferences contribute to the achievement of the outcomes?

Research designs addressing these questions have to allow for flexibility that captures the real-world variability (Zwarenstein & Treweek, 2009). Pragmatic trials are proposed to investigate the effectiveness of the intervention under the real-world conditions. In pragmatic trials, selected clients have to represent different subgroups forming the target population, implying the need to specify a set of less restrictive eligibility criteria. Multiple settings, representing those with a range of characteristics, are selected for implementing the intervention. Interventionists or healthcare professionals with diverse personal and professional characteristics are entrusted delivery of the intervention. Implementation of the intervention is not standardized but takes into consideration the clients' characteristics, needs, and life circumstances. Although differences in delivery are permitted, deviations in the provision of the active ingredients are not encouraged in order to maintain theoretical and operational fidelity and to reach accurate conclusions about its effectiveness. The comparison treatment encompasses usual care, similar intervention (e.g., low dose or one component of the same intervention) or interventions of different nature but targeting the same clinical program (e.g., behavioral versus pharmacological treatments) (Borglin & Richards, 2010; Holtz, 2007; Zwarenstein & Oxman, 2006). Partially randomized clinical trials, or preference trials, are suitable for investigating the contribution of treatment preferences to outcome achievement (Kiesler & Auerbach, 2006; Mills et al., 2006). In these trials, clients are informed of different interventions that address the presenting clinical problem and asked to indicate their preferences. Clients with a preference are allocated to the intervention of their choice, whereas those with no preference are randomly assigned to treatment. Providing treatment that is consistent with client choice reflects actual practice. Interventions that demonstrated effectiveness are ready for translation and use in day-to-day practice.

11.3   Role of intervention theory

The design of studies aimed at examining the preliminary effects, efficacy, and effectiveness of interventions rely on the theory underlying the intervention. The intervention theory identifies the characteristics of clients, interventionists, and settings that influence the implementation of the intervention and the achievement of outcomes; the intervention active ingredients and nonspecific elements operationalized in respective components, mode of delivery, and dose; and the immediate and ultimate outcomes expected as a result of the intervention. The intervention theory delineates direct and indirect relationships among these elements. As such, the intervention theory provides directions for the following:

(1) The proper operationalization of the intervention, the development of tools to assess the fidelity of treatment implementation, and the selection of strategies and methods for monitoring the implementation of the intervention across participants, as discussed in the previous chapters.

(2) The selection and specification of the comparison treatment, which can be a no-treatment control, usual care, placebo, or a different intervention to address the same presenting problem. The comparison treatment should not incorporate any of the intervention active ingredients. However, placebo and minimal treatment may have nonspecific elements that are structured in a comparable format and dose as the intervention under evaluation.

(3) The specification of client eligibility criteria, the selection of screening measures, and the plan for conducting subgroup analyses. This is based

on the client's personal and clinical characteristics posited to influence intervention implementation and outcomes. These characteristics are considered exclusion criteria in an efficacy study or form the classification variables for subgroup analyses in an effectiveness study.

(4) The clarification of personal and professional characteristics required of interventionists, the nature of their influence on intervention implementation and on outcome achievement, and the content and format for interventionists' training. These guide (1) the careful selection of interventionists in efficacy studies, and (2) the assessment of these characteristics and of the interventionist-client interactions and the examination of their effects on treatment delivery and outcomes in effectiveness studies.

(5) The identification of settings' physical and psychosocial characteristics that affect the implementation of the intervention and/or its effects on outcomes. These characteristics are controlled for by selecting comparable settings to minimize their potential influence in efficacy studies, or are assessed and accounted for in the data analysis to estimate the extent of their influence in effectiveness studies.

(6) The identification of immediate and ultimate outcomes, the theoretical definition of the outcome variables, the most accurate operationalization of the outcome variables, and the selection of relevant valid outcome measures. The consistency between the conceptual and operational definitions of the outcomes enhances construct validity and the likelihood of detecting the expected changes in the outcomes following treatment delivery.

(7) The delineation of the pattern of change in the immediate and ultimate outcomes, and therefore the points in time for assessing the outcomes before, during, and following treatment delivery. The points should be most opportune to detect the anticipated direction and magnitude of the changes. The hypothesized patterns of change in the outcomes guide the selection of the most appropriate statistical terms to include in the analysis of change in outcomes.

(8) The plan and conduct of the analyses to determine (1) the extent to which the intervention is successful in producing the anticipated outcomes, (2) the extent to which various client, intervention, setting, and intervention characteristics contribute to the expected changes in the outcomes, and (3) the extent to which the immediate outcomes mediate the impact of the intervention on the ultimate outcomes. The results of such analyses expand our understanding of the intervention effects, of factors that facilitate or hinder its effects and of the mechanisms underlying its effects. This knowledge is useful in translating the intervention into actual day-to-day practice.

Chapter 12

Testing the Acceptability and Feasibility of Interventions

Testing the acceptability and feasibility of interventions is the first and foundational phase of intervention evaluation, and is often carried out within the context of a pilot study. Acceptability and feasibility are examined for interventions that are newly designed; reconceptualized or refined in terms of content, mode of delivery, or dose; or being implemented in a newly selected target population and/or setting. Acceptability refers to clients' and clinicians' view of the treatment; it influences its uptake, implementation, adherence, and, subsequently, effects on outcomes. Clients who perceive a treatment as unacceptable may not adopt it (Eckert & Hintze, 2000). Similarly, interventionists who consider an intervention as unacceptable to clients may avoid it. Feasibility has to do with the practicality of applying a treatment. Challenges in the implementation of an intervention not only reduce the enthusiasm for the intervention, but also affect the fidelity of its implementation, and consequently its effects on outcomes. In addition to examining the acceptability and feasibility of the intervention, pilot studies can be designed to investigate the feasibility of the research methods planned for a large study aimed at evaluating the intervention efficacy. The focus is on the adequacy of the methods, that is, procedures for recruitment, screening, randomization, and data collection, as well as on challenges encountered when carrying out research activities. Results of a pilot study inform modifications or adjustments in the design of the intervention and/or the study prior to conducting the large-scale efficacy study. In this chapter, conceptual and operational definitions of acceptability and feasibility of interventions are presented, and quantitative and qualitative research methods for examining intervention acceptability and feasibility are described. Strategies for determining the feasibility of research methods, and procedures and issues in the interpretation of a pilot study's findings are discussed.

Design, Evaluation, and Translation of Nursing Interventions, First Edition.
Souraya Sidani and Carrie Jo Braden.
© 2011 John Wiley & Sons, Inc. Published 2011 by John Wiley & Sons, Inc.

12.1 Acceptability of interventions

The interest in exploring clients' acceptability of interventions has recently gained momentum with the recognition of the role it plays in the contexts of research and day-to-day practice (Bakas et al., 2009; Kazdin, 1980). In both contexts, clients have preconceived understanding, beliefs, and values about the presenting problem and its treatment. They are aware of alternative interventions to address the problem. Clients gain this knowledge from various sources including interactions with family members, friends, or healthcare professionals; the media (TV, Internet, written materials); personal or vicarious experience with the interventions; and/or participation in intervention evaluation research in which the treatment options offered in the trial are described during the process of obtaining informed consent. This understanding contributes to clients' perception and/or judgment of interventions, where they view some treatment options more favorably than others, that is, they consider the interventions as acceptable and express preference for these interventions to address the presenting problem. Assessment of clients' acceptability of and preferences for treatment and provision of the treatment option that is consistent with and responsive to clients' preferences have several benefits documented within the practice and research settings. In practice, assessment of treatment acceptability and provision of the treatment of choice constitute the essential elements characterizing client-centered care (Bakas et al., 2009). Application of client-centered care is associated with adoption and full implementation of and adherence to treatment, satisfaction with treatment, establishment and maintenance of a trusting relationship with healthcare professionals, achievement of outcomes such as resolution of the presenting problem, increased self-management ability, and improved functioning (Dana & Wambach, 2003; Hibbard et al., 2009; Kowinsky et al., 2009; Reid Ponte et al., 2003; Ruggeri et al., 2003; Sidani, 2008; Stewart et al., 2000; Wolf et al., 2008). These benefits further contribute to low health services utilization, costs to the healthcare system, and burden to self and to society (Eckert & Hintze, 2000; Naber & Kasper, 2000). In research, if participating clients (also referred to as participants) are allocated to the treatment option they perceive as acceptable and consistent with their preference, they develop enthusiasm for treatment, initiate and adhere to it, and consequently experience its beneficial effects (Borrego et al., 2007; Eckert & Hintze, 2000; Naber & Kasper, 2000; Sidani et al., 2009). In contrast, when participants are assigned to a treatment option they view as unacceptable and hence non-preferred, they experience disappointment and react by either withdrawing from treatment or not applying it fully. Such reactions reduce the chances of achieving the intended outcomes. The diverging responses of participants allocated to acceptable and preferred or to unacceptable and nonpreferred interventions decrease the statistical power to detect significant intervention effects (Halpern, 2003; Huibers et al., 2004; Sidani et al.).

Although acceptability of interventions has been, and still is being, discussed relative to clients, it can be extended to the case of interventionists. Whether providing treatment in research or day-to-day practice, interventionists may view interventions favorably or unfavorably. Their perceptions are derived from various factors including, but not limited to, their personal values and beliefs; professional orientation, role, and functions; theoretical knowledge and practical training acquired through formal and continuing education; experience; and availability and use of best practice guidelines. Interventionists' perceptions influence their judgment of treatment acceptability and subsequently its implementation. Similar to clients, interventionists who perceive an intervention as acceptable develop enthusiasm for it, offer it to clients assigned to their care, deliver it with fidelity, and encourage and support clients in its application, all of which contribute positively to achievement of intended outcomes. In contrast, interventionists who perceive an intervention as unacceptable avoid it and do not adopt it, even if effective (Severy et al., 2005). Withholding a potentially effective intervention may interfere with prompt resolution of the presenting problem and improvement in clients' health condition.

The significant contribution of intervention acceptability to uptake or initiation, application or use, adherence to or fidelity of implementation, and consequently effectiveness of treatment in producing the intended outcomes demands special attention in intervention evaluation research. Acceptability of treatment can be explored systematically at different phases of the process of designing, evaluating, and translating interventions. The inductive, experiential approach for designing interventions represents one strategy for eliciting clients', as well as interventionists' or clinicians', input relative to the acceptability of components and activities constituting the intervention, as discussed in the previous chapters. Methods for examining treatment acceptability in studies aimed at evaluating interventions are the focus of this chapter. Approaches for assessing clients' and clinicians' acceptability during the translation phase are highlighted in the respective chapter. Prior to discussing research designs and methods for determining the acceptability of interventions, it is necessary to define this concept and to clarify its indicators.

12.1.1   Conceptualization of intervention acceptability

The emerging literature on intervention acceptability is focused on clients', more so than interventionists', perception of acceptability. Different conceptualizations of acceptability have been proposed, reflecting variability in disciplinary perspectives. In medical and health sciences, acceptability is generally defined in terms of clients' satisfaction with treatment (Reimers & Wacker, 1988) or correct, consistent, and continuous use of a treatment (Carballo-Diéguez et al., 2007), such as medications (Tanaka et al., 2006), microbicidal cream (Severy et al., 2005), or an informational CD-ROM (Shapiro et al., 2007). In behavioral sciences, acceptability refers to clients' general view or attitude toward treatment (Lebow, 1987), operationalized in terms of judgments about interventions. Specifically, Kazdin (1980) defined acceptability as "the judgments about treatment procedures by nonprofessionals, lay persons, clients, or other potential consumers of treatments. Judgments of acceptability are likely to embrace evaluation of whether treatment is appropriate to the problem, whether it is fair, reasonable, and whether treatment meets with conventional notions about what treatment should be" (p. 259).

Acceptability, satisfaction, and continued use of treatment are distinct but interrelated concepts, representing aspects of the process for social validation of an intervention. Social validation addresses the value desirability, usefulness, and importance of interventions (Eckert & Hintze, 2000). It encompasses social evaluation of the significance of treatment goals, the appropriateness of the treatment procedures, and the importance of the treatment effects (Borrego et al., 2007). The aim is to determine the extent to which clients view interventions favorably and "like" them. Within this conceptualization, acceptability reflects clients' attitudes toward (Sidani et al., 2009) or perceived notions about (Andrykowski & Manne, 2006) interventions, operationalized as judgments of the appropriateness of the intervention procedures. As such, acceptability is assessed at the time of treatment decision-making, prior to actual exposure or receipt of the intervention. Satisfaction broadly refers to clients' reaction to treatment. It is often operationalized as rating or evaluation of the intervention process or procedures (i.e., components and activities of which it is comprised) and results or outcomes (i.e., effectiveness in addressing the presenting problem). The evaluation is done according to predetermined criteria that are frequently defined in terms of clients' expectations of helpfulness (Ames et al., 2008; Speight, 2005; Weaver et al., 1997). Accordingly, satisfaction is a reflection of clients' experience with treatment and is assessed following its receipt. Continued use of treatment is considered the behavioral consequence of satisfaction; clients who are satisfied with it are likely to continue its proper application in the context of daily life, as long as needed.

As a favorable attitude toward or preconceived notion about interventions, acceptability is guided by an understanding of the treatment options offered to clients to address their presenting problem and is based on careful judgments of the treatment attributes. Clients need to have a clear, accurate, and adequate understanding of each intervention under consideration before they assess its acceptability (Corrigan & Salzer, 2003; Eckert & Hintze, 2000; Wensig & Elwyn, 2003). Such an understanding encompasses knowledge of the intervention goals, nature of its components and activities, method of delivery, dose, benefits or effectiveness in addressing the presenting problem and/or in enhancing overall functioning or health, and risks or side effects (Sidani et al., 2006). This understanding contributes to judgment of the intervention's acceptability. Judgments are made relative to several treatment attributes that are classified into five categories (Borrego et al., 2007; Carter, 2007; Kazdin, 1980; Lambert et al., 2004; Miranda, 2004; Naber & Kasper, 2000; Sidani et al., 2009; Tacher et al., 2005). The categories include the following:

(1) *Appropriateness in addressing the presenting problem:* This involves clients' perception of the overall intervention's reasonableness, that is, how logical the intervention is in managing the problem.

(2) *Convenience:* It entails clients' judgment of the intervention's intrusiveness, that is, how easy the intervention is applied in the context of daily life, how long it takes to implement it, how much it interferes with daily life, or how suitable it is to one's lifestyle.

(3) *Effectiveness:* It refers to clients' perception of the extent to which the intervention is helpful in managing the presenting problem in both the short and long terms.

(4) *Risks:* Risks consist of clients' perception of the level of severity of the intervention's adverse reactions or side effects.

(5) *Adherence:* It involves clients' rating of the extent to which they are willing to follow or adhere to treatment.

In general, clients perceive an intervention acceptable if judged to be appropriate, convenient, effective, with no or minimal risks, and comfortable to adhere (Carter, 2007; Tarrier et al., 2006). This conceptualization of acceptability as an attitude toward interventions implies that acceptability can be assessed regardless or prior to experience with treatment. Accordingly, acceptability is explored to determine the value or desirability of interventions, which are main components of social validation (Eckert & Hintze, 2000). Acceptability of various pharmacological and behavioral interventions for the management of diverse problems, such as depression (e.g., Cooper et al., 2003; Gum et al., 2006), heart diseases (Janevic et al., 2003; Morrow et al., 2007), insomnia (e.g., Sidani et al., 2009; Vincent & Lionberg, 2001), and smoking (e.g., Bollinger et al., 2007; Cupertino et al., 2008) has been examined. Results of these studies point to treatment options that clients value, desire, and seek to manage their presenting problem, and therefore, are to be made available and accessible for use. For example, the perceived acceptability of complementary alternative interventions prompted healthcare professionals and organizations to adopt them and offer them to clients, and healthcare insurance companies or systems to cover their costs. The finding that clients differ in perceived acceptability of various treatment options has implications for practice. Acceptability is a key element of treatment decision-making. During the decision-making process, clients are informed of the interventions available to address the presenting problem, and are requested to consider the attributes (i.e., appropriateness, convenience, effectiveness, risks, and adherence) and hence the acceptability of each intervention prior to selecting the treatment option they desire or want to manage the presenting problem. Thus, acceptability informs the choice of treatment; therefore, it should be assessed systematically and comprehensively in order to capture it accurately, and to ensure the choice of treatment is well informed.

12.1.2 Operationalization of intervention acceptability

Different conceptualizations of intervention acceptability translated into variability in the operationalization and strategies for assessing this concept.

This variability was also prominent at the stages of designing and evaluating interventions.

12.1.2.1 Design of interventions

At the intervention design stage, acceptability is investigated for the purposes of obtaining stakeholders' input related to the relevance and appropriateness of interventions and of using this feedback to guide the development and/or refinement of interventions. The ultimate goal is to enhance the favorableness of interventions to the target population. Two approaches have been used to examine acceptability of interventions at this stage. The first is the experiential inductive approach for designing interventions, where the input of key stakeholders is sought to develop the intervention, as discussed in the previous chapters. The stakeholders include clients' representative of the target population and/or healthcare professionals involved in the care of the target population. Members of each stakeholder group are invited to participate in a discussion of strategies or techniques they perceive as acceptable and helpful in addressing the presenting clinical problem. The discussion is prefaced by a clarification of the presenting problem and proceeds with posing open-ended questions to elicit participants' input on what constitute acceptable interventions to address the problem. The questions inquire about general strategies and specific techniques participants consider appropriate and helpful in preventing or resolving the problem, and in improving the health status of clients experiencing the problem. Additional specific questions are asked to probe for the context for intervention delivery encompassing: the type of interventionist perceived as most helpful in providing the intervention to the target population; the time in the clinical problem trajectory at which the intervention is to be offered; the most convenient setting in which the intervention is to be given to reach the largest proportion of the target population; the mode of delivery perceived as suitable; and the dose viewed as adequate yet manageable. The discussion is then focused on reaching group agreement on the goals, components, activities, mode of delivery, and dose of the intervention that are acceptable to the target population. The study of MacDonald et al. (2007) illustrates the experiential inductive approach. The researchers conducted qualitative interviews with adolescents ($n = 25$) to identify smoking cessation services acceptable to this population. The results elucidated adolescents' perspective on who and what could help them quit smoking. The adolescents found it appropriate to engage with their friends in leisure activities as a diversion from smoking, or to attend with their friends a flexible smoking cessation support program facilitated by a leader who was characterized as "friendly, confidential, supportive, and respected" and offered outside the school system.

The second approach for examining acceptability of interventions at the intervention design stage embraces a consultative, deductive stance, where the input of key stakeholders is elicited regarding the appropriateness, relevance, and usefulness of newly developed or available interventions. Stakeholders include clients and healthcare professionals, and their feedback is obtained after either (1) describing the intervention to them or (2) providing them the intervention. The former procedure is applied in a group or individual interview with, or in a survey of, clients and healthcare professionals. The interview involves an interactive discussion of the acceptability of various aspects of the intervention, which gives opportunities to probe for clarification of stakeholders' perspective and to explore ideas for modifying aspects of the intervention with the goal of improving its acceptability to the target population. The interview entails the following steps: (1) reviewing the clinical problem requiring intervention; (2) providing an overview of the selected intervention, presenting its goals, components, mode of delivery, and dose; (3) describing, in detail, each aspect of the intervention including the specific activities of which it is comprised, the responsibilities of interventionists and of clients, and the setting and timing for its delivery; (4) after describing each aspect of the intervention, asking interviewees to comment on its relevance; (5) requesting interviewees to appraise the overall intervention in terms of its appropriateness and usefulness in addressing the presenting problem, and its suitability to the target client population; and (6) asking interviewees to suggest ways for modifying any aspect of the intervention and/or additional content, activities, or techniques to enhance the comprehensiveness and acceptability of the intervention.

Survey is an alternative method for gathering clients' and healthcare professionals' perception of treatment acceptability. The content and structure of the survey may vary depending on the level of details in the feedback required of or provided by respondents.When the interest is in examining the acceptability of different aspects of the intervention, the survey is designed to capture respondents' judgment of each aspect, similar to the content covered in the interview. Specifically, the survey begins by introducing the clinical problem targeted by the intervention and providing a general description of the intervention in question. It proceeds by listing the intervention aspects, including its goals, active ingredients, and/or the activities constituting the intervention and the way in which they are implemented (i.e., mode of delivery), and dose. The list of activities to be provided differs with the nature of the intervention. For educational interventions, the list consists of the topics to be discussed, whereas for physical and behavioral interventions, the list contains the series of techniques to be taught by interventionists and the exercises/assignments to be performed by clients. This list may be derived from the tool developed to assess fidelity of treatment implementation, as discussed in the previous chapters. Respondents are requested to rate the appropriateness of the intervention aspects, to suggest changes to the proposed aspects, and to identify activities that may be missing but important to enhance the intervention's acceptability. Table 12.1 presents an excerpt of such a survey to examine the acceptability of sleep education and hygiene for the management of insomnia. This type of survey for assessing acceptability of interventions is illustrated by the work of Bakas et al. (2009). These researchers requested ten experts to rate the acceptability of the Telephone Assessment and Skill-Building Kit (TASK) intervention that was designed to

Table 12.1 Excerpt of survey for examining acceptability of sleep education and hygiene

Intervention aspects	Rating of acceptability				
Activities:	0	1	2	3	4
Discuss the following topics:					
What is sleep	0	1	2	3	4
Why do we sleep	0	1	2	3	4
What regulates sleep	0	1	2	3	4
What is insomnia	0	1	2	3	4
How does insomnia develop	0	1	2	3	4
What keeps insomnia going	0	1	2	3	4
What can be done to manage insomnia	0	1	2	3	4
Mode of delivery:					
Discussion done in small group of 6–8 persons with insomnia	0	1	2	3	4
Booklet covering topics of discussion given for future reference	0	1	2	3	4
Dose:					
Discussion takes place in 1-hour session	0	1	2	3	4

Rating of acceptability: 0, not acceptable at all; 1, somewhat acceptable; 2, acceptable; 3, very acceptable; 4, very much acceptable.

assist caregivers of clients with stroke develop skills for finding information about stroke, managing survivor emotions and behaviors, providing physical and instrumental care, and dealing with one's own personal responses to providing care. When the interest is in examining the acceptability of the intervention as a whole, the survey is designed to capture respondents' judgment of its appropriateness. The survey consists of three parts. In the first part, a description of the intervention's goals, activities, mode of delivery, and dose is provided. The second part contains items and respective scales for respondents to rate the intervention's appropriateness and convenience, as detailed in a later section of this chapter. In the last part of the survey, open-ended questions are presented for respondents to comment on the overall acceptability of the intervention and to offer suggestions for altering any aspect of the intervention in order to make it attractive to the target population.

The interview and survey methods for examining acceptability of interventions at the treatment design stage have advantages and limitations. The interview permits in-depth discussion of all aspects of the intervention, where participants' perspective is explored, suggestions for modifying or changing the intervention are clarified, and agreement on its refinement is reached. However, the feedback is based on input of a select small group of participants. The survey allows quantification of the level of treatment accept-ability, contributed by a large number of clients and healthcare professionals. The information gained from the survey complements and supplements the detailed feedback provided in the interview in giving a comprehensive depic-tion of clients' and healthcare professionals' perceived acceptability of the intervention.

Feedback on acceptability can also be obtained after a trial implementation of the intervention, as originally designed, in a small-scale pilot study. In this case, the acceptability, as perceived by the interventionists delivering the in-tervention and by the clients exposed to the intervention, is assessed. This strategy for examining acceptability can be carried out using quantitative or qualitative methods, or a mix of both for data collection, and independently with interventionists and with clients. Interventionists' perception of the ex-tent to which different aspects of the intervention are acceptable to various subgroups of the target population is assessed following their training as well as their experience delivering the intervention to a small number of par-ticipants. Clients' view of the treatment aspects is explored throughout the implementation of the intervention. At the beginning of the intervention de-livery session, participating clients are informed of the need and importance of their feedback regarding the treatment acceptability, and of the procedure for getting it. The procedure entails provision of an intervention component and related activities, then requesting participants to rate the acceptability of the component and activities provided and to comment on their appropriate-ness and convenience to the target population; the procedure is repeated until all components and activities are delivered. Once the implementation of the intervention is completed, participants are asked to appraise it in terms of its overall appropriateness and usefulness in addressing the presenting problem and its suitability to the target population, to suggest ways to enhance its rel-evance and acceptability, and to identify any element or content that may be missing. This procedure for examining acceptability has been frequently used with educational interventions offered in a face-to-face format (e.g., Chung et al., 2009; Collie et al., 2007), written mode (e.g., Gwadry-Sridher et al., 2003), or computer-assisted programs (e.g., Vandelanotte & De Bourdeaud-huij, 2003; Vandelanotte et al., 2004), as well as behavioral treatment (e.g., Ames et al., 2008). For educational interventions, participants discussed the appropriateness, comprehensibility, readability, and relevance of the content covered; they identified topics of interest that were missing and commented on the format for providing the information such as the helpfulness of the group meeting or user-friendliness of the computer-assisted program. For behavioral interventions, participants were engaged in a discussion of the treatment components and activities they considered most and least helpful in addressing the presenting problem.

Examining acceptability following implementation of the intervention has the advantage of obtaining judgments that are based on actual experience, as compared to a description, of treatment. However, the acceptability rat-ings are gathered from a small number of select interventionists and clients.

Complementing these ratings with those generated from a survey of a large number of interventionists and clients contributes to a full account of the perceived acceptability of an intervention and to a meaningful refinement of treatment that enhances its favorableness or attractiveness to different subgroups of the target population.

12.1.2.2 Evaluation of intervention

Several indicators have been used, independently or in combination, to examine acceptability in intervention evaluation studies. A critical review of the indicators is presented first, followed by a discussion of the purpose and methodology for investigating acceptability in studies focusing on pilot, efficacy, or effectiveness test of interventions.

Various indicators have been suggested and actually used to determine acceptability of the intervention to the target client population. The indicators entailed enrollment rate, attrition or retention rate, uptake and adherence to treatment, continued use of the intervention, and self-report questionnaire.

Enrollment rate

Enrollment rate represents the percentage of eligible clients who consented to take part in the study, out of the total number of clients who met the study selection criteria. It is often assumed that clients with a favorable attitude toward the intervention under evaluation agree to enroll in the evaluation study, believing that their participation will provide them the opportunity to be exposed to and receive the intervention. Accordingly, a high enrollment rate is indicative of the acceptability of the intervention by a large proportion of the target population. In contrast, clients who perceive the intervention as unacceptable decline enrollment in the evaluation study. Whereas perceived treatment acceptability could contribute to clients' decision to enroll or to decline participation in an evaluation study, it is by no means the most common factor cited for refusing enrollment, and it is not directly and clearly captured in the enrollment rate, thereby invalidating the use of enrollment rate as an indicator of treatment acceptability (Andrykowski & Manne, 2006). Multiple factors related to the characteristics of participants and of study have been reported to influence enrollment in intervention evaluation research. Participants' characteristics include personal (e.g., employment status, poor health) and psychosocial (e.g., misconception or negative attitude toward research) attributes (Harris & Dyson, 2001; Heaman, 2001). Study characteristics encompass resentment of randomization (Stevens & Ahmedzai, 2004) and practical consideration (e.g., transportation, amount of time to participate) (Andrykowski & Manne, 2006). Simply reporting the number of eligible clients who enrolled and/or declined participation does not provide meaningful information on the acceptability of the intervention. However, inquiring about the reasons for clients' decision to enroll or not enroll in the study could shed some light on treatment acceptability. Content analysis of the reasons given assists in identifying clients' attitude toward the intervention, which is inferred from statements describing their perception of some aspects of treatment or their overall view of the intervention. For example, in a study designed to evaluate behavioral treatments for the management of insomnia (Sidani et al., 2007), the following reasons for declining participation suggested an unfavorable perception of the behavioral treatments under evaluation: not interested in the type of treatment, treatment may not be helpful, treatment is time consuming and requires too much work, and do not like the treatment. Eligible individuals expressing an unfavorable perception of treatment as the reason for nonenrollment represented a very small proportion (8 of 370) of those who refused participation in the study. Inferring that participants viewed the behavioral treatments as acceptable was inappropriate as no empirical evidence was available to support the inference; rather, unsolicited comments suggested that clients decided to participate because they were "in search for an alternative to sleeping pill" and/or were "desperate to get some relief." The comments implied a sense of willingness to try any treatment, regardless of its perceived acceptability. In summary, enrollment rate offers no information about acceptability of the intervention and consequently is not a valid indicator of this concept. Inquiring about reasons for enrollment or nonenrollment, with explicit questioning of the clients' overall view of the intervention under evaluation, is a promising strategy to gather qualitative data pertaining to treatment acceptability.

Attrition or retention rate
Attrition rate (also referred to as drop-out rate) is the percentage of participants who withdraw from the study, at any time point, out of the total number of eligible and consenting clients. Its corollary, retention rate, reflects the percentage of consenting participants who complete the study. Attrition and retention rates have been used as indicators of intervention acceptability (e.g., Shapiro et al., 2007) under the assumption that participants who consider the treatment inappropriate and irrelevant decide to withdraw from the study to avoid further exposure to an unacceptable intervention, whereas those with a favorable attitude to the intervention are motivated to continue with and complete treatment. Thus, a low attrition rate and/or a high retention rate operationalize high levels of intervention acceptability. The assumption underlying the use of attrition rate as an indicator of intervention acceptability is flawed because participants' decision to drop out at any point in time during the study, especially after treatment implementation (e.g., posttest or follow-up), may be affected by a host of factors that are not necessarily associated with the treatment under evaluation. Attrition has been attributed to: (1) participants' personal (e.g., age, socioeconomic status), clinical (e.g., severity of illness), and psychosocial (e.g., distress, perceived social support) characteristics; and (2) study characteristics related to burdensome research procedures (e.g., number of follow-ups, length of data collection sessions), invasiveness of research procedures (e.g., blood withdrawal), lack of flexibility in the study protocol, and poor communication or interaction skills of research personnel (Ahern & Le Brocque, 2005; Lindsay Davis et al., 2002; Moser et al., 2000). It is important to recognize that the nature and attributes of the treatments

offered in an evaluation study contribute to attrition. For instance, participants allocated to complex and inflexible treatments find them cumbersome and demanding and hence difficult to carry out with fidelity, to adhere, and to continue their use. They may decide to withdraw rather than face the struggle of implementing such treatments. In contrast, participants assigned to comparison treatments, which often are ineffective, drop out of the study due to the perceived lack of improvement in their condition and the desire to seek treatment elsewhere. Attrition rate reports the total number of participants who drop out of the study, regardless of the specific reason for withdrawal. As such, it is not a unique and precise indicator of intervention acceptability (Andrykowski & Manne, 2006). Requesting participants to state the reason for withdrawal and content analysis of their responses offer a more accurate operationalization of this concept, particularly if the responses describe their view of the intervention. In the previously mentioned study evaluating behavioral treatments for insomnia, the following reasons for withdrawal illustrated participants' perception of the intervention: did not like the type of treatment, treatment is time consuming and requires too much work, treatment is not helping, treatment interfered with daily routine, and could not handle the treatment. Treatment-related characteristics represented 8% of all reasons given for withdrawal (Sidani et al., 2007). The assumption underlying the use of retention rate as an indicator of intervention acceptability is questionable. Although treatment acceptability is a possible factor affecting participants' retention, it is not the only one. For instance, some participants decide to complete the study because of a sense of obligation to the researcher, an appreciation for and desire to contribute to knowledge development, and a need to receive compensation. Therefore, unless explicitly explored by the researcher and stated by participants as the main reason for completing the study, it would be inadequate to infer that a high retention rate is directly and solely associated with intervention acceptability. Briefly, attrition and retention rates are invalid indicators of intervention acceptability as other factors equally and significantly contribute to clients' decision to withdraw or to complete the intervention evaluation study.

Uptake, adherence, and continued use of intervention

Uptake refers to the initiation of treatment. It is operationalized in terms of the percentage of eligible and consenting clients who agree to participate in treatment (Klem et al., 2000). This initial engagement is indicated by report of participants beginning treatment such as taking the first dose of a medication, reviewing first parts of educational materials, and attending the first session of a behavioral intervention. Adherence is broadly defined as the appropriate enactment and implementation of treatment recommendations at the appropriate dose level. Continued use refers to the sustained implementation of the intervention, as needed, over time. It is illustrated with participants' review of educational guide or CD-ROM as frequently as required after study completion (e.g., McCormack et al., 2003; Shapiro et al., 2007), or consistent application of a medication (e.g., Severy et al., 2005), or behavioral intervention (Cohen et al., 2007). It is believed that participants are motivated to initiate and to implement properly an intervention they perceive as acceptable; correct implementation of the intervention is associated with the experience of improvement in the presenting problem and in overall health. This, in turn, prompts further adherence and continued use of the intervention, and contributes to a reinforcement of a favorable perception of the intervention (Eckert & Hintze, 2000; Finn & Sladeczek, 2001). The conceptualization of intervention uptake, adherence, and continued use as indicators of acceptability is behaviorally based, which is not consistent with the conceptualization of intervention acceptability adopted in this chapter. As explained in a previous section, acceptability is defined as clients' attitudes toward or preconceived notions about interventions that are expressed prior to exposure or receipt of treatment. Acceptability is operationalized in terms of clients' judgment of the extent to which the intervention is appropriate and effective in addressing the presenting problem, is convenient and has minimal risk, and the extent to which they are willing to adhere to it. As an attitude, acceptability influences performance of behaviors such as uptake of intervention, as proposed by health behavior theories such as the theory of planned behavior (Ajzen, 1991). Accordingly, uptake of treatment may not be an indicator of acceptability, but a behavioral consequence of a favorable attitude toward the intervention. Acceptability serves to motivate clients to initiate the intervention. Although acceptability could be related to adherence to and continued use of the intervention, various factors have been found to shape adherence and continued use. Most relevant factors include: (1) clients' socioeconomic status, where those with limited income or social support may not have the resources required for appropriate implementation of the intervention over time; (2) clients' ability to enact complex interventions, where they encounter difficulty following complicated and demanding treatment protocols; (3) clients' experience of treatment side effects, where those who suffer untoward reactions do not enact the treatment; and (4) clients' satisfaction with the treatment where those finding that the treatment processes and outcomes met their expectations are likely to adhere and continue to use the intervention. It can be promised that experience and satisfaction with treatment, rather than initial perceived acceptability, are meaningful determinants of adherence and continued use of the intervention. Acceptability may be altered following actual experience with treatment (Andrykowski & Manne, 2006) whereby clients having negative experience and hence dissatisfied with treatment develop a less favorable attitude or view of the intervention. Consequently, adherence and continued use cannot be considered as unique indicators or behavioral consequences of intervention acceptability; however, they can reflect behavioral consequences of satisfaction with treatment.

Self-report questionnaire

Several self-report questionnaires have been used to assess clients' perceived acceptability of pharmacological, educational, and behavioral interventions. Although the use of self-report measures is appropriate and consistent with the subjective nature of acceptability, defined as attitudes or preconceived notions about treatment, the questionnaires differed in content. Differences in content reflect differences in the conceptualization and operationalization of acceptability as well as in the nature and/or mode of delivery of the intervention under evaluation. Questionnaires measuring acceptability of pharmacological interventions focused on clients' evaluation of preselected properties of a medication or product and satisfaction with it (Severy et al., 2005). For example, Carballo-Diéguez et al. (2007) requested participants to rate a rectal microbicide, after applying it, in terms of: how much they liked it and how much they were bothered by leakage, soiling, or bloating. Foley (2005) investigated children's, parents', and dentists' perception of the acceptability and efficacy of nitrous oxide inhalation sedation for dental procedures. The questions inquired whether the children needed the sedation, coped with the sedation, found the sedation helped with administration of analgesia and with dental treatment, would have managed without sedation, and would require sedation for future dental treatment. Most questionnaires assessing acceptability of pharmacological treatments were developed with no clear conceptualization of acceptability, leading to inclusion of items tapping satisfaction with treatment; further, the content was often specific to the treatment under investigation, precluding applicability of the questionnaire to other treatments and hence, comparison of different treatments for acceptability. In addition, the psychometric properties of these questionnaires have not been investigated, raising questions about their validity in measuring intervention acceptability.

Questionnaires assessing the acceptability of educational interventions, delivered in different formats (e.g., booklet, computer-based), captured comprehensibility, readability, and usefulness of the content, as well as usability of the delivery method. Questions regarding comprehensibility, readability, and usefulness have been commonly used to examine acceptability of educational materials, regardless of the format selected for relaying the information. These questions inquire about the extent to which the information provided is: clear, easy to read and understand; presented in a logical order; interesting and relevant; and helpful in applying the treatment recommendations such as engagement in physical activity (Haerens et al., 2007; Vandelanotte & De Bourdeaudhuij, 2003), taking drugs (McCormack et al., 2003), reducing fat intake (Vandelanotte et al., 2004), management of heart failure (Gwadry-Sridher et al., 2003), smoking cessation (Etter & Etter, 2007), and HIV/AIDS prevention (Bowen et al., 2007). Questions about usability focused on the technical quality (e.g., layout, size of print) of educational booklets (Gwadry-Sridher et al., 2003) and ease of using computer (Haerens et al., 2007). Although the content of these questionnaires was rather consistent across interventions and studies, it was not derived from any particular conceptualization of acceptability.

Questionnaires assessing the acceptability of behavioral interventions are concerned with clients' rating of treatment attributes, which were derived from and extended those identified in Kazdin's (1980) definition of treatment acceptability. Embedded within social validation, this definition conceptualizes acceptability as the judgment of the appropriateness of interventions to consumers. The judgment is made relative to the following treatment attributes:

(1) Appropriateness, fairness, or reasonableness, that is, the degree to which clients like the procedures of which the treatment is comprised.
(2) Perceived effectiveness, that is, the extent of improvement in condition/presenting problem clients expect as a result of treatment.
(3) Potential side effects, that is, the disadvantages of treatment perceived by clients.
(4) Suitability, that is, the time it takes to apply the treatment and the extent of disruption it causes in clients' life.
(5) Willingness, that is, the extent to which clients are willing to implement the treatment.
(6) Cost or affordability of the treatment.

Finn and Sladeczek (2001) and Carter (2007) conducted systematic reviews of instruments measuring the acceptability of behavioral treatments used in the school system (e.g., Behavior Intervention Rating Scale) and in clinical practice (e.g., Treatment Evaluation Inventory). The review identified the treatment attributes captured by the instruments, and synthesized empirical evidence of their psychometric properties. The results indicated that the instruments focused on similar attributes of intervention acceptability and demonstrated acceptable internal consistency reliability and validity. In addition to the instruments mentioned in the two reviews, the Credibility Scale and the Treatment Perceptions Questionnaire have been administered to assess acceptability of behavioral interventions. The Credibility Scale (Becker et al., 2007) consists of items to rate the following attributes of treatment: acceptability, suitability, tolerability, expectation of positive benefit, credibility, appropriateness, reasonableness, justifiability, and discomfort. It was used to assess acceptability of different treatments for posttraumatic stress disorder (Tarrier et al., 2006). The Treatment Perceptions Questionnaire focuses on the acceptability, believability, and effectiveness attributes. It was adapted to measure acceptability of pharmacological and behavioral therapy for management of insomnia (Morin et al., 1992; Vincent & Lionberg, 2001) and anxiety disorder (Deacon & Abramowitz, 2005).

In conclusion, the self-report questionnaires represent the most appropriate method for assessing the subjective concept of treatment acceptability, defined as favorable attitude toward interventions. The instruments measuring acceptability of behavioral interventions are guided by a clear conceptualization and operationalization of acceptability. They capture various attributes of treatment that have been found to form the basis for judging acceptability. Empirical evidence supports their psychometric properties. The content of their items can be easily adapted, as needed, to examine clients' and interventionists' perceived acceptability of specific interventions in evaluation studies.

The purpose for investigating acceptability differs slightly with the primary focus of the intervention evaluation study, that is, pilot, efficacy, or effectiveness test. Consistent with the stated purpose, the methodology for examining treatment acceptability varies.

Pilot studies

In pilot studies, the focus is on gaining a comprehensive understanding of participants' view of all aspects of the intervention in order to determine those deemed acceptable and those considered inappropriate and irrelevant to the target population. Participants' feedback is obtained throughout and after a trial implementation of the intervention, as described in the previous section, using a mix of quantitative and qualitative methods of data collection. Specifically, participants are exposed to an intervention component and are asked to rate the appropriateness and convenience of the activities constituting the component, with adapted respective items of self-report questionnaires. In addition, participants are engaged in a discussion to explore particular activities perceived as inappropriate and suggest ways to enhance their acceptability to the target population. After discussing the specific components, participants are requested to judge the acceptability of the overall intervention as designed, using a self-report measure. Participants' quantitative ratings are analyzed descriptively and qualitative responses are content analyzed. Converging quantitative and qualitative findings, along with emerging themes suggesting what to modify and how, guide the refinement of the intervention. For instance, when the mean rating value and the comments converge in reflecting inappropriateness of an intervention activity and reasons underlying such a perception, then there is indication to modify it. A careful review of participants' responses may point to the changes to be made to the intervention activities, mode of delivery, dose, setting, and timing of its delivery that are most relevant to the target population. The revised intervention is further evaluated for its acceptability, feasibility, and effects on the intended outcomes. For example, Chung et al. (2009) reported that African American women found relevant the content of Taking Charge self-management program for breast cancer survivors. They also identified additional content areas of interest to this target population encompassing spirituality and faith, strength and self-preservation, and response to body image. Incorporating these topics would definitely enhance the acceptability of the self-management program to African American breast cancer survivors.

Efficacy studies

The purpose of efficacy studies is to demonstrate the direct causal effects of the intervention on the hypothesized outcomes. Any factor that could confound the causal relationship between the intervention and the outcomes is controlled for either experimentally or statistically. Treatment acceptability represents a potentially confounding factor. Acceptability shapes clients' preferences for treatment in that clients prefer treatment options they view as acceptable. Preferences have been reported to influence clients' (1) decision

to enroll in an intervention evaluation study, where those with a strong preference decline entry into a trial to avoid being randomized to the nonpreferred
intervention; (2) attrition, where participants allocated to their nonpreferred
intervention decide to drop out of treatment and of the study; (3) adherence
to treatment, where participants adhere to the treatment of their choice; and
(4) achievement of outcomes, where participants allocated to their preferred
treatment experience the expected levels of improvement in outcomes. Thus,
treatment preferences present threats to the internal and external validity
of an efficacy trial (Sidani et al., 2009). Accordingly, treatment preferences,
reflecting acceptability, have been controlled for in studies evaluating the efficacy of interventions that used experimental or randomized controlled/clinical
trial (RCT) design. In these studies, participants' preferences for the treatment
options (i.e., experimental and comparison) under investigation are assessed
by asking participants to indicate the option of their choice, at baseline before
random assignment of participants to the experimental or comparison group.
Experimental control of the potential confounding effects of preferences is
exerted by excluding participants who express a preference for either treatment option. This strategy, although possible, has rarely been applied because
it could reduce statistical power if a large number of participants express preferences resulting in a small sample size and it could limit the generalizability
of the findings to participants with no preferences found to form a small
percentage (<40%) of the target population (Sidani et al., 2009).

Statistical control of the potential confounding effects consists of catego-
rizing participants into two subgroups, (1) matched and (2) mismatched, and
representing the subgroups as a between-subject factor in the data analysis.
Participants in the matched subgroup are those randomly assigned to the
treatment option of their choice, whereas participants in the mismatched subgroup are those randomly allocated to the nonpreferred treatment option. The
extent to which preferences affected the efficacy of the intervention is determined by examining the main affect of the matched–mismatched subgroup
and its interaction with study group for significance. Statistically significant
main and interaction effects imply that outcome achievement differed for participants allocated to their preferred and nonpreferred treatment options. The
application of this strategy for statistically controlling the confounding effects
of treatment preferences is illustrated in Klaber-Moffett et al.'s (1999) study.

Effectiveness studies

The goal in effectiveness studies is to examine the robustness of the intervention effects on the expected outcomes under the conditions of the real
world of day-to-day practice. The condition of particular interest here is the
method for treatment allocation. In the practice setting, and consistent with
the emphasis on patient- or client-centered care, clients are informed of the
treatment options available to address the presenting clinical problem; requested to indicate the option of preference; and given the intervention of
choice. The preference or partially randomized clinical trial is a design that
reflects this method of treatment allocation, which will be discussed in more

detail in a later chapter. Suffice it to say here that clients' acceptability of and preference for treatment are assessed to guide assignment of participants to treatment options, where those with a preference are allocated to the option of their choice and those with no preference are randomly assigned to treatment. The application of a preference trial is illustrated with Coward's (2002) study. Reliable and valid instruments are administered to measure treatment acceptability and assess preferences (e.g., Sidani et al., 2009) in order to enhance accuracy of participants' choice and subsequent treatment allocation.

Examining the acceptability of interventions by clients and interventionists is critical to explore their viability. Interventions that are viewed as unacceptable will not be adopted, even if effective. However, acceptability alone does not determine the fate of interventions. Feasibility plays an important role.

12.2 Feasibility of interventions

Testing the feasibility of interventions is recognized as an important aim of pilot studies (Bruckenthal & Broderick, 2007; Hertzog, 2008; Lancaster et al., 2004). Despite its identified importance in early stages of evaluation interventions, feasibility of intervention implementation has not been explicitly defined. As a result, the indicators of feasibility are not clearly operationalized and guidance for conducting a feasibility test is not well delineated. In this section, a definition of feasibility is presented, followed by specification of its indicators and strategies for collecting pertinent data. The indicators are derived from elements of process evaluation, which encompasses fidelity of treatment implementation.

12.2.1 Definition of feasibility

As mentioned previously, feasibility has to do with the practicality of implementing the intervention. It refers to the adequacy of the logistics, that is, the resources and procedures required for delivering the intervention (Becker, 2008). The focus is on determining the capability of carrying out the components and activities of the intervention as planned, and on identifying difficulties in applying any aspect of the intervention. Problems in the availability, quality, and skills of human resources; in the availability and proper functioning of material resources; in the physical and/or social context; and in the clarity of the treatment protocol, interfere with the implementation of the intervention. Challenges in treatment delivery reduce clients' and interventionists' enthusiasm for the intervention. Clients may react unfavorably; they experience disappointment and dissatisfaction with treatment and unwillingness to follow its recommendations, or they decide to withdraw from treatment. Interventionists may experience frustration and modify aspects of the intervention to overcome the encountered difficulty. Therefore, achievement of expected outcomes is jeopardized. Inadequate implementation of the intervention by clients and/or interventionists results in type III error, that is, concluding that an intervention is not effective when it has not been implemented as planned. Such conclusion, although erroneous, could adversely affect decisions to further evaluate the intervention effects on the outcomes and subsequently to adopt it and offer it in the practice setting. Identifying difficulties in the implementation of the intervention in early stages of evaluation is essential. Understanding the nature of the difficulty and the factors contributing to the difficulty is a prerequisite for finding the most appropriate solution. Resolution of the difficulty is necessary to enhance the feasibility as well as the fidelity of treatment implementation when testing the efficacy of the intervention (Hertzog, 2008).

12.2.2   Indicators of feasibility

The definition of feasibility presented in the previous section suggests that all aspects of intervention implementation are to be assessed for adequacy or for challenges in their execution. This implies that feasibility is examined with the actual delivery of the intervention by skilled interventionists to a select group of clients representative of the target population, in the specified context. It involves close monitoring of the activities performed in preparation of and throughout treatment implementation. Specifically, monitoring is done using relevant quantitative and qualitative methods on the following.

12.2.2.1   Availability and quality of interventionists

The delivery of the intervention to the right clients, in the right way, at the right time requires the availability of an adequate number of interventionists with the personal and professional qualities identified in the intervention theory. Estimation of an adequate number is based on the nature, mode of delivery, and dose of the intervention; the timing within the clients' health trajectory for delivering the intervention; the clients' preferences for the location and time of intervention delivery; and the size of client sample anticipated to receive treatment. It is safe to anticipate the need for several (5-10) interventionists to provide complex, cognitive behavioral therapy, on an individual face-to-face basis, in at least six sessions, to a large sample of newly diagnosed clients, beginning within a month of diagnosis. The sessions are scheduled at different times of the day and in different geographic locations to accommodate the preferences of clients with different characteristics. For instance, our experience indicates that older women may refuse to participate in a group session scheduled at 5:00 PM in the winter (when it is dark) because of fear of slipping on ice and breaking the hip; they preferred the morning or early afternoon time. In contrast, young working clients find a session starting at 5:30 PM most convenient, giving them enough time to travel from work to the location of the session. Having several interventionists is also important to cover for vacation, sick time, and resignation.

12.2.2.2   Training of interventionists

In addition to the number of interventionists with the specified personal and professional qualities, the interventionists should be adequately prepared to provide the intervention in the right way. Therefore, training covering the theory underlying the intervention and the protocol for applying the intervention is designed to help them acquire the cognitive and behavioral skills needed for implementing the intervention as planned, as well as for recognizing and resolving challenges they may encounter in this endeavor. Thus, it is important to monitor training sessions for any issues that may arise in the relay or receipt of content, and evaluate effectiveness of training in enhancing the interventionists' skills. The issues could be related to the following:

(1) *Content of the training session:* The content may lack clarity, depth, and breadth of information on the theoretical underpinning of the intervention, or may provide limited time allotted for practical skill training, or may involve applications of skills using case studies that are not representative of all possible subgroups of the target population. Alternatively, the presentation of the content may not be clear, logical, and effective in relaying the key messages.

(2) *Design of the intervention:* The training provides an excellent opportunity to review the conceptualization and the operationalization of the intervention, following the treatment manual developed to guide its implementation. During explanation of the nature and sequence of intervention activities, difficulties or challenges in carrying out these activities with specific subgroups of the target population and in particular settings may be identified by the researchers or clinicians who designed the intervention, or by experienced interventionists who undergo the training.

(3) *Interventionists:* Some interventionists may demonstrate limited ability to grasp the theoretical foundation of the intervention and/or to acquire an acceptable level of skill performance. The issues are identified informally through observation or discussion taking place throughout the training sessions, or formally through group discussion focused on the strengths and limitations of the training sessions. The effectiveness of training is evaluated formally, using self-administered questionnaire or group discussion scheduled upon completion of training. Self-administered questionnaires contain items testing the interventionists' knowledge of the theory underlying the intervention and vignettes followed by pertinent questions assessing the interventionists' skills in managing different scenarios and in problem-solving. The group discussion is concerned with identifying aspects or elements of the training that were most and least helpful, and with exploring ways to improve training. Results of the descriptive analysis of quantitative data and content analysis of qualitative data indicate difficulties with interventionists' training and suggest strategies to resolve them prior to providing the training sessions in future application of the intervention in the research and practice setting.

12.2.2.3 Material resources

Feasibility also encompasses availability of all material resources needed for the proper implementation of the intervention. The type of resources differs with the nature of the intervention activities. They can be categorized into (1) equipment such as laptop or desktop computer, or slide projector for the presentation of educational material, or personal device assistant (PDA) for diary entries; (2) printed materials such as educational booklet, guides summarizing key treatment recommendations, or other self-help written information for distribution to participants; (3) general supplies such as pens for participants to complete in-session forms and items for demonstration of health-related skills (e.g., food item or menu to illustrate diet selection); and (4) medical supplies such as containers to collecting specimen and pedometers for participants' use. These items should be available in adequate number to cover all clients participating in the intervention concurrently, and be functioning properly. Such information is gathered (1) formally by having research staff (i.e., research assistants and interventionists) complete a checklist to facilitate preparation of the items and indicate the availability of items needed to deliver the intervention, or (2) informally during regular meetings with research staff. Necessary steps are taken to ensure preparation of the items prior to the delivery of the intervention.

12.2.2.4 Context

Context refers to the physical and social environment in which the intervention is implemented. Although the theory underlying the intervention delineates factors that could influence treatment delivery and outcome achievement, and guides the selection of the sites for intervention implementation, it is important to assess the presence of these factors in the selected sites and the extent to which the sites' characteristics interfere with the implementation of the intervention. Specifically, the physical environment is evaluated for its adequacy relative to its (1) location, which should be easy to identify by clients, within reasonable distance to most subgroups of the target population, and reachable through public transportation or has affordable parking; (2) accessibility to various subgroups of the target population, where necessary amenities are in place for clients requiring assistance (e.g., elevator for frail older clients with cardiac conditions); and (3) characteristics (e.g., layout, furniture, ambiance) known to facilitate or hinder treatment delivery. Aspects of the social environment that influence implementation of the intervention vary with its nature. In general, they include services to be offered by other departments or personnel (e.g., laboratory, information technology), and support for the intervention by other healthcare professionals caring for participating clients. A checklist can be developed and used to assess the presence or adequacy level of all factors in the physical and social environment, as specified in the intervention theory, at all participating sites. Research personnel and/or interventionists complete the checklist prior to and/or during treatment delivery, and are requested to document other environmental characteristics or difficulties encountered throughout intervention implementation. In addition, complaints reported by participating clients are noted. Results of all data analysis point to aspects in the context that do not meet the requirements for or that interfere with the implementation of the intervention. Necessary modifications are made prior to future delivery of the intervention to clients participating in research or seen in practice.

12.2.2.5 Fidelity of intervention implementation

Fidelity of intervention implementation is an important element or component of studies evaluating the feasibility, efficacy, and effectiveness of interventions, as emphasized in the previous chapters. However, it is of primary concern when testing feasibility because close monitoring of fidelity is instrumental in identifying challenges in the application of the treatment activities, in the selected mode, and the selected dose, experienced by the interventionists and the clients, as well as in understanding factors contributing to the challenges. A trial implementation of the intervention as designed provides an excellent opportunity to assess adequacy of the intervention delivery protocol and the comprehensiveness and clarity of the treatment manual in guiding actual implementation, and to recognize issues related to (1) clarity, comprehensiveness, and logical sequencing of the information given to patients (e.g., are technical words used, well explained, and understood; are the treatment recommendations stated in simple terms understandable to different subgroups of the target population; do complex treatment recommendations build on simpler ones and therefore discussed in a meaningful sequence); (2) ease with which the intervention activities are performed in the specified mode (e.g., is the number of clients in a group session adequate allowing meaningful participation by all; is the video or telephone conferencing connection stable and of good quality offering uninterrupted and clear exchange by all clients including those with vision or hearing problem; can the planned physical activities be done in the group format within the allotted space) and carried out by clients (e.g., do clients residing in rural areas have the proper equipment set up at home and the ability to operate the equipment for maintaining connection or transferring data to the intervention center; do various subgroups of the target population have instrumental and/or social support to initiate and maintain the recommended dietary regiment and physical activity program; what percentage of participants complete the homework assignments); and (3) the time it takes to deliver different components of the intervention (e.g., does the implementation of one component take longer than anticipated, thereby limiting the time to deliver remaining components). Quantitative and qualitative, observational and self-report, methods for collecting data related to fidelity of intervention implementation have been discussed in detail in the previous chapters. Qualitative data obtained from researchers' records of issues observed, interventionists' feedback on challenges encountered, and/or clients report of difficulties faced are useful in identifying barriers and facilitators to treatment delivery (by interventionists) and enactment (by clients), and in clarifying what brought up these challenges and how they influenced the fidelity of intervention implementation. Analyses of this information point to aspects of the intervention that are to be modified and the nature of the modification, with the goal of enhancing the quality of intervention

implementation in the context of research and practice. Revisions of the treatment manual are made to guide future delivery.

12.2.2.6 Reach

As an indicator of feasibility, reach refers to the extent to which various
subgroups of the target population are able to participate in the intervention.
Of particular concern are clients who may not be able to do so because of
logistical reasons related to transportation, accessibility to the site in which
the intervention is offered, to the resources needed at home to engage in
treatment, and the time at which the intervention is given. Data on reach
are gathered when inquiring about the reasons for clients' nonenrollment or
when discussing the intervention study with healthcare professionals to be
ascribed the responsibility of referring eligible clients. These professionals
are familiar with the needs and characteristics of various subgroups of the
target population attending their services and hence, are in a position to
indicate anticipated challenges. Content analysis of qualitative data obtained
from the two sources (clients and healthcare professionals) delineates the
nature of the logistical challenges. Counting the number of clients reporting
these challenges gives an estimate of their prevalence in the target population.
Logistical problems that are prevalent (e.g., reported by $\geq 30\%$ of clients) and
amenable to remediation (i.e., something can be done to address it, such as
providing the intervention in a location convenient to a group of the target
population) can be addressed prior to future delivery of the intervention.

In conjunction with determining the feasibility of the intervention, some
researchers plan to explore the feasibility of research methods planned for
future studies aimed at evaluating the efficacy or the effectiveness of the
intervention. The specific research methods to be examined and the strategies
used to collect data reflecting their feasibility are discussed next.

12.3   Feasibility of research methods

Determining the feasibility of research methods planned for a large-scale
study for evaluating the efficacy of interventions is commonly and rightfully
emphasized. Here, feasibility refers to the adequacy, effectiveness, and efficiency of the study protocol in gathering pertinent data from participants
representative of the target population that will contribute meaningfully to addressing the objectives preset for the intervention evaluation research. The
goal of testing feasibility of the study protocol is to identify (1) the research
procedures that are appropriate, can be easily or conveniently performed as
planned, and yield quality information within a reasonable time frame, and (2)
difficulties or challenges in carrying out the planned research procedures. Put
in other terms, feasibility testing is done to see where Murphy's law can strike.
Thus, the results of this testing, usually done in prior studies, give advance
warning about possible pitfalls or deficiencies in the design, methods, and logistics planned for large-scale efficacy trials. These pitfalls have the potential

to "derail" a study and/or invalidate its conclusions (Streiner & Sidani, 2010). A thorough assessment of and lucid knowledge about these possible pitfalls in terms of their nature, extent, and determinants guide the search for appropriate solutions and the revision of procedures, and the refinement of study protocol prior to the conduct of the large-scale efficacy or effectiveness trial. This is essential for enhancing the quality of the trial and hence the validity of its conclusions.

Although every step of the study protocol starting with recruitment and ending with data analysis can be subjected to feasibility testing, it is advisable to focus on those that are novel, innovative, untested, or complex and it is frequently recommended to examine the adequacy of the following complex procedures: recruitment, screening, randomization, retention, and data collection (Cohen et al., 2007; Fisher et al., McCarney, Harford & Vickers, 2006; Lancaster et al., 2004; Thomas Becker, 2008). Strategies for assessing feasibility are presented for each of these procedures.

12.3.1 Recruitment procedures

The adequacy of recruitment procedures relates to the size of the sampling pool, the effectiveness of recruitment approaches, and the recruitment time.

(1) *Sampling pool:* It is essential to accurately estimate the size of the sampling pool available at the sites involved in recruitment of potentially eligible participants. This requires obtaining the following information: (a) The number of clients at each participating site that are representative of the target population and are known to possess general eligibility criteria (e.g., English-speaking or female sex): these data can be requested from sites that maintain a database of clients who receive their services (such as hospitals, health maintenance organizations) or the number of clients responding to an advertisement for the study and expressing interest in learning about the study. (b) The number of clients who agree to the screening and who meet all study eligibility criteria, which can be extracted from a well-maintained study participant log that tracks engagement of each client in each planned research activity. The percentage of clients who meet the eligibility criteria (out of the total available/showing interest) as well as the actual number of eligible clients are indicative of the size of the sampling pool. A low percentage and/or number suggests possible difficulties accruing a large sample size required for an efficacy or effectiveness trial, which could be addressed by expanding recruitment to multiple sites serving the target population or by revising the study inclusion and exclusion criteria to be more encompassing allowing representation of different groups constituting the target population while also minimizing the influence of potential confounds.

(2) *Effectiveness of approaches:* Whether a single approach or multiple approaches are used to recruit participants, awareness of their effectiveness

in reaching large sections of the target population is necessary to guide the process of making decisions regarding which approach to use in the large-scale trial. Effectiveness is operationalized in terms of the number and characteristics of individuals who learned about the study through a particular approach. To obtain relevant data, individuals showing interest in the study are requested to indicate the source of information about the study. For example, in the study evaluating the effectiveness of behavioral treatment for insomnia, individuals who called the research office to inquire about the study were asked the question: "How did you learn about the study?" followed by a list of recruitment approaches used: advertisement in newspaper, Web site, flyer, and referral by healthcare provider. The most frequent response was advertisement, which provided empirical evidence to continue use of this strategy and to justify the need for a rather large amount of funds to cover the advertisement costs. In addition, results of descriptive analyses of the socio-demographic and clinical characteristics of clients who participated in the pilot study delineate the profile of participants. The observed sample profile is compared qualitatively to that of the target population reported in previous research or of the accessible population available at participating sites. Similarity of the sample and the population on key characteristics (e.g., age, sex, severity of illness) is indicative of the effectiveness of the recruitment approaches in reaching various sections or groups of the target population. For example, in the study of behavioral treatments for insomnia, the sample consisted of middle-aged (mean = 55 years) women (66%) with moderate level of insomnia severity (mean score on the Insomnia Severity Index: 17); this profile is typical of persons with insomnia. Dissimilarity in the profile of the sample and the population raises questions about the adequacy of the recruitment approaches and requires investigation of the reasons underlying it. This involves reviewing pertinent literature and/or discussing with expert researchers and clinicians, as well as key informants or clients representing the targeted community or population, possible reasons for the dissimilarity, and relevant approaches for recruiting nonrepresented groups of the community or population. The most effective and relevant approaches are used in the large-scale trial.

(3) *Recruitment time:* The time it takes to recruit participants in the pilot study is another area to examine feasibility, which may be a function of the effectiveness of the recruitment approaches. The focus is on the period to accrue the total number of participants required for the pilot study. It is operationalized as the length of time (e.g., number of weeks or months) from the start of recruitment to the enrollment of the last participant, or the average number of participants recruited within a unit of time (such as week or a month). This information is gathered from the study's administrative records that document the date on which the planned research activities (as specified in the study protocol) are performed. Data on the recruitment time is most useful in delineating the time frame and hence, in justifying the budget for the large-scale efficacy or effectiveness trial.

12.3.2 Screening

Adequacy of screening focuses on the practicality of the screening procedures and the appropriateness of the inclusion and exclusion criteria. Practicality of screening procedures relates to the following:

(1) Ease with which screening is done, that is, do the procedures run smoothly or unduly increase burden on research staff and participants, and how long does the screening take to complete?

(2) Time at which screening is scheduled relative to recruitment, consent, and baseline data collection, that is, is screening done as soon as possible following recruitment to identify ineligible clients and prevent them from participating in unnecessary research activities?

(3) Validity and utility of the questions or instruments used for screening, that is, is the content of the screening measures easy to understand by clients of different backgrounds, are the measures reliable and valid, do they have well-established cut-off scores resulting in acceptable sensitivity and specificity which are necessary to accurately identify eligible and noneligible clients?

(4) Ethical conduct of screening, that is, is the screening done after obtaining, at the minimum, oral agreement of interested clients, and within a context that ensures the right for self-determination (i.e., right to not answer a question), privacy, and confidentiality.

Data on the practicality of the screening procedures are collected informally by (1) observing or recording the actual conduct of screening with participants, which provides information on the average length it takes to complete the screening and on difficulties encountered in administering the screening measures (such as misunderstanding of items, participants' refusal to answer a question they perceive as intrusive, redundancy in the items or questions posed which is burdensome); (2) eliciting feedback of research personnel on challenges faced in applying the screening procedures; and (3) reviewing complaints about the content, the length, or the timing of screening voiced by participating clients. Formal evaluation of the sensitivity and specificity of screening measures can be planned in conjunction with testing the feasibility of data collection (discussed in a later section). Cognitive interviewing techniques are used to determine participants' understanding of the content and response options of screening measures. Participants' responses to the screening measures and to well-established diagnostic criteria are compared to examine the sensitivity and specificity of the screening measures in the target population.

Appropriateness of inclusion and exclusion criteria relates to their relevance or suitability in selecting a sample of clients that are representative of the target population. The questions to be addressed when evaluating the appropriateness of the eligibility criteria include: Are the eligibility criteria stringent or "too strict" to the point they limit the pool of potential participants and the ability to accrue the required sample size and obtain a representative sample, within a reasonable time frame? Or, are the criteria less restrictive to the point that potential confounding characteristics are introduced? Data addressing these questions are obtained from the database maintained for all individuals who agree to undergo screening and documenting their responses to items/questions related to eligibility criteria. Descriptive analysis of the latter responses is done to examine the percentage of clients who do not meet each criterion and hence, are deemed ineligible. The results indicate if a large ($\geq 50\%$) percentage of clients are indeed ineligible and the most common reasons for ineligibility (i.e., the specific criterion or criteria that most clients do not meet). The reasons are carefully reviewed to determine the centrality of the criteria in defining the target population and in introducing possible confounds, and consequently to make informed decision to confirm or modify the inclusion and exclusion criteria for the efficacy or effectiveness trial. For instance, in a study evaluating the quality of nursing care on outcomes for patients admitted to complex continuing in-hospital units, the following selection criteria were preset: 21 years of age or older, fluency in spoken and written English, no cognitive impairment, and admission for the following high-volume conditions: congestive heart failure, diabetes, and chronic obstructive pulmonary disease. Of the 61 patients recruited for the study, 52% were found ineligible because of language barrier and cognitive impairment. These two criteria are critical for participation in the study (i.e., patients had to be able to provide informed consent, and understand and respond to self-report measures) and therefore should not be altered. However, the preselected conditions, although considered high volume, were not representative of all those with which admitted patients presented. Consequently, this inclusion criterion was expanded to conditions affecting other body systems (e.g., kidney, blood vessels, skin), without jeopardizing the validity of the conclusions reached in the large-scale study.

12.3.3 Randomization

Two aspects of the randomization procedure are tested for feasibility: (1) logistics and (2) acceptability. Logistics relate to the ability to apply the randomization procedure as planned. This aspect is of particular concern when randomization is entrusted to a central office. The office's services are evaluated for organization (e.g., what clients' data are needed, what is the best means for relaying the data, how clearly is the information on participants' assignment to study group presented) and timeliness (i.e., how long does it take to reach/contact the office to feed in clients' data and to get a response from the office). The evaluation is often done informally, through discussion at regularly scheduled research staff meetings, or by reviewing pertinent complaints made by research staff. Acceptability of the randomization procedure is operationalized as the attitude toward allocation to treatment on the basis of chance held by clients and clinicians responsible for referring clients to the evaluation study. The attitude influences clients' and clinicians' behavior related to enrollment in the study. A positive attitude reflecting acceptability of randomization entices clinicians to refer clients and clients to enroll in the study. A negative attitude indicating unacceptability of the notion of random assignment to treatment groups contributes to clinicians' decision to not refer clients and clients' decision to decline enrollment in the study. In studies relying on clinicians' referral as the recruitment strategy, it is worth monitoring their referral pattern closely by generating a database to document, at a minimum, the clinical site from which clients are referred, and if possible and ethically allowable, the name of the clinicians initiating the referral. The data are analyzed descriptively and periodically (e.g., every month) to identify sites or clinicians with low referral rates (i.e., a small number of clients relative to the total number of clients recruited through this strategy). Meetings can be held with clinicians at these sites to explore the reasons for low referral rate, with specific probing about their perception of and reaction to randomization. The themes of the discussion reflect if and the extent to which unacceptability of randomization is an issue, which, in turn, assists in planning the efficacy or effectiveness trial. The plan consists of either (1) changing the design of the trial to one that does not require randomization at the individual level (e.g., use cluster RCT instead) where participating sites are randomly assigned to treatment groups; or (2) excluding the site from further participation in the study and replacing it with one where a more positive attitude toward randomization is prevailing. Empirical evidence indicative of clients' attitude toward randomization is derived from the reasons clients give for declining initial (i.e., once they learn about the study, particularly when random assignment is mentioned at the time of recruitment) or continued (i.e., during or after the process of obtaining consent when chance allocation to treatment is explained in detail) enrollment in the study. A tally of the reasons for refusal to participate indicates the percentage of clients who find randomization as unacceptable. In community-based participatory research, key informants or community leaders engaged in the study design represent a source of information about the target population's attitude toward randomization. The published and gray literature also provides evidence of the target population's acceptability of randomization. For example, patients with cancer resent randomization; they perceive it as unfair and they feel it reduces their sense of control (Jenkins & Fallowfield, 2000; Stevens & Ahmedzai, 2004). King et al. (2005) reported that 26% to 88% of participants in studies evaluating different medical and surgical treatments accept random assignment to the experimental or comparison group. In situations when a large proportion (30%) of clients resent randomization, alternative research designs should be considered for the large efficacy or effectiveness trial. Such designs are discussed in the later chapters but are exemplified by waiting list control group and preference trials. Maintaining randomization as the procedure for assigning participants to treatment groups in the large-scale trial may have untoward consequences: (1) increased effort, time, and costs to recruit a large number of clients to offset the percentage of those who resent randomization and decline enrollment, and (2) self-selection bias where the sample of participants represent only clients accepting random assignment to treatment, which limits the applicability of the study results to all subgroups of the target population.

12.3.4 Retention

It is wise to incorporate strategies to enhance retention and thus minimize attrition in intervention evaluation studies, and most important to pilot test the adequacy of these strategies. The focus is on examining the extent to which the strategies can be applied as planned, contribute to retention, and are well received by participants. The proper application of the strategies at the preselected point in time is essential for their effectiveness in retaining participants. Difficulties are recognized by research staff responsible for their implementation. The types of difficulty encountered vary with the nature of the strategies used; examples include: participants' inability or refusal to identify and provide contact information of persons who know the whereabouts of hard to reach participants; challenges in being flexible to accommodate participants' needs and make their involvement convenient; and delays in sending and/or receiving incentives. The difficulties and ways to address them are usually discussed during regularly scheduled research staff meetings. Although the direct and unique contribution of each strategy used for retention cannot be assessed in a pilot study, the extent to which the strategies, taken together, are effective in enhancing retention can be implied from the study retention or attrition rate. Retention rate is the percentage of consenting participants who completed the study, whereas attrition rate is the percentage of consenting participants who withdraw at any point during the study. These rates can be compared, qualitatively, to those reported in previous studies evaluating the intervention in the same or comparable target population. Similarity in the retention/attrition rates across studies provides evidence supporting the effectiveness of the strategies used in the pilot in improving retention or reducing attrition. Effectiveness of specific retention strategies can be also determined by reviewing results of methodological studies designed to compare the effects of different strategies on retention/attrition rates. For example, Sullivan et al. (1996) found that a three-phase retention protocol contributed to a higher retention rate in a longitudinal study of a postshelter advocacy intervention targeting women experiencing abuse. The retention protocol involved the following strategies: establishing trust; acquiring detailed information on participants' address and contacts as well as the best time to call; providing reminders; using strategies most relevant to individual participants to contact them (e.g., phone call, visit to home, letter); and using participants' social network to reach them at follow-up. Participants' perception of the relevance and appropriateness of the retention strategies can be informally assessed by: (1) asking key informants or community leaders about the target population's view of the strategies used and to suggest those considered appropriate; and (2) content analyzing and tallying reasons for attrition or unsolicited comments offered by participants, with special attention given to responses reflecting level of satisfaction with the strategies. For instance, some individuals who participated in the study evaluating the behavioral treatments for insomnia expressed dissatisfaction with the incentive provided to promote retention. Seven participants withdrew because in their opinion, "the compensation is not enough." Synthesis of the evidence obtained in a pilot study indicates the strategies that can be easily applied, appropriate to the target population, and effective for use in the large-scale efficacy or effectiveness trial to enhance retention.

12.3.5 Data collection

Data collection and measures are other research methods tested for feasibility in a pilot study. The data collection measures are evaluated for comprehension (i.e., ease of understanding the instructions, items' content, and response option), relevance (i.e., applicability of the content to the target population), variability of responses, and time it takes to complete them. Two methods can be used to assess comprehension and relevance of measures. The first involves cognitive interview techniques, comprising semistructured individual or group interview with participants. Participants are asked to read each item, reiterate the content captured in the item (by answering the question: What does this mean to you?), read the response options, explain what the options mean, and think aloud when formulating their response and selecting the most appropriate response. Participants' responses identify words, phrases, sentences, or response options that are misunderstood or misinterpreted by most (>50%) respondents (Oremus et al., 2005). The semistructured interview could address relevance of the item content to the target population, in addition to comprehension (Eremenco et al., 2005; Nápoles-Springer et al., 2006). The second method for assessing comprehension and relevance is partially based on, but less formal than, cognitive interviewing techniques. It involves having participants complete the measures and comment on any word or content and response options that are unclear and/or irrelevant. Items and response options found difficult to understand or not appropriate are identified and have to be revised prior to using the measures in the large-scale efficacy or effectiveness trial. Failure to do so reduces the quality of the data (i.e., high rate of missing data) and increases error of measurement, which, in turn, adversely affects the statistical power to detect significant intervention effects, precision of parameter estimates, and the validity of study conclusions (Sidani & Braden, 1998). Variability of responses to measures of all concepts of interest, and in particular those capturing the intervention outcomes, is examined to detect possible floor or ceiling effects. Participants' responses are analyzed descriptively; attention is given to the frequency distribution with the expectation that all possible response options have been selected. The length of time it takes to complete the measures at each occasion of measurement (e.g., pretest, posttest, follow-up) is assessed prospectively by noting the start and end time of the data collection session and calculating the total administration time. The longer the time, the higher the likelihood of response burden; response burden negatively influences the quality of data.

The data collection procedure is examined for its ease of implementation, promptness, and logistics. Questions to guide evaluation of feasibility include: How easy is it or what difficulty is encountered in administering the measures in the selected format (e.g., interview, computer-based) and/or in obtaining specimen? How do participants react to data collection (e.g., how many refuse to answer a question or to provide the specimen)? Is the sequence of steps for data collection (e.g., self-report followed by specimen collection) logical and easy to follow? Are materials, supplies, or equipment available in good functioning condition, when needed? Can the data collection take place in the selected location, at the specified time intervals, and within the specified time frame? Are the collected specimen managed properly and sent for analysis as delineated in the study protocol? What contributes to delays in data collection? Are research personnel consistent in implementing the data collection procedure, adhering to the study protocol? What factors prevent strict adherence to the study protocol? Answers to these questions are obtained through (1) discussion of issues encountered in carrying out the data collection procedure at regular research staff meetings, (2) concerns or complaints expressed by participants and relayed to research personnel, and (3) close monitoring (direct observation or audio-recording) of research staff in-action. The nature of issues and factors contributing to them are clarified to facilitate the generation of strategies to manage adequately and/or to prevent their occurrence in the large-scale efficacy or effectiveness trial. Challenges in the appropriateness, promptness, and consistency of data collection procedure in the large-scale trial influence the quality and consistency of data, and hence introduce error, thereby reducing statistical power and/or precision of parameter estimates.

In addition to testing the feasibility of recruitment, screening, randomization, retention, and data collection procedures, pilot studies have been and still are designed to estimate the size of intervention effects. Effect sizes are computed as the standardized difference in the main outcomes between the experimental and comparison groups, or as the standardized difference in the main outcomes measured at pretest and posttest within the experimental group. Effect sizes are then used in the power analysis done to calculate the sample size required to achieve adequate power to detect significant intervention effects in the efficacy or effectiveness trial. This practice is no longer highly recommended because the estimates of effect sizes based on the small number of participants in a pilot study are known to be negatively biased, that is, they underestimate the magnitude of the intervention effects expected for the target population (Hertzog, 2008).

12.4   Design of pilot study

As recommended, the research methods selected for the pilot study should be consistent with the stated study purpose, providing relevant data to appropriately address the objectives. Accordingly, the following designs are considered for pilot studies concerned with:

(1) *Examining the acceptability of interventions:* Cross-sectional designs are used to assess clients' perceived acceptability of the intervention of interest, whether the intervention is described or provided in a trial implementation to participants. Alternatively, a preexperimental pretest–posttest one-group design in which outcomes are measured before and after implementation of the intervention is appropriate for addressing acceptability. Either design (i.e., cross-sectional or preexperimental) involves a mix of quantitative and qualitative methods for collecting relevant data to develop a comprehensive and in-depth understanding of the target population's perception of the intervention.

(2) *Examining the feasibility of interventions:* Feasibility can be evaluated in conjunction with acceptability of the intervention in a preexperimental design in which the intervention is delivered to a small number of participants. Quantitative and qualitative data are gathered to obtain a complete picture of aspects of the intervention that can be implemented as designed, difficulties or issues in implementation, and modifications that are needed to enhance the appropriateness of the intervention to the target population and to facilitate its delivery.

(3) *Examining the feasibility of research methods:* To address this purpose, the design selected for the pilot study should mimic/be the same as the design selected for the efficacy or effectiveness trial, be it experimental or quasi-experimental, involving a comparison group and repeated measurement of outcome data reflecting long-term follow-up. Qualitative data are collected, as discussed earlier, to supplement and/or complement quantitative data in identifying what works, what does not work, what should be modified, and how to enhance the design and conduct of the large-scale efficacy trial.

The following section details the plan for a pilot study aimed at evaluating the acceptability and feasibility of an intervention, using a preexperimental mixed methods design. In this design, the intervention is provided to a group of participants representing the target population. Quantitative data pertaining to the following variables of interest are collected at the specified schedule:

- Acceptability of the intervention as perceived by clients and interventionists, prior to implementation of the intervention
- Fidelity of intervention implementation by clients and interventionists, throughout the treatment period
- Clients' satisfaction with the intervention, immediately after receiving its components
- Immediate and ultimate outcomes, before and after treatment delivery

Qualitative data are obtained on:

- clients' and interventionists' view of treatment during and immediately after the intervention implementation period;
- interventionists' report of challenges and issues in, as well as the ease of, the delivery of the intervention;
- clients' and interventionists' perspectives on elements of the intervention that are useful in achieving the outcomes, suitable for application in day-to-day life, and/or need refinement; and
- clients' and interventionists' reports on how the intervention affects the outcomes and on experience of unanticipated effects.

Although the proposed preexperimental design includes one intervention group, the number of outcome measurements can vary to improve inferences about preliminary effects of the intervention. The traditional preexperimental design involves assessment of the outcomes at pretest and posttest, that is, immediately before and after intervention delivery, respectively. The pretest measurement scores serve as a reference for determining intervention effects forming the baseline values against which the posttest outcome scores are compared. Differences in the outcomes observed from pretest to posttest, in the hypothesized direction (i.e., increase or decrease in the scores over the two occasions of measurement, based on the interpretation of scores), and of the anticipated magnitude (e.g., small, medium, high) are indicative of preliminary treatment effects.

Alternatively, outcome measurement can be done repeatedly before and after implementation of the intervention. This repeated measure design provides empirical evidence that is consistent with the counterfactual claim for causality, where participants serve as their own control. Assessment of the outcomes on at least two occasions prior to the intervention represents the control condition during which participants receive no treatment. Therefore, no changes in the outcomes are anticipated over this time period. However, changes in the outcomes are expected following treatment delivery, which reflect the preliminary effects of the intervention. Posttest changes in immediate outcomes are hypothesized to be maintained at follow-up outcome assessment (e.g., 3 and 6 months post treatment), supporting sustainability of intervention effects. Whereas no or minimal changes are observed for ultimate outcomes at posttest, the hypothesized pattern of change is expected to take place at follow-up. If repeated assessment of the outcomes prior to treatment is not possible for conceptual (e.g., unstable or differences in conditions under which the assessment is done or anticipated changes in clients' status over time despite lack of treatment) or logistic (e.g., inability to identify and access eligible clients on time), then the pilot study is designed to incorporate a comparison group of participants who do not receive the intervention under evaluation. Assignment to the comparison and intervention groups is done on the basis of chance (i.e., randomly) or convenience. The comparison group serves as reference, whereby changes in the pretest-to-posttest outcomes are compared between the comparison and the intervention groups. It is expected to observe no changes in the outcomes for the comparison group and changes in the outcomes in the hypothesized direction and magnitude for the intervention group. Between-group differences in outcome changes indicate preliminary effects of the intervention.

In summary, the first phase in intervention evaluation is concerned with determining its acceptability, ensuring its feasibility, and devising the most appropriate methods for evaluating its effects on the expected outcomes. Pilot studies assist in identifying challenges in implementation of the intervention and in conduct of its evaluation. Gaining a thorough understanding of these challenges and their determinants is critical for improving the design and hence, the validity of studies aimed at investigating the intervention efficacy.

Chapter 13

Examining the Efficacy of Interventions

Interventions found acceptable and feasible are subjected to efficacy test-ing, which is the next logical phase in the intervention evaluation process. The primary concern in efficacy testing is to demonstrate the causal rela-tionship between the intervention and the hypothesized outcomes. A causal relationship implies that the intervention's active ingredients are solely and uniquely responsible for producing improvement in the outcomes observed after implementation of the intervention. Thus, changes in the outcomes are attributable, with confidence, to the intervention and not to any other factor that may be operating in the context of intervention delivery. Several concep-tual and methodological factors can contribute to the outcomes, and therefore present plausible alternative explanations for the causal relationship between the intervention and the outcomes. These factors should be controlled in order to maintain the validity of conclusions or inferences pertaining to the causal effects of the intervention on the outcomes. Control of these factors is exerted experimentally or statistically. Experimental control consists of eliminating or minimizing their potential influence on the implementation of the intervention and/or on the outcomes; this is accomplished by incorporating some features into the design of an efficacy trial (Shadish et al., 2002). Statistical control involves assessment of these factors, when feasible, and accounting for or partialling out their influence on the outcomes in the data analysis aimed at examining the causal effects of the intervention on the outcomes (Schafer & Kang, 2008). Whereas both types of control may be required in a particular intervention evaluation study, experimental control is commonly applied in an efficacy trial.

In this chapter, key factors that provide plausible alternative explanations for the causal relationship between the intervention and the outcomes are identified and the nature of their influence is explained. Design features that control, experimentally or statistically, the potential effects of these factors are discussed.

Design, Evaluation, and Translation of Nursing Interventions, First Edition.
Souraya Sidani and Carrie Jo Braden.
© 2011 John Wiley & Sons, Inc. Published 2011 by John Wiley & Sons, Inc.

13.1 Factors affecting the causal relationship between intervention and outcomes

Of the criteria for demonstrating the causal relationship between the intervention and the hypothesized immediate and ultimate outcomes mentioned in Chapter 11, showing that alternative explanations for this relationship are implausible is key in efficacy trials (Cook et al., 2010; Schafer & Kang, 2008; Shadish et al., 2002; Worrall, 2002). This means ruling out the contribution of conceptual and/or methodological factors to the improvement in the outcomes observed following the implementation of the intervention.

13.1.1 Conceptual factors

Conceptual factors are related to the characteristics of clients who are exposed to and receive treatment; the characteristics of interventionists who implement the intervention; and the characteristics of the environment in which the intervention is applied. As delineated in the intervention theory, these factors could influence, directly or indirectly, the achievement of expected outcomes.

Clients' personal and clinical characteristics affect outcome achievement directly and/or indirectly. The direct influence of client characteristics on outcomes confounds the intervention effects. The characteristics may be highly associated with the outcomes and affect the experience of anticipated improvement in the outcomes. Therefore, the effects (i.e., hypothesized changes in the outcomes) observed following implementation of the intervention are attributable to the client characteristics and not necessarily to the intervention. For example, McEwen and West (2009) found significant associations between smokers' characteristics and abstinence within 3-4 weeks of initiating replacement therapy. Specifically, older clients and men had higher chances, whereas clients with high levels of nicotine dependence had lower chances, of achieving short-term abstinence. The indirect influence of client characteristics on outcomes takes two forms. First, client characteristics moderate the intervention's effects, that is, they affect the direction or strength of the causal relationship between the intervention and the outcomes (Bennett, 2000). Operationally, moderators strengthen or weaken this causal relationship, indicated by differences in the outcome levels achieved by different subgroups of the target population; the subgroups are differentiated on the basis of their possession of or level on the client characteristics. Patterns of differences between subgroups in outcome levels include (1) observation of hypothesized outcome levels in one subgroup but not in another subgroup of the target population; (2) the outcome does not occur to the same level in the different subgroups; or (3) the outcome changes in different directions in the different subgroups such as an increase in one subgroup, a decrease in one subgroup, and no change in one subgroup. For example, Brown (1992) found smaller effect sizes for the outcomes of education in older adults ($\geq$40 years) as compared to younger adults with diabetes. Johnson et al.'s (2007) results indicated that dispositional phenotype (operationalized as depression and hostility) moderated the effects of two smoking prevention school programs; the programs were effective in preventing smoking progression in youth with high levels of depression or hostility. The second form of the indirect influence of client characteristics on outcomes is mediated: the clients' characteristics may interfere with clients' uptake, engagement, adherence, and/or satisfaction with treatment, which, in turn, affect outcome achievement. This indirect influence is illustrated with the proposed contribution of preferences for treatment to outcome achievement; specifically, clients assigned to the intervention of their choice tend to engage in recommended treatment activities (Macias et al., 2005) and to experience the anticipated improvement in outcomes (Swift & Callahan, 2009).

Interventionists' personal and professional qualities exert an indirect influence on outcomes. Interventionists' qualities (1) shape their interpersonal skills and ability to initiate and maintain a trusting therapeutic relationship or working alliance with clients, and (2) affect their implementation of the intervention. Working alliance may confound or mediate the causal effects of the intervention on outcomes. Clients who develop a positive relationship with interventionists are motivated to engage in and apply the treatment recommendations, and therefore experience the anticipated improvement in outcomes. Alternatively, these clients gain an understanding of the nature and importance of the intervention activities, which promotes adherence to and satisfaction with treatment, and subsequently outcome achievement, as reported by Fuertes et al. (2007), Kim et al. (2006), and Joyce et al. (2003). Interventionists' qualities may interfere with the delivery of the intervention as designed and in a consistent manner across clients. Some qualities such as advanced knowledge of the presenting problem and the needs and values of the target population enhance treatment implementation and consequently outcome achievement; other qualities such as unfavorable attitude toward the intervention limit the appropriate application of treatment and therefore production of anticipated outcomes. For example, McGilton et al. (2005) found no significant difference in the dose of the communication intervention provided by regulated (i.e., registered nurses and licensed practical nurses) and unregulated (i.e., healthcare aides) nursing staff to clients with speech impairment; however, the researchers reported higher levels of comfort in communication in regulated than unregulated nursing staff, which translated in experience of closer relationships with clients assigned to their care. Nonetheless, these improvements in nursing staff's interactions with clients were not related to the anticipated positive changes in clients' satisfaction with care and perceived sense of well-being. Client characteristics (i.e., level of cognitive and communication impairment) and factors in the inpatient settings (i.e., workload and noise) influenced nursing staff's implementation of the communication intervention at the prescribed dose and hence improvement in client outcomes.

Characteristics of the environment or setting in which the intervention is implemented encompass physical and psychosocial features, and have an indirect influence on outcomes. They affect interventionists' ability to deliver treatment with fidelity, and clients' ability to enact, adhere, or respond to treatment. Consequently, achievement of outcomes is jeopardized.

For instance, McGilton et al. (2005) conducted group interviews with nursing staff to explore their perception of setting factors that interfere with the implementation of the intervention. Content analysis of the staff's qualitative responses suggested that balancing multiple demands (e.g., assisting other clients and families, answering phones, looking for supplies) limited the time available to provide the communication intervention, and noise in patients' rooms (due to roommates' loud TV or radio) interfered with engagement in a meaningful interactive communication with patients over the prescribed time period. Sobieraj et al. (2009) found that gender of the parent present during implementation of music therapy to children undergoing simple laceration repair affected the children's participation and response to treatment (i.e., level of distress). Children's level of distress was higher in the presence of the father than the mother. The researchers attributed this difference to the coping strategies used by the parents, where fathers tended to use strategies that increase distress such as reassurance and criticism, whereas mothers tended to use more effective strategies such as distraction and humor.

13.1.2 Methodological factors

Methodological factors of various nature present threats or biases that affect the validity of the causal relationship between the intervention and the outcomes. Validity refers to the approximate truth or accurate reflection of reality. In efficacy studies, the concern is in obtaining results that accurately capture the occurrence, direction, and magnitude of the intervention effects (i.e., the extent to which the intervention is responsible for producing the observed improvements in the outcomes), and hence in making valid inferences (i.e., reaching valid conclusions) about the efficacy of the intervention under evaluation. Four types of validity have been delineated:

(1) *Statistical conclusion validity:* Validity of inferences about the correlation or covariation between the intervention and the outcomes; it is an issue of accuracy in results of statistical analyses.
(2) *Internal validity:* Validity of inferences about whether the observed covariation between the intervention and the outcome reflects a causal relationship from the intervention to the outcomes, as those variables are manipulated or measured; it is an issue of confounding, that is, the extent to which the observed effects are attributable to the intervention and not to other factors.
(3) *Construct validity:* Validity in which inferences can be made from operations in a study to the theoretical constructs or concepts those operations are intended to represent; it is an issue of intervention implementation and measurement of outcome concepts.
(4) *External validity:* Inferences about whether the causal intervention-outcome relationship holds over variations in persons, settings, treatment variables, and measures; it is an issue of generalizability of findings (Shadish, 2010).

A threat or bias is any element of the planned research protocol or any situation occurring during the conduct of the study that contributes to distorted findings related to the causal effects of the intervention. Distorted findings yield erroneous inferences about the intervention effects; they indicate that the intervention is efficacious when in reality it is not (type I error) or the intervention is not efficacious when in reality it is (type II error). Threats to statistical conclusion, internal, construct, and external validity are identified in Table 13.1, along with a description of their effects on the intervention study findings.

13.1.3 Addressing conceptual and methodological factors

Awareness of conceptual and methodological factors and understanding the nature of the mechanisms underlying their potential contribution to the observed outcomes are critical for elucidating how they distort the findings and offer alternative explanations of the causal relationship between the intervention and the outcomes. This, in turn, assists in devising and/or selecting the most appropriate strategies to prevent and/or control, either experimentally or statistically, the factors. In studies aimed at evaluating the efficacy of interventions, the conceptual factors are commonly controlled for experimentally by (1) carefully selecting participants on the basis of strict eligibility criteria that exclude those with characteristics that directly or indirectly affect outcome achievement, and include those who are most likely to enact and adhere to treatment and/or to respond favorably to it (Rothwell, 2005); (2) randomizing eligible consenting participants to the experimental and comparison groups to control for any between-group imbalances in participants' characteristics that potentially confound the response to treatment; (3) carefully selecting interventionists, providing them with intensive training, and demanding their strict adherence to the standardized intervention protocol; and (4) choosing sites with features that facilitate the implementation of the intervention and allow control of any environmental factor (by making them constant across participants) which can influence treatment delivery and/or outcome achievement. Strategies for preventing and/or addressing specific threats to statistical conclusion, internal, construct, and external validity are mentioned in Table 13.1. How these strategies can be incorporated and integrated into an experimental study or randomized controlled/clinical trial for evaluating the efficacy of interventions is discussed in the next section.

13.2 Design features of an efficacy study

The experimental design or randomized controlled/clinical trial (RCT) is considered the most appropriate for an efficacy study aimed at examining the causal relationship between the intervention and the outcomes. As explained in the previous chapters, the experimental design or RCT has features that contribute to the control of factors known to threaten the validity of the

Table 13.1 Threats to validity in intervention evaluation research

Type of validity	Threat	Effects of threat	Strategies to minimize/address threat
Statistical conclusion	Low statistical power, related to small sample size and preset p-value at low level (e.g., $p \leq .01$)	Low statistical power increases probability of type II error, that is, concluding the experimental and comparison groups' posttest outcomes do not differ when in reality they do	Conduct power analysis to determine sample size required to detect significant intervention effects, while also accounting for anticipated response rate and attrition rate typical for the target population or the intervention under evaluation (available from relevant literature)
	Violated assumptions of statistical tests, that is, participants' data do not meet the assumptions for the statistical tests used to determine effects of the intervention on the outcomes (e.g., normal distribution)	Inappropriate use of statistical tests results in inaccurate results (e.g., finding no significant intervention effects with skewed outcome data)	Examine the data before running the analyses to determine if the data meet the assumptions for the statistical tests to be performed. Identify assumptions not met and address them appropriately, for example: 1. Nonnormal distribution: Determine reasons (e.g., outliers, data-entry error, actual responses) Correct data-entry error Conduct sensitivity analysis (i.e., run the statistical tests with and without outliers) Use statistical tests that do not require normal distribution–avoid transformation of nonnormally distributed data as it creates problem with interpretation of results 2. Unequal group variance: Use formula of the same statistical test that adjusts for inequality of variance

| Fishing and error rate problem, which is likely when performing multiple tests or comparisons on the same data set | With a large number of tests/comparisons, a significant group difference may be observed but it is due to chance. This increases probability of type I error, that is, concluding the experimental and comparison groups' posttest outcomes differ when in reality they do not | Use multivariate tests that compare experimental and comparison groups on all outcomes simultaneously (such as structural equation modeling).

Conduct univariate tests to determine the specific outcome on which the groups differ and adjust the preset p-value to account for multiple testing (e.g., Bonferroni adjustment)

Specify and conduct planned comparisons only to minimize the number of tests to be performed. The planned comparisons are based on theory and hypotheses guiding the study (e.g., compare pretest to 3-month follow-up for long-term outcomes only and pretest to immediate posttest for immediate outcomes only) |
| Low reliability of measures, related to measurement error associated with measurement properties or application of instruments' assessing outcomes | Low reliability of measures leads to interindividual variability in responses/scores that is not associated with the outcome concept being measured and/or intervention effects. This increases within-group variance (i.e., error variance in statistical tests comparing experimental and comparison groups), and hence decreases the statistical power to detect significant intervention effects | Select and use instruments that demonstrated acceptable internal consistency reliability with Cronbach's α coefficient $\geq.7$ for newly developed measures and $\geq.8$ for established measures

Maintain consistency in the context of measure administration across participants and occasions of measurement

Pilot test measures for clarity, comprehension, and relevance of content to the target population, and adopt the measure as necessary

Examine reliability of measures before analyzing the data to determine intervention effects; identify source of measurement error and remedy as necessary

Use multi-item measures when possible and compute total scores; total scores are more reliable than individual items, since error inherent in each item is counterbalanced and reduced) |

(Continued)

Table 13.1 *(Continued)*

Type of validity	Threat	Effects of threat	Strategies to minimize/address threat
			Provide intensive training to observers responsible for collecting outcome data until interobserver or rater agreement of ≥ 80% is reached
			Conduct frequent but random check on observers' performance throughout the study period and provide remedial training as needed
			Check equipment for proper functioning and calibrate equipment for outcome data collection prior to each use
	Low reliability of treatment implementation associated with lack of standardization in the implementation of the intervention	Low reliability of treatment implementation leads to variability in the type and/or dose of the intervention that participants in the experimental group are exposed to/receive, and hence enact	Provide intensive training to interventionists to enhance their understanding of the intervention nature and dose, and their skills in implementing the intervention
		Variability in type and/or dose of intervention yields variability in responses to treatment/outcomes achieved posttest	Provide interventionists with treatment manual that details the activities and steps to be undertaken when implementing the intervention
		Increased variability in outcomes within the experimental group, which increases error variance and decreases statistical power to detect significant intervention effects	Request interventionists to follow treatment manual when delivering the intervention to all participants assigned to the experimental group
			Monitor interventionists' implementation of the intervention to participants through videotaping, audio recording, direct observation, or interventionists' self-report on a checklist (as fits the context of treatment delivery) regularly, throughout the study period
			Obtain data on participants' exposure/receipt of the prescribed intervention dose (e.g., attendance at intervention sessions), enactment and adherence to treatment recommendations (e.g., diary or checklist of recommendations performed)

Random irrelevancies of the experimental setting due to factors in the environment in which the intervention is delivered	Environmental factors influence the implementation of the intervention by preventing or facilitating its delivery as designed and in a standard manner across participants, resulting in outcome achievement, which reduces the power to detect significant intervention effects	Account for variability in treatment implementation, based on interventionists' and participants' data in data analyses (e.g., dose-response analysis), in addition to traditional intention-to-treat analysis Select the environment that is most suitable for delivering the intervention Experimentally control factors in the environment by making or keeping them constant when providing the intervention to all participants assigned to the experimental group Monitor and document any changes that may occur in the environmental factors throughout the study period Account for these changes in the data analysis and/or interpretation
Random heterogeneity of participants, that is, differences in personal or clinical characteristics across participants	This heterogeneity is of primary concern when observed in characteristics that are correlated with the outcome. As such, the characteristics influence participants' response to the intervention, where participants differ in their response. This, in turn, results in increased variance in the outcome within the experimental group and hence error variance, which decreases the power to detect significant intervention effects	Identify, based on the intervention theory or previous empirical evidence, personal and/or clinical characteristics that are correlated with the outcome Control these characteristics experimentally by specifying them as exclusion criteria, or, measure these characteristics and control their influence on the outcome statistically by either exploring differences in outcomes between participants with different levels on the characteristics (i.e., subgroup analyses) or residualizing the effects of the characteristics on the outcomes (i.e., covariate) before running the analyses to examine intervention effects (e.g., analysis of covariance or hierarchical linear models/growth curve analysis)

(Continued)

Table 13.1 (*Continued*)

Type of validity	Threat	Effects of threat	Strategies to minimize/address threat
			Stratify/block the participants based on their levels on the identified characteristics (e.g., high versus low), then randomly assign participants within each block to the experimental or comparison group (i.e., randomized block design), then determine the effects of the intervention and the characteristics on the outcome, using factorial analysis of variance or hierarchical linear models
Internal	History refers to the occurrence of an event, not related to any aspect of the study during the implementation of the intervention, or in the period between implementation of the intervention and outcome assessment following treatment (e.g., unexpected life event, change in nursing care model)	Events could influence participants' reaction or response to the intervention, either positively or negatively. The outcomes observed postintervention implementation can be attributed to the event, rather than the intervention Event could affect the implementation of the intervention and subsequently outcome achievement	Incorporate a comparison group in which participants do not receive the intervention under evaluation and collect outcome data at the same points in time as those scheduled before and after treatment delivery to participants in the experimental group (Buckwalter et al., 2009). The assumption here is that the event affects all participants' outcome equally or in the same way and level. Posttest outcome comparison between experimental and comparison groups will determine the effects of the intervention above and beyond the influence of the event on the outcome
			Monitor occurrence of contextual events during implementation of the intervention
			Collect data on occurrence of life events from participants
			Explore the contribution of reported contextual or life events on treatment implementation and/or outcome achievement using appropriate data analytic technique (i.e., quantitative or qualitative)

Maturation refers to changes in physical function, knowledge, cognitive or reasoning ability, psychosocial function, or experience that take place over the study participation period

Maturation affects participants' response to the intervention either
(1) favorably, yielding positive outcomes as hypothesized; thus, the outcomes are attributable to the maturation changes rather than the intervention, or
(2) unfavorably, yielding no change or negative outcomes, which "mask" the real causal effects of the intervention

Incorporation of a comparison group could assist in determining the effects of the intervention above and beyond the maturational changes, provided the changes are comparable across all participants

Testing refers to changes in responses to outcome measures that are due to the repeated administration of the same measures

With repeated administration of the same measures before and after treatment delivery, participants may alter their responses (e.g., because they remembered an earlier inaccurate response); this is likely to happen with short time interval between administrations. Changes reflecting improvement in outcome can be mistaken for the intervention effects

Use alternative forms of the same outcome, if available, at the different times of data collection (e.g., five randomly selected items of the State-Trait Anxiety Inventory measuring state anxiety)
Use of the Solomon four-group design, where one experimental and one comparison group provide outcome data on pretest and posttest, and one experimental and one comparison group complete posttest outcome measures only. Differences in the posttest outcome measure between the two experimental and the two comparison groups indicate the extent to which testing influenced outcome achievement

(Continued)

Table 13.1 *(Continued)*

Type of validity	Threat	Effects of threat	Strategies to minimize/address threat
	Instrumentation refers to changes in the instrument (equipment or observer) measuring the outcome	Changes in the calibration of equipment and in the level of experience of an observer recording data are associated with changes in the levels of the outcome from pretest to posttest. The observed changes in outcomes are erroneously attributed to the intervention	Recalibrate the equipment for outcome data collection prior to each use Provide adequate initial training to observers responsible for collecting outcome data and continued remedial training throughout the study period Conduct frequent but random check on observers' performance throughout the study period
	Statistical regression to the mean involves pretest to posttest changes in the level of the outcomes for participants with extreme values on the outcome. The exact reason for the changes are not clear	Participants with extreme (high or low) levels on the outcome at pretest tend to show a change (decrease or increase, respectively) in their outcome levels at posttest, whereby their posttest outcome levels are closer to the mean value observed for their respective group or the total sample at posttest When the changes in outcome levels take place for participants in the experimental group and in the same direction as the hypothesized intervention effects, then they confound the intervention effects	Adjust, statistically, for pretest extreme values on the outcomes; e.g., consider pretest outcomes as covariate in analysis of covariance, or conduct subgroup analyses to examine direction and magnitude of change in the outcomes for participants categorized as having high or low pretest outcome values Conduct sensitivity analyses to determine the intervention effects for the total sample and for cases without extreme values on pretest outcomes

Selection refers to differences in the characteristics, assessed at pretest, of participants assigned to the experimental and comparison groups, related to (1) lack of randomization, (2) inadequate implementation of randomization	When the changes in outcome levels take place for participants in the experimental and comparison group, then they may lead to increased within-group or error variance, and hence reduced power to detect significant intervention effects	Ensure appropriate implementation of the randomization procedure
	Differences in pretest characteristics (personal, clinical, or level on outcome) may be directly associated with the achievement of outcomes at posttest, or indirectly related to posttest outcomes, mediated by the extent of treatment implementation. Therefore, the posttest outcomes are attributable to pretest characteristics rather than the intervention effects	Compare the experimental and comparison groups on all variables measured at pretest, while adjusting the p-level for repeated tests
		Identify variables showing significant differences between the experimental and comparison groups, as well as significant correlation with the outcomes measured at posttest
		Account for the identified variables in the statistical analysis by (1) using them as covariates to control for them prior to determining the intervention effects, (2) examining their direct and interactive effects on the posttest outcomes, or (3) generating a propensity score which reflects the set of variables that predict assignment to the experimental and comparison groups, and including the propensity score as a covariate in the analysis aimed at determining intervention effects (Shadish, 2010)

(Continued)

Table 13.1 (Continued)

Type of validity	Threat	Effects of threat	Strategies to minimize/address threat
	Mortality, also referred to as attrition, occurs when participants drop out at any point in time after consenting (i.e., they do not complete the study). Attrition is related to a variety of factors including characteristics of participants, of treatment conditions, and of research study	Attrition threatens the validity of conclusions about the intervention effects in several ways: (1) Decreased sample size available for analysis, which reduces the power to detect significant intervention effects (2) Differences in the characteristics of participants who complete the study and of those who drop out; thus, completers may not be representative of the target population (3) Differences in the number and characteristics of participants who withdraw from the experimental group and from the comparison group; this results in differences in the pretest characteristics of participants assigned to the groups, leading to potential confounding of the intervention effects (referred to as differential attrition) (Ahern & Le Brocque, 2005; Dumville et al., 2006; Valentine & McHugh, 2007)	Prevent attrition by applying any, preferably a combination of the following retention strategies: creating an identity for the study (e.g., logo) training research staff in communication skills and in strategies for handling participants' issues developing trusting relationships with participants through clear communication of expectations related to their involvement in research activities, clarification of key points (e.g., randomization), promoting a sense that participants can access research staff as needed, and showing interest in the "person" (e.g., calling to inquire about participants' status if they do not show up for a planned research activity, responding to participants' inquiry promptly, respecting participants' time, emphasizing usefulness of the study) maintaining regular contacts (e.g., postcards, newsletters, holiday greetings) with participants at regular interval in-between data collection time points expressing appreciation for participants' involvement verbally (e.g., thanking them) and nonverbally (e.g., provision of incentives) making involvement in study convenient and rewarding by allowing flexibility to address participants' needs (e.g., time for providing intervention should fit their schedule) maintaining an accurate system to track participants (Given et al., 1990; Lindsay Davis et al., 2002; Ribisl et al., 1996; Sullivan et al., 1996; Weinert et al., 2008)

Compute attrition rate (percentage of eligible consenting participants who withdraw from the study) to determine extent of attrition for the total sample (should be < 20%; Valentine & McHugh, 2007) and for each of the experimental and the comparison group

Compare participants who withdraw to participants who complete the study on variables measured at pretest to determine the profile of completers to whom the results would be applicable

Compare completers assigned to the experimental and comparison groups on variables measured at pretest to examine the initial comparability of these two groups

Impute posttest outcome values for participants who withdraw (e.g., last observation carried forward, respective group's mean value; McKnight et al., 2007) and conduct intention-to-treat analysis to examine intervention effects using the data (original and imputed) obtained from all participants randomized to the experimental and comparison groups. By using all randomized participants, comparability of the two groups on variables measured at pretest is maintained, thereby minimizing the potential for selection bias that may occur because of differential attrition (Porter et al., 2003)

Create an instrumental variable that reflects the profile (based on pretest variables) of participants likely to complete the study, and account for this variable in the analysis aimed at determining intervention effects (Leigh et al., 1993)

(Continued)

Table 13.1 *(Continued)*

Type of validity	Threat	Effects of threat	Strategies to minimize/address threat
	Contamination or diffusion of the intervention occurs when the experimental intervention or some of its components are disseminated to participants randomized to the comparison group. This could happen when (1) participants in both groups are in close proximity, which facilitates comparison and/or participants' access to the intervention (e.g., clients attending the same clinic) or (2) interventionists provide both the experimental and comparison treatments, or (3) some components of the intervention are widely disseminated and easily accessible to participants in the comparison group (e.g., through Web)	Participants in the comparison group who become aware of the experimental intervention or some of its components may apply it and experience improvement, to various extent (based on the components they enact), in the outcomes. Such improvement reduces the magnitude of the difference in the posttest outcome between the experimental and comparison groups; therefore, the intervention is claimed to be ineffective	Make the unit of assignment to the experimental and comparison groups more aggregated (e.g., clinic, hospital, community) than individual participants. This separates participants in the two groups and prevents communication among them, that is, use cluster randomized trial (Cook et al., 2010) Assign different interventionists to provide the experimental and the comparison group Explain to participants the importance of not sharing intervention-related information with other persons within their usual network Request and constantly remind interventionist responsible for delivering both experimental and comparison treatments, to follow the treatment manual when implementing them and explain the importance of avoiding "slippage" of any intervention components to the comparison group Monitor the fidelity of implementation of the intervention and comparison treatments by interventionists and participants (using strategies discussed in Chapter 10) Account for participants' exposure to intervention components and/or dose in the data analysis—component and dose-response analysis (Sidani & Braden, 1998)

Compensatory equalization of treatments occurs when healthcare professionals, administrators, or community leaders consider it unacceptable to withhold desirable and potentially useful treatments from participants in the comparison group; they attempt to compensate by providing widely disseminated components of the intervention, or by enhancing usual care

As mentioned above, participants in the comparison group receiving some components of the experimental intervention or enhanced usual care experience improvement in the outcomes, thereby reducing the magnitude of the difference in the posttest outcome and increasing the likelihood of incorrect conclusions about the intervention effects

Monitor closely elements of usual care or of the comparison treatment using observational or self-report strategies discussed in Chapter 10
Account for participants' exposure to intervention components and dose in the data analysis, and for the nature of the comparison treatment received, in the interpretation of findings (i.e., similarity in treatment received explains the observed nonsignificant differences in posttest outcomes)

(Continued)

Table 13.1 (*Continued*)

Type of validity	Threat	Effects of threat	Strategies to minimize/address threat
	Reactivity to treatment assignment by participants allocated to the less desirable (i.e., comparison) treatment. Participants learn about the experimental and comparison treatments under evaluation through public advertisement of the study, recruitment, and informed consent process. Once randomized to the comparison treatment, they realize that they received what they believe or is considered by their significant others or healthcare providers the less effective treatment	Participants receiving the less desirable or effective treatment react by either: (1) attempting to reduce or reverse the difference in outcomes (compensatory rivalry) through seeking treatment or showing acceptable levels on outcome; as a result, the difference in posttest outcomes between the intervention and comparison groups is minimal implying the intervention is ineffective; (2) reacting unfavorably to the allocated treatment such as with anger and by "giving up" (resentful demoralization); as a result, participants withdraw from the study (attrition) or respond in a way that reflects worsening of the outcome; the latter response widens the difference in posttest outcomes between the experimental and comparison groups, which leads to the erroneous conclusions that the intervention is effective	Avoid, when possible, public dissemination of the nature of the experimental and the comparison treatments. Consider delayed treatment design which has been suggested to minimize attrition related to unfavorable reaction to treatment assignment (Pruitt & Privette, 2001). This type of crossover design involves randomly assigning participants to the immediate group, which receives the experimental intervention following pretest data collection, or the delayed group, which receives the same experimental intervention following posttest data collection on all participants. Whereas this design mimics what may happen in clinical practice (e.g., clients put on a waiting list for treatment), it has been recently criticized for inducing expectancies that translates into spontaneous but limited improvement in outcomes

| Construct | Inadequate preoperational explication of constructs refers to unclear conceptualization of variables, specifically outcomes. This is related to the lack of theoretical foundation for the intervention and its effects, and lack of explicit theoretical definitions of concepts | Unavailability of explicit theoretical definitions of concepts, particularly outcomes, results in unclear specification of the attributes defining the concepts, and therefore inappropriate operationalization. The latter may lead to the selection of measures in which content is not congruent in representing all domains of the outcome concept or reflects potentially confounding concepts. Accordingly, the measures used cannot capture the intended intervention effects, leading to erroneous conclusions that the intervention is not effective | Have a clear conceptualization of the outcomes that provides explicit theoretical and operational definitions of the outcome concepts Use the theoretical and operational definitions to guide the selection of outcome measures, which content should reflect all identified domains of the outcome concepts and be relevant to the target population Select appropriate outcome measures that demonstrated content and construct validity, acceptable reliability, and relevance to the target population (i.e., has been used in the target population or populations with characteristics similar to those of the target population) |
| | Method bias refers to systematic error of measurement related to the use of one instrument to measure each outcome (monooperation bias) or of one method of data collection (monomethod bias) | Systematic error in the responses to outcome measures introduces an artifactual increase or decrease in the outcome levels, yielding an overestimation or underestimation of the intervention effects | Use multiple measures of the same outcome, if available (e.g., one global item and multidimensional measure of a symptom), and/or different methods for collecting data on outcomes that are manifested in various dimensions (e.g., physiological, physical, behavioral, self-report), or that are rated by different sources (e.g., client, family, healthcare provider). Selection of outcome measures and methods should attend to the need for minimizing response burden, which negatively influence the quality of the obtained data |

(Continued)

Table 13.1 (Continued)

Type of validity	Threat	Effects of threat	Strategies to minimize/address threat
	Evaluation apprehension refers to changes in participants' verbal or behavioral responses to the outcomes related to their awareness that they are being evaluated	Participants' awareness of being evaluated makes them change their verbal and behavioral responses to outcome measures; the change is consistent with their desire to be seen competent or in a favorable way. Such alternations can mask the hypothesized intervention effects	Emphasize to participants that there are no "right or wrong" answers (Padsakoff et al., 2003) Provide adequate training for research staff responsible for collecting observational data in nonjudgmental manner Assess social desirability and control its influence on the responses to outcomes prior to examining the effects of the intervention
	Experimenter expectancies refers to the researchers' expectations regarding the effectiveness of the intervention in that they anticipate its success in achieving the hypothesized, beneficial outcomes	Favorable expectations influence research assistants' observations (if asked to rate behavioral outcomes), interventionists' and research staff's interactions with participants (positive interactions contribute to development of a trusting relationship and subsequently to satisfaction with treatment and with research experience that translates into a desire to please the researchers, and reported improvements in outcomes), and researchers' plan for data analysis. Additional analyses are done to identify significant intervention effects for some outcomes, in some subgroups of participants—this is well illustrated with the sentence: "if you torture data long enough, they will confess" (Fleming, 2010)	Provide adequate training to research staff and interventionists in the skills required to assume their responsibilities and to interact with participants that maintain interest in the study and that do not provoke extreme (negative or positive) reactions Apply, when feasible, the principle of blinding research staff to the treatment to which participants are allocated, specially when the research staff are to observe participants' responses at posttest; in cluster randomized trials, "rotate" research staff responsible for outcome data collection across participating sites and across occasions of data collection, without informing them of the sites' allocated treatment Have a statistician conduct the data analysis as planned and consider the results of any additional analysis as exploratory, requiring confirmation in future studies (rather than definitive indicators of intervention effects in subgroups of clients)

Interaction of different treatments refers to the participants' exposure or receipt/enactment of additional treatments for the same presenting problem (also called cointervention). The additional treatments could be given as part of usual care which cannot be withheld, or could be sought by participants for various reasons (e.g., dissatisfaction with assigned treatment)	When additional treatments are implemented by participants in the comparison group and if effective, they reduce the magnitude of the difference in posttest outcomes between the experimental and comparison groups; hence, erroneous conclusions that the experimental intervention is not effective When additional treatments are implemented by participants in the experimental group, and if effective, then (1) improvements in outcomes are erroneously attributed to the experimental intervention, or (2) they interact with the experimental intervention, potentially strengthening its effects, yielding overestimate of the intervention effects (often not replicated in subsequent studies) and lack of clarity as to the specific treatment or combination of treatments responsible for producing the observed effects	Preset the study eligibility criteria to exclude participants currently receiving treatment for the presenting problem Request participants taking treatment for the presenting or any other problem to not change their treatments and/or doses during the study period Collect data on nature and dose of additional treatments participants may be taking during the study period Account for the additional treatments taken when analyzing the intervention effects (i.e., consider such treatments as covariates or explore their direct and moderating influence on the outcome)

(Continued)

Table 13.1 (*Continued*)

Type of validity	Threat	Effects of threat	Strategies to minimize/address threat
External	Interaction of selection and treatment involves the situation where participants in the study represent a select subgroup of the target population and their response to the intervention is unique to the select subgroup. This is the case when clients who enroll in and/or complete the study differ from clients who decline enrollment in and/or withdraw from the study	Participants who enroll in and/or complete an intervention evaluation study often differ on some personal and clinical characteristics as well as perceived acceptability of the treatment under evaluation, from nonparticipants and dropouts. Their profile is not necessarily representative of the different subgroups of the target population; however, it could influence their response to the intervention, in that they demonstrate improvement or no change in the outcome. Therefore, the findings are not applicable to other subgroups of the target population presenting with a different profile	Make participation in the intervention evaluation study attractive to different subgroups of the target population (e.g., flexibility in scheduling research activities and treatment delivery) Provide detailed description of the participants' profile which is useful in delineating the target population subgroup to whom the results are applicable or who would benefit from the intervention
	Interaction of setting and treatment involves the situation where the sites (e.g., organization) in which the intervention is implemented represent a select type not reflective of all settings in which the intervention could be provided	The sites selected for participation in the study are often chosen because they have physical and psychosocial environmental features that facilitate the implementation of the experimental intervention, and subsequently the achievement of hypothesized outcomes. The findings are not replicated in sites with different or less than optimal environmental features	Include in the study sites that differ in the environmental features that facilitate implementation of the intervention Compare fidelity of treatment implementation and outcome achievement across sites Provide detailed description of the environmental features of sites showing highest fidelity of treatment implementation and outcome achievement which is useful to determine the characteristics of the sites to which the findings are generalizable

causal relationship. By eliminating or minimizing these factors, changes in the outcomes observed following implementation of the intervention can be attributed to the intervention only. However, establishing a causal relationship requires, in addition to the application of relevant design features, a theory that specifies the nature of the relationship between the intervention and the outcomes (Towne & Hilton, 2004). The intervention theory, as discussed in Chapter 5, identifies characteristics of clients, interventionists, and settings, representing the conceptual factors, that affect the implementation of the intervention and the achievement of the outcomes; clarifies elements of the intervention (components, activities, dose, mode of delivery) that produce the outcomes; and explains the mechanism underlying the intervention effects on the ultimate outcomes by specifying the interrelationships among the intervention, immediate outcomes, and ultimate outcomes. As such, intervention theory is instrumental in guiding the design of an efficacy study, in identifying the conceptual factors to control, in planning and conducting data analysis, and in interpreting the findings.

The following is a discussion of the key features of an experimental design or RCT and related points to consider when planning and executing an efficacy study. Kraemer et al. (2002) described the characteristics of a well-designed RCT in terms of (1) a sample that is well justified, representative of the target population, and of sufficient size; (2) presence of at least one comparison group, in addition to the experimental group, with clear protocol for each to permit replication of treatment delivery; (3) randomization of participants to comparison and experimental groups to avoid selection bias; (4) well-chosen outcomes assessed with blinded research staff to minimize researchers' and participants' expectancies; (5) analysis done on all randomized participants (i.e., intention-to-treat) and a priori specified subgroup analyses and estimate of effect size; and (6) application of valid test for statistical inference. The features are discussed in an order consistent with the expected sections of a study proposal and the steps of a research study.

13.2.1 Careful selection of participants

In an efficacy study using the RCT design, participants are carefully selected to ensure enrolling clients that are representative of the target population, yet do not have characteristics that are known to confound the intervention effects. The target population is often defined in terms of particular medical diagnosis such as cardiac disease or type 2 diabetes; most importantly, it should be identified relative to the experience of the presenting health-related problem and its determinants that are the target of the intervention under evaluation such as women with breast cancer experiencing fatigue with chemotherapy, or older (>65 years) adults with insomnia related to inability to maintain sleep. As mentioned previously, personal and clinical characteristics of participants can influence the implementation and/or enactment of the intervention, and/or the immediate and ultimate outcomes; thus, they offer alternative explanations of the intervention effects. The intervention theory clarifies the nature of the presenting problem and its determinants as well as prominent client characteristics that affect, directly or indirectly, the outcomes. It guides the prespecification of the criteria for selecting participants.

The criteria are categorized into inclusion and exclusion criteria. Inclusion criteria are a set of characteristics that are reflective of those defining the target population. They ensure that persons who take part in the efficacy study belong to the target population and experience the presenting problem amenable to treatment by the intervention under evaluation. Exclusion criteria are used to control for participants' characteristics that are hypothesized to interfere with the implementation of the intervention and/or to be directly associated with the immediate or ultimate outcomes expected of the intervention. These characteristics could be related to (1) demographic profile, such as proficiency in the language used for communicating the treatment recommendations and for completing the outcome measures; (2) health or clinical condition, such as presence of comorbid conditions that may limit engagement in the intervention activities or for which the intervention is contraindicated; (3) current treatment for the same presenting problem or for any comorbidities which can moderate (strengthen or weaken) the intervention effects; and (4) psychological status, such as cognitive impairment and severe levels of psychological dysfunction that precludes or limits participants' engagement in and enactment of the intervention activities. For some efficacy trials, the following additional criteria are preset for selecting participants: (1) participants' and their healthcare providers' agreement to maintain constant the dose and schedule for current treatment received to manage the presenting problem or comorbidities throughout the study period (Pincus, 2002), and (2) participants' tendency to comply with treatment (Rothwell, 2005).

To ensure that participants meet all the eligibility criteria, all clients showing interest in taking part in the study are subjected to screening, using where available, validated measures of the characteristics constituting the inclusion and exclusion criteria. The content of the measures should be congruent with the defining attributes of the characteristics. The measures include the following:

(1) Single items or questions inquiring about possession of a characteristic that reflects a general eligibility criterion, such as language proficiency, current treatment (type and dose), and experience of the problem; the items, often generated for the purpose of the study, should be pilot tested for comprehension and clarity.

(2) Multi-item self-report instruments assessing characteristics manifested in different domains and indicators such as the Mini Mental State Exam (Folstein et al., 1975) to determine participants' level of cognitive impairment, and the Insomnia Severity Index (Morin, 1993) to measure the severity of insomnia (e.g., participants with moderate and high levels of insomnia are targeted). Well-validated measures with high sensitivity, specificity, and established cutoff scores are used to accurately identify participants that meet or do not meet the eligibility criteria. If available,

validated short versions of the measures are used to minimize response burden.

(3) Relevant instruments (or equipment) to assess objective characteristics such as blood pressure or oxygen saturation. The instruments should have demonstrated precision and accuracy.

(4) Letters from the participants' healthcare providers are required to determine agreement to fix the schedule and dose of current treatments and the intervention under evaluation is not contraindicated.

(5) Assessment of participants' tendency for compliance is done in what is called "run-in" period. Participants are requested to adhere to some aspect of the study, such as diary, during the period. Only participants who show an acceptable, preset level of adherence (e.g., >70%) are included in the efficacy study (Rothwell, 2005).

Although screening is scheduled once recruited individuals show interest in taking part in the efficacy study, the specific location and time for administering the screening measures are determined by their level of intrusiveness. Simple items assessing eligibility criteria reflecting general characteristics may be administered over the telephone or secure Web site, but only after obtaining initial consent. Multi-item measures assessing participants' clinical condition, current treatment, psychological status, and tendency to comply may be considered intrusive and, thus, are administered in a face-to-face session held in a private setting, after obtaining written informed consent. Depending on the advice of the institutional research board or research ethics committee, the consent should cover agreement to the screening only, since individuals who do not meet all eligible criteria are excluded from the study. Participants' responses to screening measures indicate whether they are eligible (i.e., have all inclusion criteria and none of the exclusion criteria) and which specific criteria led to their exclusion.

The selection of participants on the basis of the strictly preset eligibility criteria "guarantees" the exclusion of individuals who have characteristics that potentially confound the intervention effects and the inclusion of participants who are homogeneous in terms of their personal and psychological, and most importantly, their clinical characteristics, particularly those related to the presenting problem (Hyde, 2004). The sample homogeneity is believed to contribute to the initial comparability of the experimental and comparison groups prior to intervention implementation (i.e., pretest), and hence to the comparability of their response to the intervention. That is, participants with similar initial characteristics are expected to respond in the same way to the intervention implying that they demonstrate the same pattern (i.e., direction and amount) of change in the outcomes following treatment implementation. This comparability in response to the intervention reduces the variability in the outcomes within the experimental group. When the outcomes measured following treatment implementation (posttest) of the experimental group are compared to those of the comparison group (i.e., did not receive the intervention under evaluation), the difference in the means of the two groups is large, thereby increasing the power to detect significant intervention effects (Sidani & Braden, 1998). In addition, because potentially confounding factors are controlled (by excluding participants with these factors), the observed changes in the outcomes are validly attributable to the intervention.

It is important to note that the application of strict inclusion and exclusion criteria reduces the percentage of recruited participants that meet the eligibility criteria. Kotwall et al. (1992) reported that 46.1% of women with breast cancer were found ineligible for entry into efficacy trials of medial treatments. Similarly, Grapow et al. (2006) estimated that many RCTs include ≤10% of screened participants. Stirman et al. (2005) pointed that the stringent eligibility criteria preset for efficacy trials of psychotherapy results in exclusion rates of 68% for depressive disorders, 64% for panic disorders, and 65% for generalized anxiety disorders. This has implications for recruitment. Multiple strategies are required to recruit a large number of members of the target population from several sites in order to obtain an adequate sample size. In addition, sufficient resources should be planned for screening this large number of individuals.

13.2.2 Control of experimental condition

Although various aspects of the efficacy study are under the researchers' control (e.g., implementation of treatment), this feature of the experimental design or RCT has to do primarily with the setting or environment in which treatments are offered, with the interventionists responsible for delivering the intervention, and with the research staff responsible for collecting outcome data. The control is exerted by carefully selecting the setting and the interventionists, and by adequately training therapists and research staff or data collectors.

The setting is selected on the basis of the physical and psychosocial features, hypothesized in the intervention theory to affect implementation of the intervention. The features that are known to interfere with the delivery of the intervention and/or with participants' response to treatment are clearly delineated and controlled. The control involves (1) selecting settings that do not have the features, (2) eliminating the features from the particular environment in which the intervention is given, or (3) maintaining the features constant across all participants receiving the intervention when the first two strategies are not possible, such as keeping the room temperature at the same level when having all participants listen to relaxing music to avoid any potential discomfort which may affect the achievement of the intended outcome of decreased pain levels. The features proposed as essential to facilitate the implementation of the intervention are clarified and their particular indicators are specified to guide the careful selection of setting. It is often the case that most appropriate settings are located in research intensive organizations such as universities or university affiliated institutions (e.g., hospitals, clinics, health centers), which are highly qualified facilities with adequate resources and research-oriented culture that promote high fidelity of treatment implementation, and consequently achievement of the anticipated outcomes (Bottomley, 1997).

The interventionists also are selected on the basis of well-defined criteria reflective of professional preparation and experience, interpersonal skills, as well as theoretical knowledge of and skills in delivering the intervention, specified in the intervention theory. The interventionists' characteristics are assessed informally during the hiring interview, or formally by administering relevant measures where available. The selected interventionists are given intensive training in the theory underlying the intervention and the skills for carrying out the intervention activities. Interventionists with specific qualities and intensive training are adequately prepared to implement the intervention as designed and in a standard way, which enhances fidelity and consistency of treatment delivery across participants, and consequently achievement of anticipated outcomes. In addition, they are instructed to maintain the same style of interpersonal interactions and the same demeanor with all participants in order to standardize the nature and level of therapeutic relationship or working alliance and, therefore, to minimize its influence on outcomes.

The research staff are also trained in the protocol for data collection. The training should assist them in understanding the theoretical and operational definitions of the concepts of interest, the principles and recommendations for obtaining the information with the selected methods of data collection (e.g., appropriate ways or tips for conducting telephone interviews), and the specific instructions for administering particular measures, such as interpretation of scores on screening measures. Opportunities for applying the skills are offered, particularly when the measures to be used are observational (e.g., assessment of pain in infants), and remedial training is given until the research staff achieve an acceptable level ($\geq 80\%$) of interrater reliability. Such training enhances accuracy of the data. It is commonly recommended to withhold information on the efficacy study hypotheses, the nature of the experimental and the comparison treatments, and participants' assignment to treatment, of research staff, also known as "blinding" (Keirse & Hansens, 2000). When research staff are unaware of which participants receive what treatment, they do not develop expectancies or prejudice that could shape their perception, observation, or judgments when collecting outcome data, particularly following implementation of the intervention (Kaptchuk, 2001).

13.2.3 Selection of comparison group

The presence of a comparison group in an efficacy trial is an essential design feature for making valid inferences about the causal relationship between the intervention and the outcomes (Pincus, 2002; Watson et al., 2004). The comparison group is a subgroup of the sample recruited for the study; it comprises participants who meet all study eligibility criteria and complete all outcome measures at the points in time specified for the study, but do not receive the experimental intervention under evaluation. Thus, participants in the comparison group are comparable on personal and clinical or health characteristics, as well as baseline outcome variables measured before implementation of the intervention, to participants in the experimental group. They provide outcome data prospectively and concurrently with those in the experimental group. This simultaneous outcome data collection and comparison on outcome achievement between the two groups are critical for establishing causality. Causality is inferred if the following are observed: (1) no significant difference between the two groups on the outcomes assessed prior to the implementation of the intervention; (2) participants in the experimental group show the expected changes in the outcomes after treatment delivery; (3) participants in the comparison group show no changes in the outcomes; and (4) there is a significant difference between the two groups on the outcomes measured after implementation of the intervention. This pattern of findings indicates that expected changes in the outcomes occur following implementation of the intervention and do not occur when it is not implemented, which supports the temporality and covariation criteria for causality, and increases confidence in attributing the outcomes to the intervention. However, changes in the outcomes may be observed in the comparison group. These changes could be related to history, maturation, or testing, which are threats to internal validity and weaken the confidence in inferring a causal relationship between the intervention and the outcomes.

Alternatively, these changes could reflect the effects of treatments or care that participants in the comparison group may receive. Consequently, it is important to select the appropriate comparison treatment condition in an efficacy study. Different comparison treatment conditions have been used in efficacy trials of medical, educational, and cognitive behavioral interventions. These include the following:

(1) *No-treatment control condition:* In a no-treatment control condition, participants do not receive any treatment for the presenting problem, and those who may be taking treatment are requested to withhold it for the duration of the study. This condition creates a situation that generates the evidence for demonstrating the criterion of covariation for inferring causality. It is most suitable for an efficacy study of a newly designed intervention (Borkovec, 1993). Nonetheless, the no-treatment control condition presents not only an ethical dilemma because treatment is withheld, but also methodological problems. Participants need an explanation regarding the reason for not receiving treatment (to which they are entitled!) and are likely to withdraw from the trial in order to seek treatment elsewhere, yielding high levels of differential attrition; that is, a larger number of participants drop out of the comparison than the experimental group (Barkauskas et al., 2005; Kazdin, 2003).

(2) *Waiting-list control condition:* This is another type of no-treatment condition, with a modified crossover, where the control group participants' treatment is delayed. That is, participants assigned to the waiting-list-control condition are not given the intervention under evaluation at the same time as it is delivered to those in the experimental condition, but

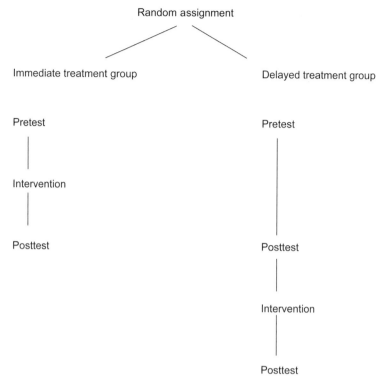

Figure 13.1 Waiting-list control design.

are offered the intervention following posttest outcome data collection (Figure 13.1) as suggested by D'Agostino (2009). This design addresses the ethical dilemma of withholding treatment and mimics the reality of day-to-day practice where clients are put on a waiting list for treatment. Another advantage of this condition is the ability to replicate the effects of the intervention in the comparison group, following delayed treatment delivery (Borkovec, 1993). However, participants in the delayed treatment group may withdraw from the study prior to receiving treatment to seek care elsewhere, especially if the presenting problem is severe and prone to rapid deterioration (Borkovec, 1993). They may develop some expectations resulting in some improvement in the outcomes observed prior to receiving treatment; the improvement, even if small, alters the magnitude of the differences between the two groups in the outcomes assessed at posttest, jeopardizing the ability to detect significant intervention effects.

(3) *Placebo condition:* The term placebo refers to an inert, innocuous treatment that has no inherent power to produce a given effect (Stewart-Williams & Podd, 2004). In medicine, placebo treatments consist of preparation or pills, even surgical procedures, that look exactly like the experimental treatment under evaluation and contains nonmedicinal substances such as sugar (Sidani & Stevens, 2000); they lack the active ingredients that characterize the experimental treatment. In the behavioral sciences,

placebo interventions are designed in a similar way in that they are structurally equivalent to the experimental intervention but do not incorporate the active ingredients that distinguish the experimental intervention. Structural equivalence means that the placebo intervention is comparable to the experimental intervention in the following aspects: mode of delivery (e.g., individual or group format for giving treatment); dose such as total number of sessions, duration of each session, and frequency of session delivery (e.g., six sessions of 60 minutes each, given once a week); setting in which it is delivered (e.g., same organization and room characteristics); attention given to participants during the session where a rationale for the treatment is provided (which is important to maintain credibility of the placebo treatment received and to avoid disappointment due to getting the less desirable treatment); a discussion of issues (that are not directly related to the presenting problem) is initiated; and homework exercises or planned activities (such as problem-solving) are assigned. The placebo intervention is implemented by trained, skilled interventionists (Baskin et al., 2000; Kazdin, 2003). Although placebo treatments are theoretically expected to have no effects on the outcomes of the experimental intervention, they have been found to induce what is called placebo response or effects, manifested in either favorable outcomes such as improvement in participants' condition or unfavorable outcomes such as development of side effects. Since by definition a placebo treatment is inert, several mechanisms have been proposed to explain the placebo effects. The placebo effects have been attributed to: (1) natural resolution of the presenting problem such as pain after surgery (Hamunen & Kalso, 2005); (2) motivation resulting from perception of a positive therapeutic relationship or working alliance with the interventionist; (3) expectancy of improvement associated with the belief that the treatment is credible and effective (Finnis et al., 2010); (4) classical conditioning where improvement is anticipated with the mere fact of receiving treatment (Stewart-Williams & Podd, 2004); and (5) neurobiological mechanisms including endogenous opioids (Van Die et al., 2009). The assumption underlying the use of a placebo treatment in efficacy trial is that well-designed placebo treatments, which are structurally equivalent to the experimental intervention and hence incorporate the same nonspecific elements of the intervention, affect participants assigned to the experimental and comparison groups equally; therefore, any difference between the two groups observed in the outcomes measured at posttest are attributable to the intervention's active ingredients (Van Die et al., 2009), thereby supporting the causal effects of the intervention. Results of earlier meta-analyses comparing the effects of active and placebo treatments (mean effect size = .55) and of active treatment and no-treatment (mean effect size = .76) lead to the conclusion that the placebo or nonspecific elements of psychological treatments exert much less of an effect than previously believed (Bowers & Clum, 1998). However, recent empirical evidence challenges this conclusion. Baskin et al. (2000) found a larger mean effect size for structurally nonequivalent (.46) than for structurally equivalent (.14) placebo treatment, and Van Die et al. (2009) reported that 65–80% of the response to antidepressant is duplicated in participants receiving placebo pill. Accordingly, the utility of placebo treatment in isolating the unique impact of the intervention's active ingredient is questionable, as the nonspecific elements of the intervention forming placebo treatment may interact with, rather than have simple additive effects as previously assumed, the intervention's active ingredients in producing the outcomes. In addition, developing a placebo treatment that is structurally equivalent to active educational and behavioral interventions and is credible, is problematic. Participants who do not view placebo treatment as credible refuse to be randomized (Barkauskas et al., 2005) and those who may not experience improvement in the outcomes despite adherence to placebo treatment may withdraw, leading to potential differential attrition.

(4) *Usual care or treatment-as-usual condition:* In this condition, participants continue to receive the usual care, services, or specific treatments to address the presenting problem. Barkauskas et al. (2005) describe two situations for providing usual care as a comparison treatment in efficacy trials. In the first, only participants assigned to the comparison condition continue to receive usual care, whereas those assigned to the experimental treatment do not. Differences in the posttest outcomes between the two groups are assumed to reflect the unique effects of the experimental intervention. In the second situation, which is commonly resorted to when it is unethical to withhold usual care, participants in the experimental and the comparison groups continue treatment-as-usual, and the experimental intervention is given only to the former group. Differences in the posttest outcomes between the two groups indicate the contribution of the experimental intervention in addition to or above and beyond usual care. Despite its advantages, usual care condition generates methodological issues that should be carefully addressed during study conduct. The issue relates to the variability in the definition and implementation of usual care (Barkauskas et al., 2005; De Maat et al., 2007). The nature of usual care is often unclear and in some instances, it comprises components or activities reflecting active ingredients of the experimental intervention, resulting in overlap of treatments. Usual care is often individualized, where the specific treatments given are responsive to the needs and preferences of individual clients; therefore, the types of treatment received vary across participants assigned to this comparison treatment. Similarly, the dose of treatments-as-usual may differ across participants. Overlap in components and activities of the experimental and comparison treatments, as well as variability in the implementation of usual care contribute to a reduction in the magnitude of the between-group difference in posttest outcomes which, coupled with an increased within-comparison-group variance, decrease the power to detect significant intervention effects. To address the methodological issues, it is highly recommended to confine the efficacy trial to one setting

or site that provides standardized usual care, guided by clearly defined best practice/clinical guidelines, and where healthcare professionals are willing/agreeing to maintain usual care consistent across clients and constant over time. When this recommendation is not feasible, it becomes critical to monitor fidelity of implementation of experimental and comparison treatments, as highlighted in a later section. Data on what constitutes usual care are helpful in clarifying the distinction in the nature of the experimental and comparison treatments, and in interpreting the results.

13.2.4 Allocation of participants to groups

In efficacy trials, randomization or random assignment is the method used to allocate eligible, consenting participants to the experimental or comparison group. It is considered the most crucial feature of the experimental or RCT therapeutic for controlling selection bias (Porter et al., 2003; Towne & Hilton, 2004) and therefore for establishing the causal relationship between the intervention and outcomes (Watson et al., 2004). Randomization involves the application of chance-based procedures for allocating participants to the experimental or comparison treatment group. The chance-based procedures eliminate human influence, whether unconscious or deliberate, on assignment to groups (Kaptchuk, 2001). Thus, each eligible participant has an equal chance of receiving or not getting the experimental intervention, without the interference of the participants themselves, the healthcare professionals referring participants to the efficacy study, the interventionists, or the research staff. Randomization is believed to enhance the comparability of participants on all measured and any unmeasured characteristics, before treatment implementation (Kaul & Diamond, 2010). It leads to a situation in which participants with given characteristics or idiosyncrasies assigned to one group will, on the average, be counterbalanced by participants with comparable characteristics or idiosyncrasies assigned to the other group (Cook & Campbell, 1979). The end result is an even or balanced distribution of participants with similar characteristics that could be associated with the outcomes, between the experimental and comparison groups. This initial group comparability reduces the variability in the outcomes assessed at posttest that is not attributable to the intervention, and hence increases the chance of detecting significant, unbiased intervention effects (Borglin & Richards, 2010; Chatterji, 2007; Sidani, 2006). That is, if participants in the two groups have similar characteristics, and those who receive the experimental intervention show the expected improvement in the outcomes while those in the comparison group report no change in the outcomes; then the observed between-group differences in the posttest outcomes can be confidently attributed to the intervention and not to any participants' characteristics (Watson et al., 2004).

   Different randomization procedures are available, including: (1) flip of a coin, which is no longer recommended as it can result in an unbalanced number of participants assigned to the experimental and comparison groups, and the resulting group assignment can be tempered with (e.g., the research staff can flip the coin repeatedly until the desirable treatment is allocated to a particular participant); (2) table of random number, which could also be tempered with; (3) preparing sealed opaque envelopes enclosing a piece of paper on which group assignment is written and opened in the presence of participants; (4) computer-generated list of random numbers, given by a centralized office to research staff at the time of randomization (Davies, 1999; Padhye et al., 2009; Watson et al., 2004). The computer-generated allocation codes can block or stratify participants on key characteristics (such as age or sex) to ensure a balanced distribution of participants with similar characteristics between the experimental and comparison groups (Dumbridgue et al., 2006). The sealed envelopes and the computer-generated codes for randomization maintain concealment of treatment allocation from research staff (i.e., research staff are unaware of group assignment) and are less prone to human influence on participants' allocation to treatments.

In situations when randomization cannot be done at the individual participant level to avoid contamination or diffusion of the experimental or the comparison group, it can be performed at the level of the site participating in the study. This design is referred to as quasi-experimental or cluster-randomized trial and is considered an appropriate alternative to the RCT for determining intervention efficacy (Taljaard et al., 2009). The clustering of participants within sites requires use of statistical tests that account for within-cluster correlation in outcomes, such as hierarchical linear models (Kraemer et al., 2009). Such within-cluster correlation reflects the observation that participants in the same cluster (e.g., site) are more likely to experience the same outcome than those in different clusters.

The timing at which participants are informed of the treatment to which they are assigned should be carefully considered. If done before collecting outcome data at pretest, then participants' awareness of the allocated treatment could affect their responses to the outcome measures. Specifically, participants allocated to the undesirable treatment (e.g., comparison treatment) may get disappointed and alter their responses, or may withdraw from the study, potentially creating an imbalance in the pretest outcome levels or other personal and clinical characteristics, between the two groups. These differences result in selection bias, which defies the purpose for which randomization is done, as illustrated with the results of Shapiro et al. (2002). Therefore, it is recommended to inform participants of their treatment assignment after collecting data at pretest.

It is important to note that randomization increases the likelihood, but does not guarantee, initial group comparability on baseline characteristics. Thus, participants in the experimental and comparison groups may differ on any characteristic or outcome variable measured at pretest. Although such a difference is due to chance, it may be observed for a characteristic known to be correlated with and confound the outcomes (Peduzzi et al., 2002). Further, comparability is achieved at the group, and not the individual participant level. As stated by Cook and Campbell (1979), random assignment "does not, of course, remove the idiosyncrasy from any one unit" (p. 340). This statement implies that randomization does not control or eliminate interindividual differences in the characteristics assessed at pretest. Therefore, these characteristics may still exert their influence on achievement of outcomes following implementation of the intervention. Accordingly, it is advisable to compare participants in the experimental and comparison groups on all characteristics measured at pretest, even when they are randomized, and to control for the potential confounding influence of characteristics showing statistically significant differences between the two groups and statistically significant correlation with posttest scores, when conducting the statistical analyses to determine the intervention effects (Porter et al., 2003). The characteristics are considered as covariates in an analysis of covariance (Padhye et al., 2009) or hierarchical linear models (Raudenbush & Bryk, 2002; Sidani, 2006).

13.2.5　Standardized treatment implementation

Standardized implementation of the experimental and comparison treatments is useful for valid inferences about the causal relationship between the intervention and outcomes (McGuire et al., 2000; Towne & Hilton, 2004). To be effective in producing the intended outcomes, the experimental intervention should be implemented in a standardized and consistent manner across participants assigned to this group. This means that the same intervention components and activities are given in the same way and at the same dose to all participants. Standardization and consistency are believed to reduce variability in treatment delivery and consequently variability in the response to treatment exhibited by participants in the experimental group. This is reflected in decreased within-group or error variance in posttest outcomes, and consequently increased power to detect significant intervention effects. Similarly, standardized and appropriate application of the comparison treatment is essential for maintaining the distinction, and preventing any overlap, with the experimental intervention. Difference in the nature of the experimental and comparison treatments generates the difference in the posttest outcomes between the two groups, which forms the basis for inferring causality.

Strategies for enhancing standardized and consistent implementation of the intervention were discussed in detail in the chapter on intervention fidelity. The same strategies for monitoring integrity of intervention delivery can be used to assess application of the comparison treatment.

Participants' adherence to allocated treatment received attention in efficacy trials. Participants' tendency for compliance is often preset as a selection criterion, so that those who enroll in the study are compliers. Strategies for enhancing adherence, such as self-monitoring and providing feedback or incentives, are incorporated in the study protocol. Monitoring adherence is planned and relevant data are obtained using objective and subjective measures, from different sources (e.g., participants, significant other). Nonadherence is a threat to validity. It results in variability in treatment enactment and consequently in outcome achievement. This, in turn, increases within-group or error variance and decreases the statistical power to detect significant intervention effects (Jo, 2002).

13.2.6 Outcome measurement

Immediate and ultimate outcomes are measured at least once before and after implementation of the intervention, in the experimental and comparison groups in order to capture changes in the outcomes. The outcomes assessed before treatment (pretest or baseline) serve as reference for comparison with those measured following treatment (posttest) and for delineating the pattern, that is, direction (i.e., increase, no change, or decrease) and magnitude of change (i.e., how large). The pattern is important to determine the extent to which participants in the experimental group experience the expected changes in the outcomes, and participants in the comparison group report no changes. The instruments used to measure the outcomes should be reliable and valid in order to accurately capture the changes in outcomes. Unreliable measures introduce error, which is manifested in unexplained variability in the outcomes assessed at posttest. Unexplained variability contributes to high error variance, which reduces the statistical power to detect significant intervention effects (McClelland, 2000). Invalid measures do not capture the outcomes expected of the intervention, or the anticipated changes in the outcomes, leading to incorrect conclusion (i.e., type 2 error) that the intervention is not effective. For a more detailed discussion of outcome measurement in intervention evaluation research, refer to Chapter 7 in Sidani and Braden (1998).

13.2.7 Outcome data analysis

Traditionally, intention-to-treat analysis was considered as the most appropriate approach for outcome data analysis in efficacy trials. This approach was, and still is, thought by many to provide valid estimates of the causal effects of the intervention on the outcomes, because it includes in the analysis all randomized participants whether or not they completed the study. As such, the initial comparability of the experimental and comparison groups is maintained, thereby controlling for selection bias and the influence of any potentially confounding baseline characteristic. To be able to conduct the analysis, outcome data are imputed for participants who dropped out of the study, using the mean of their respective group at posttest or the last observation carried forward in repeated measure design (Jo, 2002; Porter et al., 2003). With the realization that the intention-to-treat analysis tends to dilute the effects of the intervention for participants who do not receive treatment, other analyses have been suggested, such as per-protocol and as-treated analyses (Sheiner & Rubin, 1995). The extent to which these two analyses provide valid estimates of the intervention effects has not been clearly established. It is important to note that statistical tests, most frequently used to analyze outcome data (such as analysis of variance, hierarchical linear models), examine the direct effects of the intervention on each of the immediate and ultimate outcomes.

Additional analyses are required to test the indirect effects of the intervention on ultimate outcomes, mediated by immediate outcomes.

The experimental control exerted in efficacy trials is important for demonstrating the causal relationship between the intervention and the outcomes. Making valid inferences that the intervention's active ingredients are solely and uniquely responsible for producing improvements in the outcomes is prerequisite for the viability of the intervention; however, it is not sufficient for its application in the real world of day-to-day practice. The experimental control represents a strength of efficacy studies; yet, it also is its limitation: the carefully selected participants, context or setting, and comparison treatment; the highly qualified interventionists; the clearly defined intervention implemented in a standard and consistent manner; and chance-based allocation of treatments; are not reflective of day-to-day practice. Thus, the results of efficacy trials are not generalizable to practice and do not provide answers to practice-related question: Who most benefit from the intervention, given in what mode and at what dose? Effectiveness studies address these questions.

Chapter 14

Determining the Effectiveness of Interventions

For an intervention that demonstrated efficacy to be applied in the real world of practice, it has to successfully pass the test of effectiveness. This test aims to determine the extent to which the intervention's causal effects are reproduced under the real-world conditions that are characterized by variability in the personal and clinical or health profile of clients receiving and enacting the intervention; the physical and psychosocial features of the setting or environment in which the intervention is given; and the personal and professional qualities of interventionists or healthcare professionals delivering the intervention. Such variability in context yields variability in the implementation of the intervention, and consequently in the achievement of the intended immediate and ultimate outcomes. Determining the causal effects of the intervention under these conditions cannot be done in isolation of, by ignoring, and/or by controlling the factors that influence its implementation and outcomes; rather, this influence is of relevance to clinicians, organizations, and policy makers contemplating the adoption and use of the intervention to benefit their clientele (Sox et al., 2010). Therefore, the contribution of client, setting, interventionist, and intervention characteristics to outcome achievement is of concern in studies designed to evaluate the effectiveness of interventions. The experimental control exerted in the randomized controlled/clinical trial (RCT) limits the utility of this design in examining effectiveness. Alternative research designs, including practical or pragmatic trials, have been suggested as suitable for testing the effectiveness of interventions.

In this chapter, the distinction between efficacy and effectiveness is highlighted to clarify the importance of demonstrating effectiveness prior to translating interventions into the practice setting. The limitations of the RCT design in evaluating effectiveness are discussed. The features of alternative designs, with a particular focus on pragmatic clinical trials (PCT), are described. The strengths and limitations of the PCT are reviewed.

Design, Evaluation, and Translation of Nursing Interventions, First Edition.
Souraya Sidani and Carrie Jo Braden.
© 2011 John Wiley & Sons, Inc. Published 2011 by John Wiley & Sons, Inc.

14.1 Efficacy versus effectiveness: A brief review

Efficacy and effectiveness are qualities related to the intervention's effects, that is, both efficacy and effectiveness are concerned with demonstrating the extent to which the intervention produces the intended outcomes. However, the two qualities differ in the specific emphasis and subsequently the context or conditions under which the intervention effects are evaluated.

As mentioned in the previous chapters, the emphasis in an efficacy test is on demonstrating the causal relationship between the intervention and the outcomes. A causal relationship implies that the intervention, and not any other factor, produces the outcomes. Specifically, the intervention's active ingredients are solely and uniquely responsible for the changes in outcomes observed following treatment implementation. The purpose of an efficacy study is to isolate the causal intervention effects from confounding factors. Therefore, the intervention is evaluated under "ideal" controlled conditions that permit the manipulation of the intervention implementation and the elimination of factors that could influence treatment implementation and/or outcome achievement. The features of the RCT make it appropriate for exerting the required experimental control under which the intervention is most likely to show benefit. Accordingly, results of an efficacy study using the RCT design address the question: Does the intervention work under ideal circumstances (Zwarenstein & Oxman, 2006)?

The emphasis in an effectiveness test is on demonstrating the reproducibility of the intervention effects when the intervention is implemented under the less controlled conditions of the natural or practice setting. These conditions encompass: (1) clients presenting with different personal profiles; complex clinical status; different manifestations, determinants, and levels of the clinical problem amenable to treatment by the intervention under evaluation; beliefs and attitudes toward health, the presenting clinical problem, and treatment; perceived acceptability and preferences for treatment; and desire to participate in treatment-related decision-making and in treatment enactment; (2) healthcare professionals having different personal attributes, professional qualities, interpersonal and technical skills in implementing the intervention, and preferences for treatment modalities; and (3) settings with various physical features, human resources, care-delivery models (such as client-centered care), and policies. These conditions present a context that interferes with the implementation of the intervention, yet cannot be easily controlled. These contextual characteristics can facilitate or impede the fidelity of treatment delivery, where healthcare professionals may provide some components of the intervention, at different dose levels, to be responsive to clients' needs, values, and preferences, and in concordance with available material and human resources; and where clients enact some treatment recommendations, at different dose levels, based on their functional abilities and perceptions of the intervention. Differences in the fidelity of treatment implementation are associated with variability in the pattern of changes in the outcomes among clients. The overall purpose of an effectiveness study is to understand the contribution of client, interventionist, setting, and intervention characteristics to outcome achievement. Such an understanding provides answers to questions of relevance to clinical and policy makers. The questions include: How is the intervention applied in practice? What conditions are required to facilitate its implementation? What adaptations to the intervention can be made to fit these conditions yet maintain its effectiveness? Which client subgroups, presenting with which personal and clinical characteristics, benefit, to what extent, from the intervention delivered in what mode and at what dose? What mechanism is responsible for producing the intervention ultimate outcomes? How effective is the intervention in producing beneficial outcomes compared to alternative interventions, available and/or used, to address the same presenting clinical problem (Holtz, 2007; Sidani & Braden, 1998)? Research designs that embrace flexibility required to account for variability in treatment implementation and in contextual factors are needed to address the questions meaningfully. The RCT design has limitations that preclude its use in effectiveness studies (Zwarenstein & Treweek, 2009), as discussed next.

14.2 Limitations of the RCT design in effectiveness research

The key features of the RCT, careful selection of clients, interventionists, and settings, randomization, and manipulation of the intervention delivery, ascribe this design the strength of controlling factors that could confound the effects of the intervention on the outcomes. The control of potential confounds rules out alternative plausible explanations of the causal relationship between the intervention and the outcomes. This strength in achieving high internal validity (i.e., validity of inferences about causal effects) comes at the expense of low external validity, that is, limited generalizability of the RCT findings across clients and settings. In addition to limited generalizability that restricts the utility of the RCT results in guiding practice, the critique of the RCT has also entailed the specific methods and procedures applied in this design. Below is a detailed discussion of the RCT weaknesses, which render it of very limited usefulness in evaluating effectiveness of interventions.

14.2.1 Unrepresentativeness of the sample

Nonconsent bias and stringent eligibility criteria contribute to the unrepresentativeness of the RCT sample of the target population. Nonconsent bias is associated with the number of clients enrolling in the RCT and the difference between participants and refusers. A large number of clients tend to decline entry into an RCT for various reasons. Recent trends indicate that between 25% and 45% of eligible clients decline enrollment in RCTs evaluating different interventions such as cancer therapy (Jenkins & Fallowfield, 2000), and pharmacological and/or behavioral treatments for insomnia (Edinger et al., 2007; Jacobs et al., 2004; Pallesen et al., 2003; Savard et al., 2005). Reasons for refusal relate to personal, psychological, or lifestyle characteristics of clients (Heaman, 2001) or to concerns about the study design, in particular random assignment to treatment (Stevens & Ahmedzai, 2004). King et al. (2005) estimated the percentage of clients who accept randomization to range between 26% and 88%; a lower percentage is observed when clients have clear, strong preferences for the treatments under evaluation (Klaber-Moffett et al., 1999; Macias et al., 2005). Significant differences in the socio-demographic profile, clinical or health status, and preferences for treatment have been reported for clients enrolling and clients declining entry into RCT (e.g., Dwight-Johnson et al., 2001). Nonconsent bias yield a small sample of clients presenting with personal and clinical characteristics that are not representative of the subgroups with different profiles forming the target population (Borglin & Richards, 2010; Hyde, 2004; Kaptchuk, 2001; Lehman & Steinwachs, 2003; Scriven, 2008; Stone & Pocock, 2010).

Stringent eligibility criteria are preset in an RCT to control for client characteristics with potential confounding effects on the outcomes. This results in the exclusion of a large percentage of clients. For instance, it has been estimated that more than 60% of clients belonging to the target population are excluded from RCTs of behavioral interventions for depressive, panic, and anxiety disorders (Stirman et al., 2005), and that less than 50% of screened clients enter trials in general (Grapow et al., 2006; Pincus, 2002). Consequently, the sample of clients included in the RCT is homogenous in baseline characteristics. Homogeneity of the sample characteristics is conducive to homogeneity in clients' response to the intervention. Therefore, the sample represents some subgroup of the target population and the observed intervention effects are relevant or applicable only to clients with the same profile. Yet, clients seen in the practice setting may present with the same clinical problem, but different sets of personal and clinical characteristics that formed exclusion criteria for the RCT. Ignoring the latter characteristics' influence on the intervention outcomes does not address the question of relevance to practice: Which clients, presenting with which characteristics, benefit most from the intervention and, therefore, limits clinical decision-making (Nallamothu et al., 2008; Pincus, 2002; Sidani & Braden, 1998).

14.2.2 Highly select setting

Careful selection of the setting in which the intervention is implemented limits the generalizability of the RCT findings. It is usual to choose sites with characteristics that facilitate delivery of the intervention as designed, specifically those related to material and human resources. Thus, the sites tend to be highly specialized, with advanced technology, highly qualified healthcare professionals, and a general orientation of openness and receptivity to innovation (Bottomley, 1997; Zwarenstein & Treweek, 2009). In addition, specialized sites tend to provide services to clients with complex needs, representing a select subgroup of the target population. This situation raises question about the applicability of the intervention and the reproducibility of its effects in less-specialized context.

14.2.3 Limited applicability of interventions

The interventions evaluated in an RCT are discrete, standardized, and implemented with fidelity by intensively trained interventionists who are hired for
the study. The intervention consists of a clearly defined and distinct set of
components and activities, given in a specific mode or format, at a specified
dose (Nallamothu et al., 2008). Multicomponent interventions, involving interventionists' and clients' engagement in various activities over an extended
period, and clients' enactment of demanding treatment recommendations requiring major changes in lifestyle, are complex and difficult to implement
without adequate resources (Dzewaltowski et al., 2004; Lindsay, 2004). Their
integration in day-to-day practice is hard and costly, as it requires adjustment
of the healthcare professionals' workload or caseload so that they can provide the intervention, as designed, to clients assigned to their care. Further,
the implementation of such interventions takes place within the context of
interpersonal interactions through which a trusting therapeutic relationship
may develop between the interventionist and the client. Although such a relationship may motivate the client to engage and enact treatment recommendations, it is either ignored or its effect is isolated (by using placebo treatment for
comparison) in an RCT (Lindsay, 2004). Yet, interactions between healthcare
professionals and clients form the essence of day-to-day practice; they are
the medium through which treatment is delivered. Long-standing trusting and
working relationships develop between professionals and clients with chronic
conditions. The extent to which such interactions or relationships influence the
implementation of the intervention and the achievement of outcomes is of interest. Related information may guide the selection and training of healthcare
professionals entrusted the delivery of the intervention.

In an RCT, the intervention is standardized and implemented with fidelity.
This implies inflexibility in that all components and activities are consistently
applied with all clients, in a rigid sequence, in the same mode or format, and
in a predetermined fixed schedule, regardless of the individual clients' needs,
values, and preferences. Although standardization and fidelity of implementation are important for inferring a relationship between the intervention and
the outcome, they are not congruent with what goes on in day-to-day practice.
With the current emphasis on a client-centered approach to care, and within
the context of a long-standing therapeutic relationship between healthcare
professionals and clients, there is a need to attend to clients' needs, and be
responsive to clients' values and preferences. This translates into the ne-
cessity to apply the intervention in a way that best fits the clients' condition.
Therefore, variability in intervention implementation is the norm in day-to-day
practice. Accordingly, standardized intervention protocols that are carried out
in a fixed format are not relevant or compatible with, and hence cannot be
integrated in practice (Bamberger & White, 2007; Davidson, 2006; Haaga,
2004). The information needed to guide treatment-related decisions is about:
(1) the critical components that accurately reflect the active ingredients, the
most suitable mode of delivery, the optimal dose, and the most appropriate

schedule that should be offered in order to produce the intended intervention effects; (2) the range of components, dose, mode of delivery, and schedule that can be implemented yet still yield beneficial outcomes; and (3) the aspects or elements of the intervention that can be tailored, and how tailoring can be done, with the goal of meeting the needs of clients presenting with diverse personal and clinical profiles.

Last, the RCT focuses on isolating the intervention effects on the outcomes. Concurrent treatments for the same presenting problem or for comorbid conditions are either discontinued or ignored (Pincus, 2002). However, in day-to-day practice, such is not the case. Clients are expected to enact all treatments' recommendations simultaneously. The question of clinical importance relates to the extent to which other treatment influence (1) clients' enactment of the intervention: clients may find it difficult and burdensome to apply a complex therapeutic regimen, which may alter their performance of all treatments; and (2) the expected outcomes of the intervention: other treatments may have additive or interactive effects on the outcomes, or the combination of treatments may result in severe adverse reactions or unanticipated beneficial or harmful effects.

14.2.4 Irrelevance of comparison treatment

Inclusion of and the nature of the comparison treatment selected in an RCT affect the inferences about the effects of the intervention under evaluation, as well as the relevance of the RCT findings to practice. Inclusion of a comparison group is believed to provide the evidence supporting some criteria for causality, covariation, and congruity, and to assist in ruling out some threats to internal validity, primarily history and maturation. However, it does not eliminate all biases (Pincus, 2002) and may contribute to some biases, most notably differential attrition, negative reactivity, and compensatory equalization. Clients assigned to the comparison treatment, perceived as less desirable and ineffective, are disappointed and dissatisfied; therefore, they may withdraw and/or seek treatment outside the study context. Clients who withdraw may differ from those who complete the study; the resulting participants form a particular subgroup of the target population, thereby limiting the generalizability of the observed intervention effects. Clients who obtain treatment outside of the study context and do not disclose it may demonstrate improvement in the outcomes; even if small in magnitude, such an improvement reduces the size of the intervention effects. Interventions with small effects may not be viewed favorably in day-to-day practice.

Different types of comparison treatments can be selected in RCTs. Of these, the no-treatment control and the placebo treatment are frequently used to isolate the specific or unique intervention effects. However, comparison of the intervention to any of these treatments is of limited relevance to practice because no-treatment or placebo treatments are not viable interventions offered in day-to-day practice. Rather, in practice, clients are given alternative treatments that have shown, empirically or experientially, to be effective to variable extent, in addressing the presenting problem. Accordingly, clinical and policy decision-makers want information on comparative effectiveness of interventions, that is, how does the intervention fare in comparison to available treatments in current use (Holtz, 2007). They may be willing to adopt and integrate interventions that demonstrate superiority, and of course, that are not resource intensive or costly to implement.

14.2.5 Limited utility of randomization

Randomization, the essential feature of RCTs, long believed to eliminate selection bias and hence the confounding influence of baseline client characteristics, is being questioned on scientific and practical grounds. The following points have been advanced, based on theoretical arguments and relevant empirical evidence:

(1) Randomization does not guarantee a secure valid inference about the causal relationship between the intervention and the outcomes (Cook et al., 2010). Random assignment of participants to the experimental and the comparison groups *may* enhance the comparability of participants in the two groups on characteristics measured at pretest, thereby reducing selection bias. This is all that it does, nothing else! Randomization does not address other, equally important, threats to validity such as nonadherence to treatment protocol. Also, it may contribute to attrition in that participants randomized to the less desirable or the nonpreferred treatment are disappointed and withdraw from the study (Borglin & Richards, 2010; Lindsay, 2004; Sidani et al., 2003). Emerging empirical evidence supports this argument. Several meta-analytic studies were conducted to compare the effect sizes for the same intervention, given to the same target population, obtained in RCTs and non-RCTs (i.e., observational designs). The results indicated that the mean effect sizes for RCTs were similar to the mean effect sizes for non-RCTs (e.g., Concato et al., 2000; Ferriter & Huband, 2005). These findings suggest that well-designed nonexperimental studies that minimize or appropriately account for threats to validity (such as attrition, statistical control of confounding client characteristics) produce results that approximate those of RCTs (Kaptchuk, 2001; McKee et al., 1999; United States Government Accounting Office, 2009; Worrall, 2002). Thus, the important role traditionally ascribed to randomization in ensuring high internal validity and preeminence of quality, is questionable.

(2) Randomization does not guarantee initial group equivalence (Cook et al., 2010; Watson et al., 2004). Random assignment only increases the probability (but does not ensure) that participants allocated to the experimental and the comparison groups are comparable on characteristics measured at pretest. Further, this initial group equivalence is maintained at the group level, not at the level of individual participants. Interindividual differences in baseline characteristics are not controlled; yet they can still influence outcome achievement. This point is supported by results

reported by Sidani (2006) and Heinsman and Shadish (1996). Sidani examined the effect size for demographic and outcome variables assessed at pretest for the experimental and comparison groups in 100 randomly selected reports of RCTs. She found that the absolute main effect size was .24 for demographic and .20 for outcomes variables. These findings indicated a small, and potentially clinically meaningful, difference in the two groups' characteristics, raising questions about the success of randomization in maintaining initial group comparability. In addition, Sidani and Heinsman and Shadish found a significant low–moderate, positive correlation between the effect sizes for outcomes measured at pretest and those measured at posttest, suggesting that baseline variables continue to exert their influence on the intervention effects, despite randomization.

(3) Randomization is not acceptable to clients and healthcare professionals (Bamberger & White, 2007) and is not part of day-to-day practice (Towne & Hilton, 2004). Rothwell (2005) estimated that less than 10% of clients agree to have their treatment chosen at random. Similarly, healthcare professionals are not trained to give treatment on the basis of chance. Thus, clients and healthcare professionals expect careful consideration of alternative interventions, and selection and application of those most appropriate to clients' context. Random assignment is not at all helpful in elucidating this process, which is critical for guiding treatment-related decision-making in day-to-day practice.

14.2.6   Limited relevance of findings

The results of an RCT are based on an intention-to-treat, group-level analysis. In intention-to-treat analysis, participants randomized to the experimental group who comply or do not comply with the intervention are lumped into one group and compared, on outcomes, to those in the comparison group who do not receive the intervention under evaluation, but may have sought alternative treatments. As such, intention-to-treat provides an estimate of the causal effect of "treatment assignment," and not the actual treatment (West & Thoemmes, 2010). Thus, the results are of limited utility in determining the extent to which the intervention produces improvement in the outcomes. Most commonly, the statistical tests used in the RCT data analysis examine differences in the outcomes between the means of the experimental and comparison groups. The focus is on the *average* causal effects of the intervention. Individual clients' responses to treatment are ignored and lumped into "error variance" (Hyde, 2004; Nallamothu et al., 2008; Pincus, 2002). However, individual differences in response to the intervention are of most relevance to practice, where clients presenting with diverse personal and clinical profiles are cared for and may exhibit different responses to the intervention that deviate from the average response reported for the RCT (Lehman & Steinwachs, 2003). Knowledge of which clients with what characteristics respond in what way to the intervention is critical to guide treatment-related decision-making in the context of day-to-day practice (Sidani & Braden, 1998). The concern in an RCT is on statistical significance, that is, demonstrating that the observed intervention effects are reliable and do not occur by chance. Less attention is given to clinical meaningfulness (Hyde, 2004; Pincus, 2002), operationalized in terms of the percentage of clients who benefit from the intervention and the extent (or magnitude) of improvement experienced by these clients.

Overall, the adoption of the RCT as the "gold standard" design for evaluating interventions is based on intuitive attractiveness rather than compelling evidence (Kaptchuk, 2001). Critical review of the reasoning underlying the RCT and emerging empirical evidence dispute the utility of the RCT design in determining effectiveness. The RCT features are simplistic in that they do not capture the complex nature of causality in the practice setting, where multiple interacting factors, in addition to the intervention, are responsible for producing the immediate and ultimate outcomes in diverse clients and settings (Donaldson & Christie, 2004; Towne & Hilton, 2004). Alternative designs are needed for intervention effectiveness research.

14.3 Alternative designs for evaluating effectiveness

The limitations of the RCT in examining and providing evidence of effectiveness generated the need and search for alternative designs. The current state of science converges on proposing practical or pragmatic clinical trials or PCT as a general research approach suitable for investigating effectiveness. This approach does not identify a particular design with clearly specified methods and procedures, as the most appropriate for evaluating the effectiveness of intervention. However, it delineates the features of a study aimed at evaluating effectiveness, which are described next.

14.3.1 Overall function or goal

A PCT is generally characterized as a real-world test of an intervention in a real-world population (Maclure, 2009; Oxman et al., 2009). The overall goal is to determine the extent to which the intervention "works," that is, produces the beneficial outcomes, when applied in normal or usual practice (Thorpe et al., 2009; Zwarenstein & Treweek, 2009) by healthcare professionals with different preparation, experience, and expertise; with the range of clients usually seen in practice; and within settings with variable material and human resources. The focus is on generating results that are relevant to clinical and policy decision-makers, and that are applicable to usual practice (Borglin & Richards, 2010; Nallamothu et al., 2008; Tunis et al., 2003).

14.3.2 Broad representative sample

The sample of clients participating in a PCT has to be representative of all subgroups of the target population seen in practice. This feature implies that client selection is based on less stringent or less restrictive eligibility criteria than those specified for an RCT aimed at examining efficacy. Eligibility is determined by "broad" inclusion and few exclusion criteria (Glasgow et al., 2005; Nallamothu et al., 2008; Tunis et al., 2003; Zwarenstein & Treweek, 2009). Pincus (2002) proposed to eliminate exclusion criteria in order to enhance the representativeness of the sample, except of course, those criteria reflecting characteristics of clients for whom the intervention is contraindicated. Accordingly, the sample includes clients presenting with diverse personal profiles, as well as different levels of severity of the presenting problem, beliefs about the problem and its treatment, levels of perceived treatment acceptability, treatment preferences, levels of motivation and willingness/ability to adhere to treatment recommendations, comorbid conditions, and concurrent treatments for the same presenting problem or for the comorbid conditions.

14.3.3 Selection of different settings

Different settings are selected for participation in a PCT (Glasgow et al., 2005; Nallamothu et al., 2008; Tunis et al., 2003). This feature ensures representation of settings in which clients with diverse personal and clinical characteristics (i.e., representative sample) are seen in large numbers; a range of material resources is available for implementation of the intervention; healthcare professionals with different personal (e.g., interpersonal style) and professional (e.g., preparation, expertise) characteristics are entrusted the delivery of the intervention, independently or collaboratively. In addition, the settings may vary in organizational culture reflected in general policies, vision and mission, and values and perspectives, which are translated into the adopted approach to care, as well as orientation to research and openness and willingness to integrate innovations.

14.3.4 Comparison of clinically relevant alternative treatments

In practice, it is considered unethical and professionally unacceptable to deny treatment to which clients are otherwise entitled, and/or to give "sham" (i.e., placebo) treatment. Thus, the no-treatment control and placebo treatments are not clinically meaningful comparisons for determining the effectiveness of interventions. Clinical and policy decision-makers want to know the effectiveness of the intervention as compared to alternative, clinically relevant, treatments available and in use in the practice setting. It also is advisable to have interventions that are feasible and inexpensive (Grapow et al., 2006; Nallamothu et al., 2008; Tunis et al. 2003), that is, they can be easily implemented by healthcare professionals with different expertise and within the reality of day-to-day operations often described as having limited resources and high workload or caseload. In the context of a PCT, the intervention is applied flexibly as it would take place in usual practice (Thorpe et al., 2009; Zwarenstein & Treweek, 2009). Thus, healthcare professionals responsible for implementing the intervention are involved, independently or in collaboration with clients, in the selection and application of the intervention components, activities, mode of delivery, and/or dose that are most suitable to the individual clients' condition. Variability in clients' enactment and adherence to treatment recommendations are acknowledged as part of what happens in practice; no additional remedial strategies that extend or expand those usually provided by healthcare professionals are suggested to promote client adherence to treatment.

14.3.5 Assessment of relevant health outcomes at follow-up

In a PCT, the interest is in outcomes that are of relevance to clinical and policy decision-makers, as well as clients (i.e., individuals or communities) (Tunis et al., 2003). Involvement of different stakeholder groups in the identification of outcomes they value is suggested as a means for selecting relevant outcomes to be investigated (Sox et al., 2010). The range of outcomes include (1) clinical end points, related to the objective and subjective manifestations and level of severity of the presenting problem targeted by the intervention; development of complications, adverse reactions, or side effects; and mortality; (2) functioning, related to performance of usual physical activities, self-management, and social roles, as well as psychological well-being; (3) perceptual related to health-related quality of life and satisfaction with treatment and with care; and (4) financial, related to the cost of applying/using the intervention and the costs incurred by clients enacting treatment recommendations. In addition, PCTs are designed to evaluate the short- and long-term effectiveness of the intervention. Short-term effects are assessed following implementation of the intervention; however, examination of long-term effects requires measurement of outcomes at regular intervals that are not in excess of usual practice (e.g., at regularly scheduled visits to healthcare professionals), over an extended follow-up period (Thorpe et al., 2009). It is expected that the PCTs results point to the clinical significance of the intervention effects (Tunis et al., 2003), reporting not only on the magnitude of the effects but also the percentage of clients who demonstrated clinically important or meaningful and socially validated improvements in the outcomes (Hark & Stump, 2008; Jacobson et al., 1999).

14.3.6 Allocation to treatment

Randomization may not be feasible (Glasgow et al., 2005) or even desirable in PCTs, which aim to evaluate the effectiveness of interventions within the context of usual practice. In practice, chance does not play a role in treatment allocation. Treatment is given on the basis of a defined set of clinical characteristics (also referred to as prognostic factors) with which clients present. All clients are cared for and no one is denied treatment. Clients in some settings are provided the intervention under evaluation and clients in other sites are offered an alternative treatment for addressing the same presenting problem. Allocation to treatment in PCTs can capitalize on these features of day-to-day practice. For instance, an interrupted time series design is used when all clients receive the intervention; quasi-experimental design is useful when groups of clients are formed in parallel where some receive the intervention and others get an alternative treatment; and regression discontinuity design is applied when allocation to treatment is based on clients' level on a particular characteristic or prognostic factor. The following research designs are considered rigorous alternatives to the RCT for evaluating the effectiveness of interventions (Glasgow et al., 2005; Holtz, 2007; Nallamothu et al., 2008; United States Government Accountability Office, 2009):

(1) *Observational design:* Specifically, the interrupted time series design involves obtaining outcome data on repeated occasions before and after introducing the intervention into the practice setting, and comparing the trend in the outcome variable observed prior to, and the trend observed following introduction of the intervention. Complicated statistical techniques are used to (1) project the pattern of change in the outcomes (based on pretreatment data) expected if the intervention was not provided, and (2) compare the projected pattern to the actual trend of change in outcomes observed following the intervention. Significant difference in the hypothesized direction, between the projected and actual posttreatment trends provides the evidence supporting the effectiveness of the intervention. In addition, statistical techniques are used to examine or control for the influence of potentially confounding variables. It is important to clarify that the outcome data are obtained at the aggregate level, such as inpatient hospital unit, outpatient health clinic, or community at large, from routinely monitored outcomes such as adverse events and mortality (Burns & Grove, 2005; Rossi et al., 2004; United States Government Accountability Office, 2009).

(2) *Quasi-experimental design:* Specifically, this type of design involves parallel groups, an experimental group in which clients receive the intervention under evaluation, and a comparison group in which clients receive an alternative treatment. Alternative treatments consist of usual care (which should be clearly defined and its implementation monitored to account for any variability), minimal treatment (i.e., an intervention found to have minimal impact on the presenting problem), the intervention given at low dose, or another intervention with established efficacy addressing the presenting problem (De Maat et al., 2007). The comparison group comprises clients representative of the target population who are not offered the intervention. Allocation to the intervention or alternative treatment is done at the individual client level or site level. It is not based on self-selection if at all possible. The latter is exemplified with clients put on a waiting list for treatment or sites not taking part in the PCT for evaluating the intervention effects. Controlling potentially confounding variables (such as client characteristics and sites) is recommended by proponents of this design, prior to determining effectiveness. Assignment to treatment could be done on the basis of individual clients' level on a selected variable measured at pretest, as is characteristic of the regression discontinuity design.

The variable reflects a characteristic that defines the need for intervention and that is assessed with a valid measure that has a well-established cutoff point. Clients with scores indicating the required level (e.g., above or below cutoff point) on the variable are assigned to the intervention, whereas the others serve as comparison. Posttest outcomes are compared between the two groups after controlling for the selection variable to determine the effectiveness of the intervention. For more details on quasi-experimental designs, refer to Rossi et al. (2004) and Shadish et al. (2002).

(3) *Combination of designs:* A combination of observational and quasi-experimental designs can be used in a PCT. This may be useful to determine the effectiveness of the intervention in achieving a range of outcomes, some of which are monitored on a regular basis and pertinent data are readily available in well-maintained databases over extended time periods preceding and following the introduction of the intervention. For example, evaluation of an innovative discharge planning, implemented collaboratively by members of the interprofessional healthcare team, on older clients' functional status, self-care ability, length of hospitalization, complications, satisfaction with care, and discharge destination (e.g., home, other facility) could be conducted by (1) enlisting several hospitals for participation in the study to ensure representation of settings providing services to the target population and availability of a large pool of potentially eligible clients; (2) selecting a number of sites to receive the intervention (e.g., on the basis of the size of the target population), whereas the remaining sites are requested to serve as comparison and continue to provide discharge planning as usual; (3) giving training in the implementation of the innovative discharge planning to teams of healthcare professionals in the intervention sites; (4) collecting pertinent self-report outcome data from older clients admitted to all sites before and after receiving discharge planning offered at the respective sites, (5) obtaining relevant data on average length of hospitalization, rate of complication, satisfaction with care, and discharge destination for inpatient units participating in the PCT reported on a monthly or quarterly basis in the 1-to-2 years preceding and following the training. Appropriate statistical techniques are used to examine differences between the intervention and the comparison groups in the pattern of change in outcomes measured at the individual client level (e.g., hierarchical linear models that account for clustering of clients within sites) and at the inpatient unit level.

14.3.7 Additional features

The design of a PCT evaluating the effectiveness of interventions is strengthened by incorporating contextual and process analyses. The overall purpose of these analyses is to address, in a meaningful way, the variability generated by selecting clients, healthcare professionals, and settings of diverse characteristics, by examining different treatments given at different doses, and by assessing a range of outcomes assessed at different levels. Contextual and process analyses are guided by the intervention theory that identifies key contextual and process variables, and delineates the nature of their impact on the outcomes expected of the intervention (Bamberger & White, 2007; Glasgow et al., 2005; Thorpe et al, 2009; United States Government Accountability Office, 2009).

14.3.7.1 Contextual analysis

The aim of contextual analysis is to understand the contribution of client, healthcare professional, and setting characteristics to the implementation of the intervention and/or changes in the outcomes. The intervention theory specifies particular characteristics posited to have a direct or an indirect impact on treatment delivery by healthcare professionals, enactment and adherence to treatment by clients, and outcome achievement. The conceptual definitions of these attributes advanced in the intervention theory direct the selection of appropriate instruments to measure pertinent client (e.g., sex, severity of presenting problem), healthcare professional (e.g., profession, years of experience), and setting (e.g., location, organizational culture) characteristics, prior to the implementation of the intervention. The direct influence of these characteristics is investigated by conducting the following:

(1) Subgroup analyses, where differences in the implementation of the intervention and in levels of posttest outcomes, or of changes in outcomes from pretest to posttest are examined across subgroups of clients defined in terms of their levels on the selected characteristic (e.g., men versus women; low, moderate, and high levels on the presenting problem severity); of healthcare professionals distinguished relative to the selected characteristic (e.g., profession such as psychology versus nursing; years of experience such as junior ($\leq$5 years) and senior ($>$5 years); of setting differentiated in terms of the selected characteristic (e.g., urban, suburban, and rural; reservation versus openness to adoption of innovation), and/or,

(2) Hierarchical linear models, where variability in treatment application, represented as the actual intervention components and/or dose received by clients, and the pattern of change in the outcomes observed across all time points (i.e., pretest, posttest, follow-up) are examined in relation to individual client characteristics, healthcare professional attributes, and setting features. The advantage of hierarchical linear models is the ability to test the effects of all characteristics, assessed and operating at different nested levels (i.e., clients nested within interventionists within settings), simultaneously (Raudenbush, 2001; Raudenbush & Bryk, 2002).

The indirect impact of client, healthcare professional, and setting characteristics is often proposed as moderated, whereby the attributes moderate the effects of the intervention on the outcomes. Moderators represent variables that affect the occurrence, direction, or strength of the causal relationship between the intervention and the outcomes (Holmbeck, 1997). This implies that the outcomes observed at posttest or changes in the outcomes occur, or differ in direction (e.g., increase, no change, decrease) and in strength (i.e., extent or magnitude) in clients having certain levels on the moderating characteristics, or having received treatment from healthcare professionals with specific attributes, in settings with particular features. Moderated relationships are tested with:

(1) interaction terms, that is, interaction of the client, healthcare professional, or setting characteristics with the receipt of the intervention; these interaction terms are then incorporated in regression analysis. In such analysis the outcomes at posttest are regressed onto the client, healthcare professional, or setting characteristics, the variable representing the receipt of the intervention (i.e., treatment condition to which clients are assigned), and the characteristic–by–intervention receipt interaction terms;

(2) hierarchical linear modeling, where the parameters reflecting the association between the individual client slopes that quantify the pattern of change in the outcomes over time and the selected characteristics measured at a higher level, operationalize the moderated relationship; and/or

(3) multigroup analysis, usually done with statistical packages for structural equation modeling, where differences in the parameter of the path linking the intervention to the outcomes are examined across subgroups of clients defined in terms of their level or status on the selected characteristic (Holmbeck, 1997; Kraemer et al., 2002; Raudenbush & Bryk, 2002).

Quantitative contextual analysis can be complemented and/or supplemented with qualitative data analysis. Qualitative data are useful when (1) relevant validated measures of hypothesized client, healthcare professional, and setting characteristics are not available, (2) the nature of these characteristics' impact is not yet clearly delineated, or (3) several characteristics are interrelated and interact in influencing implementation of the intervention and/or achievement of outcomes, making it difficult to examine the complexity of their interactive effects statistically. Qualitative investigation of the characteristics' contribution is accomplished in individual or group interviews with clients and healthcare professionals. The focus of the interviews is on the factors that facilitated or hindered the implementation of the intervention, and/or that necessitated variability in treatment delivery, and the nature of the interrelationships among these factors. A grounded theory methodology is appropriate to clarify how client, healthcare professional, and setting characteristics interact in affecting treatment implementation and/or outcome achievement.

Results of contextual analysis specify the conditions under which the intervention is implemented as originally intended, and the intervention works or is effective in producing beneficial outcomes. They also provide explanations for modification in treatment delivery and for individual client or client subgroup differences in the intervention effects. As such, they guide the translation and application of the intervention in the context of day-to-day practice.

14.3.7.2 Process analysis

The purpose of process analysis is twofold: (1) to determine the extent to which the intervention is implemented with fidelity, and (2) to examine the extent to which the proposed mechanisms operated to mediate the effects of the intervention on the ultimate outcomes. The intervention theory specifies the intervention components and activities that operationalize its active ingredients, the dose at which it should be provided, and the mode or medium through which it is given to achieve its beneficial effects; in addition, the intervention theory delineates the variables that are responsible for producing the ultimate outcomes. Strategies and procedures for examining fidelity of intervention implementation, operationalized in terms of healthcare professionals' application of the intervention's components and activities, and clients' enactment of and adherence to treatment recommendations have been discussed in detail, in Chapter 10. Investigation of mechanisms underlying the intervention effects is guided by the intervention theory (Nock, 2007). It takes two forms. The first focuses on illuminating the specific elements and/or components of the intervention that are responsible for inducing changes in the outcomes, and the second is concerned with elucidating the mechanisms through which the intervention affects the outcomes.

Three approaches can be used to illuminate the specific elements and/or components of the intervention responsible for inducing changes in the outcomes. The first involves dismantling complex interventions into its constituting components and examining the effectiveness of these components, provided independently or in combination. For instance, the behavioral intervention for the management of insomnia can be dismantled into its three components: (1) sleep education and hygiene, (2) stimulus-control therapy, and (3) sleep-restriction therapy. In a PCT, each of these components, a combination of two components (e.g., sleep education and hygiene and stimulus-control therapy, or sleep education and hygiene and sleep-restriction therapy), and all three combined components are given to different groups of clients. Comparison of outcomes across client groups indicates the intervention component(s) that are most and least effective (Nock, 2007; Oakley et al., 2006). The least effective ones are discarded (thereby improving efficiency of treatment) and the most effective ones are translated for application in day-to-day practice.

The second approach, which can be used in evaluating the intervention as a whole or its components, focuses on distinguishing the contribution of the intervention's specific elements or active ingredients from nonspecific or common factors. The intervention theory identifies and defines the specific and nonspecific elements. Examples of nonspecific elements include: working alliance between healthcare professionals and clients, and mode of treatment delivery such as face-to-face group session, where group dynamics may create a supportive relationship among clients that promotes outcome achievement. The nature of the nonspecific elements directs the selection of methods and procedures for investigating their contribution to outcomes. For instance, validated self-report instruments are used to measure clients' and healthcare professionals' perception of working alliance, which impacts on outcome is analyzed with regression-type techniques, as discussed in Chapter 9. The influence of mode of treatment delivery is examined by implementing the same intervention active ingredients in different formats (e.g., self-help working booklet versus group session) to different groups of clients, and comparing the groups' outcomes. Results of such analysis clarify the active ingredients of the intervention and point to the most appropriate way for delivering them intact, nondiluted, with efficiency. This information is critical for translating the intervention and adapting it to fit local contexts but without jeopardizing its purity and, hence, its effectiveness. The third approach rests on using qualitative research methods to illuminate specific components and/or elements responsible for inducing changes in the outcomes. Individual or group interviews with clients and with healthcare professionals are scheduled following treatment delivery to explore their perception of the aspects of the intervention that contributed to changes in the outcomes. This qualitative approach to process evaluation is illustrated by Leung et al.'s (2005) study.

Quantitative and qualitative approaches are applied to elucidate the mechanisms through which the intervention affects the outcomes. The quantitative approach entails (1) identification of the mediating variables that operationalize the mechanisms proposed in the intervention theory and the specification of the relationships linking the implementation of the intervention to these mediating variables and the latter ones to the outcomes; (2) selection of instruments that reliably and validly measure the mediating variables, guided by their conceptual definition advanced in the intervention theory; (3) collection of data on the mediating variables at the hypothesized time; and (4) application of mediational analysis, using relevant statistical approaches. Examples of mediators are: client satisfaction with treatment and immediate outcomes such as self-efficacy. Mediators are experienced (e.g., satisfaction with treatment) or changes in the levels of mediators (e.g., increased self-efficacy) are observed during or soon after implementation of the intervention but prior to the occurrence of the expected changes in the ultimate outcomes (Kraemer et al., 2002). Mediational analysis is applied to examine the indirect effects of the intervention on the ultimate outcomes. The intervention is operationalized by treatment group membership (i.e., treatment condition received) and/or its dose; the mediator and ultimate outcomes are represented by the scores on respective measures observed at one point in time or by changes in the level of these variables over time (i.e., change score between two points or slope reflecting the pattern of change over time). The mediational analysis tests the direct path linking the intervention with the mediators and the direct path linking the mediators with the ultimate outcomes; the direct path between the intervention and the ultimate outcomes, if tested, should be nonsignificant and small in magnitude to support mediation (Kraemer et al., 2002). Statistical packages for structural equation modeling are useful in determining, simultaneously, the indirect treatment effects reflecting the proposed mediated relationship between the intervention and the ultimate outcomes. For details on how to conduct mediational analyses, refer to Spencer et al. (2005), Jo (2008), and Cheong et al. (2003).

The qualitative methods involve individual or group interviews with clients and with healthcare professionals. The interviews focus on elucidating their perception of the adequacy of intervention implementation, satisfaction with the intervention, view of the usefulness of the intervention in enhancing outcomes, and description of how the intervention affected outcomes (Schumacher et al., 2005; Sidani & Braden, 1998). The studies reported by McCommon et al. (2009) and Adolfson et al.'s (2008) exemplify this type of process analysis.

Results of process analysis expand our understanding of changes in intervention outcomes. They shed light on "how and why" the intervention works. This knowledge promotes clinical and policy decision-makers' appreciation for and support to incorporate the intervention in practice.

The results of contextual and process analyses depict the complexity of interrelationships among client, healthcare professionals, setting, and intervention characteristics, as well as clarify their influence on the intervention outcomes and the mechanisms responsible for producing the beneficial outcomes. This complex network of relationships is consistent with multicausality and reflects the reality of practice. As such, the findings of PCTs indicate the effectiveness of the intervention and provide answers to questions of relevance to practice. Nonetheless, the conduct of PCT requires large samples of clients, healthcare professionals, and settings; careful monitoring and documentation of different treatments given at different doses; extensive data collection to capture all variables of interest; and sophisticated statistical techniques to account for clustering of clients within healthcare professionals within sites, and to examine direct and indirect effects of a multitude of variables. This increases the amount of resources, time, and funds needed and/or expanded to complete the PCT within a reasonable time frame (Nallamothu et al., 2008; Tunis et al., 2003). Last, the PCT features do not take into consideration clients' preferences for treatment, which is an important element of practice and is emerging as a potential threat to the validity of intervention evaluation studies, as discussed in Chapter 15.

Chapter 15

Preferences for Treatment

Clients' preferences for treatment are implicated as potential threats to internal and external validity of studies evaluating the efficacy and the effectiveness of interventions. Results of a large number of studies targeting clients with physical (e.g., pain, angina) or psychological (e.g., depression, panic attack) conditions showed that the majority (60-100%) of participants expressed clear preferences for treatment options offered within the context of the study. Clients with preferences may decline enrollment in an intervention evaluation study in which participants are randomized to treatments, potentially yielding a sample that is not representative of the target population. Clients with preferences who enter the trial may react, favorably or unfavorably to the allocated treatment, which influences their response to treatment and potentially confounds the intervention effects. The importance of treatment preferences necessitates the investigation of their contribution to clients' enactment of the intervention and experience of improvement in outcomes.

In this chapter, a conceptualization of treatment preferences is presented. The mechanisms underlying the influence of treatment preferences on external and internal validity of an intervention evaluation study are clarified. Research designs that account for participating clients' preferences are described and their advantages and disadvantages are discussed.

15.1 Conceptualization of treatment preferences

Treatment preferences represent clients' choices of treatment for the presenting problem. They reflect the specific intervention or treatment option clients want to receive to address the problem (Stalmeier et al., 2007). Preferences result from an interaction of clients' understanding of and attitudes toward the treatment options available for managing the problem (Corrigan & Salzer, 2003; Wensig & Elwyn, 2003). Attitudes toward treatment represent clients' appraisal of the treatment options as acceptable or unacceptable (Van Der Berg et al., 2008). They are based on a careful consideration of treatment

---

Design, Evaluation, and Translation of Nursing Interventions, First Edition.
Souraya Sidani and Carrie Jo Braden.
© 2011 John Wiley & Sons, Inc. Published 2011 by John Wiley & Sons, Inc.

attributes. Treatment attributes are characteristics of interventions related to appropriateness in addressing the presenting problem, effectiveness, severity of side effects, and convenience (Sidani et al., 2009). Acceptable interventions are those perceived as appropriate, effective, convenient, and having minimal side effects of low severity. Clients develop preferences for treatment options they view as acceptable. Preferences are influenced by a host of factors and contribute to engagement in and adherence to treatment, and subsequently outcome achievement (Kiesler & Auerbach, 2006; Lang, 2005; Mills et al., 2006; Tacher et al., 2005).

15.1.1 Factors influencing treatment preferences

Clients' personal, clinical, and psychological characteristics, clients' beliefs about the presenting problem and its treatment, and treatment character-istics have been found to influence expressed preferences for treatment. Some of these factors are interrelated, exerting an indirect association with preferences:

(1) *Personal characteristics:* Age, gender, level of education, ethnicity, and employment status were associated with the expression of a clear choice. Results of King et al.'s (2005) meta-analysis showed that younger persons, women, the well educated, White, and employed were likely to indicate that they have (as compared to not having) a preference. Preliminary evidence supports an indirect relationship between personal characteristics and preferences for specific treatment options, mediated by clients' beliefs about the presenting problem and its treatment, as well as their appraisal of the treatment attributes. Hacklett et al. (2005) explained that older women with breast cancer tend to select less painful and less invasive treatment options. Givens et al. (2007) found that African, Asian, and Hispanic Americans do not believe in the biological causes of depression and therefore do not consider medication as an appropriate treatment.

(2) *Clinical characteristics:* Perceived severity of the presenting problem was associated with treatment preferences. Clients reporting severe levels of the problem have a preference for invasive, intensive interventions such as surgery over nonsurgical treatment for heavy menstrual bleeding (Vuorma et al., 2003) and for pelvic organ prolapse (Heit et al., 2003), and medication over counseling for depression (Bedi et al., 2000; Cooper et al., 2003; Gum et al., 2006).

(3) *Psychological characteristics:* Emotional distress influences clients' pref-erences for specific treatment options for managing the presenting problem. For instance, Hazlett-Stevens et al. (2002) found that persons screened positive for posttraumatic stress disorder, compared to those who did not, expressed preference for active over no-treatment for re-current panic attacks. Persons reporting low levels of psychological func-tioning preferred counseling, rather than medication, for the treatment of depression (Cooper et al., 2003). Men perceiving low levels of anxiety

chose monitoring over active treatment for prostate cancer (Mills et al., 2006).

(4) *Beliefs about the presenting problem and its treatment:* Beliefs about the causes and consequences of the presenting problem, as well as expectations about treatment, were related to perceived acceptability and hence expressed preferences for treatment. Riedel-Heller et al. (2005) reported that clients who considered work and/or life stress as the causes of depression judged stress-reduction therapy as a relevant intervention for this clinical problem; in contrast, those believing in organic causes of depression rated medication as relevant. In addition to personal beliefs about treatment, healthcare professionals' beliefs about treatment, reflected in their recommendations for treatment, affect clients' preferences. For example, physicians' recommendations affected women's preferences for surgical treatment for breast cancer (Lam et al., 2005; Temple et al., 2006).

(5) *Treatment characteristics:* Previous experience with treatment and appraisal of treatment attributes were related to preferences. Clients who previously applied a particular intervention and found it useful in addressing the presenting problem, tend to select it as the treatment of preference (Gum et al., 2006; Jansen et al., 2001). In contrast, clients dissatisfied with a particular intervention tend to prefer the alternative treatment option offered within the context of a study (Awad et al., 2000). The treatment attributes commonly appraised and found to shape preferences were those operationalizing acceptability of treatment, that is, appropriateness in addressing the presenting problem, effectiveness, severity of side effects, and convenience (for a definition of these attributes refer to the Chapter 14). Results of several studies showed that clients express a preference for treatment options they rate as (1) appropriate for managing the clinical problem they experience (Lambert et al., 2004) and suitable for their lifestyle (Rowe et al., 2005); (2) effective in addressing the presenting problem in the short and long terms (Cochran et al., 2008; Mulhall & Montorsi, 2006); (3) less likely to have severe side effects (Arega et al., 2006; Landy et al., 2005); and (4) convenient or easy to apply in daily life (Cochran et al., 2008; Lambert et al., 2004). In summary, clients have preferences for treatment options they view as acceptable.

15.1.2 Consequences of treatment preferences

Preference for treatment is a key element of treatment-related decision-making and subsequently uptake, engagement in, adherence to, and satisfaction with treatment. Whether based on a collaborative or client-centered care model, eliciting clients' preferences is an important step of the decision-making process. Assessment of preferences is done after informing clients of the treatment options available for addressing the presenting problem; the information covers the name of the intervention, its purpose, components, activities, mode of delivery, dose or schedule, reported effectiveness (synthesized from empirical evidence), and risks or side effects. Clarification of any aspect of the treatment is made, as needed, in order to ensure that clients' choice is well informed. Clients are requested to indicate the treatment option they want to receive to address the presenting problem (Sidani et al., 2006). Clients are given the intervention that is consistent with their preference. This, in turn, generates a sense of personal control, enthusiasm, and motivation to begin treatment and enact its recommendations at the prescribed dose. Appropriate enactment of treatment contributes to initial experience of improvement in outcomes, in particular in the immediate outcomes, which enhances satisfaction with treatment. Satisfaction contributes to continued application of treatment, and consequently to the achievement of beneficial levels on the ultimate outcomes (McLaughlin & Kaluzny, 2000; Sidani, 2008; Wensig & Grol, 2000; Wolf et al., 2008).

The influence of treatment preferences on the implementation of the intervention and the achievement of outcomes presents an alternative plausible explanation of changes in outcomes observed following treatment delivery in intervention evaluation studies. Therefore, it is important to understand the mechanisms through which treatment preferences affect the validity of causal inferences in efficacy or effectiveness trials, and methodological strategies to address the potential threats of preferences. These are described next.

15.2 Mechanisms underlying influence of treatment preferences in intervention research

Although empirical evidence shows that most ($\geq$60%) clients have preferences for treatments addressing the presenting problem, clients' choices have been ignored in intervention evaluation research. The preferences of clients participating in a randomized controlled/clinical trial (RCT) to determine efficacy or in a pragmatic clinical trial (PCT) to examine effectiveness are not of concern. Generally, preferences are not assessed and not accounted for at the time of assignment to treatment and/or in the analysis of the intervention effects. However, the conceptualization of treatment preferences, as well as empirical evidence, acknowledge the role of preferences in evaluation research: they present threats to validity (Howard & Thornicroft, 2006; McPherson & Britton, 2001; TenHave et al., 2003). Specifically, preferences affect clients' decision to enroll in a study thereby limiting external validity, and influence attrition, adherence to treatment, and outcome thereby weakening internal validity (Sidani et al., 2003, 2009).

15.2.1 Influence of treatment preferences on external validity

Treatment preferences limit external validity by reducing clients' enrollment rate, yielding a sample of participants that is unrepresentative of the subgroups of which the target population is comprised. Clients indicating interest in taking part in an intervention trial are aware of different treatment options that are available and used to manage the presenting problem. They gain this knowledge from different sources including written materials (e.g., pamphlet, brochure, health-related Web sites), media (e.g., radio and TV show, articles in newspapers), verbal discussion with friends, relatives, and/or healthcare professionals, and personal experience with treatment. The gathered information, regardless of its accuracy, shapes clients' attitudes toward treatment. Favorable attitudes toward, reflecting acceptability of, a particular treatment option translates into a preference for that option. Unfavorable attitudes are represented in unacceptability or dislike for particular treatment options. In intervention research, at the time of recruitment or during the informed consent process, clients are informed of the experimental and comparison treatments offered in an efficacy or effectiveness trial. They are also told of the procedure for allocating them to treatment. Whether the procedure consists of randomization (as is typical in an efficacy RCT) or is based on another principle (as is the case in an effectiveness PCT), clients are not involved in treatment selection. Accordingly, individuals with strong preferences may decline enrollment in the trial because they are not willing to take the risk of being assigned to the nonpreferred treatment (Ellis, 2000; McPherson & Britton, 2001; TenHave et al., 2003). The relationship between treatment preferences and enrollment is well supported empirically. Concern of being assigned to the least preferred intervention was the reason given by individuals who refuse to participate in an RCT of adjuvant therapy for breast cancer (Stevens & Ahmedzai, 2004), school-based sex education (Oakley et al., 2003), brief physiotherapy intervention for back pain (Klaber-Moffett et al., 1999), and comprehensive treatment for mental health problems (Macias et al., 2005). When a rather large percentage of persons have strong preferences and decline entry, as reported by Klaber Moffett et al. (45%) and Macias et al. (30%), the rate of enrollment in the trial is reduced. With limited resources for extending recruitment, the accrued sample size is smaller than required and potentially inadequate to achieve statistical power to detect significant intervention effects.

The obtained sample may comprise participants who are not representative of all target population's subgroups. When clients with strong preferences decline enrollment because they do not want to take the risk of receiving the least preferred treatment, then these nonparticipants differ from participants. Participants consist of clients who may not have strong preferences and are willing to be randomized. In addition, empirical evidence indicates that persons with preferences and expressing unwillingness to be randomized differ from individuals with no preferences and expressing willingness to be randomized on socio-demographic and clinical characteristics. In addition, persons with preferences differ from those with no preferences on personal, clinical, and psychological characteristics, as well as beliefs about the presenting problem, as reported in the previous section. Such differences between participants and nonparticipants on these characteristics, preferences for treatment, and willingness to be randomized limit the generalization of the intervention evaluation study findings to the target population (Lambert & Wood, 2000; Millat et al., 2005). In particular, the applicability and the reproducibility of improvement in outcomes to clients with diverse profiles and views of treatment seen in day-to-day practice are questionable.

15.2.2 Influence of treatment preferences on internal validity

Clients with preferences for either the experimental or comparison treatment enter the efficacy or effectiveness trial because they view their enrollment as the only opportunity to receive the treatment option of their choice. Even if they are aware of and understand random assignment to treatment, they recognize that they have a 50% chance of being allocated to the preferred option (Bradley, 1993). However, clients with preferences who participate in the trial react differently to the allocated treatment; their reaction affects their uptake of, engagement in, adherence to, and response to treatment.

Participants' reaction differs depending on the treatment option to which they are allocated, be it the experimental or the comparison treatment. They may be assigned, by chance or other mechanism, to the treatment of their choice or to the nonpreferred or least preferred option. Participants assigned to their preferred treatment are satisfied with the treatment they receive and react favorably. Their enthusiasm motivates them to initiate treatment and actively engage in it; they enact the treatment recommendations appropriately and adhere to them adequately, at the preset dose level. With correct enactment and sufficient adherence, participants experience the expected improvement in the immediate outcomes, and with continued implementation of the intervention they demonstrate beneficial changes in the ultimate outcomes. In contrast, participants allocated to the nonpreferred or least preferred treatment option react unfavorably; they are disappointed because they are deprived of treatment of choice. Dissatisfied with treatment, participants may decide to withdraw from the study or experience a sense of demoralization. Participants' withdrawal or attrition represents a major threat to the validity of the inference about the causal effects of the intervention. As explained in Chapter 13, attrition decreases the sample size and subsequently statistical power to detect significant intervention effects, whereas differential attrition adversely affects the comparability of participants in the experimental and comparison groups on characteristics assessed at pretest. Characteristics showing between-group differences confound the intervention effects. Participants experiencing a sense of demoralization have low motivation to enact and/or adhere to treatment recommendations, which, in turn, results in no or minimal improvement in the immediate and ultimate outcomes (Halpern, 2003; Huibers et al., 2004). The distribution of satisfied and dissatisfied participants within the experimental and comparison groups may bias the estimates of the intervention effects. When the number of satisfied and dissatisfied participants is balanced (or comparable) across the experimental and comparison groups, then the levels on outcomes observed at posttest vary within each group, that is, within each of these two groups, satisfied participants show the expected improvement and dissatisfied participants experience no change in the outcome. This increased within-group variance in

posttest outcomes decreases the power to detect significant intervention effects. When the number of satisfied and dissatisfied participants is unbalanced
(or unequal) across the experimental and comparison groups, then the levels
on posttest outcomes differ between the two groups, resulting in invalid inferences about the causal effects of the intervention (Sidani, 2006). For instance,
if most dissatisfied participants happen to be in the experimental group, then
they may not demonstrate the expected changes in the outcomes and the
intervention is erroneously claimed to be ineffective. If most satisfied participants are located in the experimental group, then they may report high
levels on the posttest outcomes, which are reflected in a large between-group
difference leading to overestimation of the intervention effects.

Preliminary empirical evidence provides initial support for the influence of
treatment preferences on attrition, adherence to treatment, and outcomes.
Two systematic reviews examined the effects of preferences on attrition.
Swift and Callahan (2009) conducted a meta-analysis of 26 trials that have
accounted for participants' preferences for pharmacological, psychoeduca-
tional, and behavioral interventions for the management of psychological
problems such as depression. They found lower attrition rates for participants
assigned to the preferred treatment option. In contrast, King et al. (2005)
reported no difference in attrition rates for participants receiving medical
treatments on the basis of chance (i.e., randomization) or preference. The
inconsistency in the results of the two systematic reviews can be explained
by differences in the target population and the nature of interventions investigated in the primary trials. Four studies focused on the influence of preferences on treatment adherence. Despite variability in the operationalization
of adherence, the studies' findings showed that participants allocated to the
treatment option of choice reported higher levels of adherence than those
randomly assigned to treatment. The former group of participants attended
a large number of the planned intervention sessions (Bedi et al., 2000; Hitchcock Noël et al., 1998; Janevic et al., 2003), and engaged in most intervention
activities (Macias et al., 2005). Three systematic reviews synthesized results
of studies that evaluated the effects of preferences on outcome achievement.
King et al. (2005) found that seven of the 19 trials of medical treatments
reported a significant difference in outcomes between participants randomly
assigned to treatment and those allocated to the treatment of preference.
In five (of seven) studies, the expected beneficial outcomes were observed
in participants who received the treatment of choice more so than randomized participants. The Preference Collaborative Review Group (2009) analyzed data obtained in eight trials evaluating treatments for back and neck
pain. Results indicated greater improvement in outcomes for participants randomly allocated to the preferred, as compared to the nonpreferred, treatment. Similar findings were reported by Swift and Callahan (2009). Although
the magnitude of the influence of treatment preferences on outcomes was
small (mean effect size = .15; Swift & Callahan; The Preference Collaborative
Review Group), the consistent results across the three systematic reviews
affirm the role that treatment preferences play in making valid inferences

about the efficacy and/or the effectiveness of interventions. Accordingly, it is important to account for treatment preferences in intervention evaluation research.

15.2.3 Research designs accounting for treatment preferences

Two general approaches can be used to account for treatment preferences, and hence improve the validity of causal inferences in intervention evaluation research. The first consists of assessing treatment preferences and controlling, statistically, their effects on outcomes. This first approach can be implemented in an RCT. The second involves assigning participants to the experimental and the comparison groups on the basis of chance or preference, and comparing their outcomes. This second approach is applied in the partially randomized clinical trial (PRCT) or the two-stage PRCT design. The features of these trials have been described by Sidani et al. (2009) and are reviewed briefly next.

Randomized controlled/clinical trial. Accounting for treatment preferences in an RCT involves the following steps:

(1) Participants are informed of the treatment options under evaluation, using a comprehensive but easy to understand description of each option, as proposed by Sidani et al. (2006).

(2) Participants are requested to rate the acceptability of each treatment option and to indicate their preference, using a validated measure such as the one developed by Sidani et al. (2009). Participants' expressed preferences are clearly identified and recorded.

(3) Participants are randomized to treatment, as is usually done in an RCT. Outcome data are collected as planned.

(4) At the stage of data analysis, participants randomized to each treatment options are categorized into two subgroups. The first subgroup, matched, represents participants who received the treatment option of their choice. The second subgroup, mismatch, comprises participants who received the nonpreferred or least preferred treatment option. Thus, in an RCT involving one experimental and one comparison group, four groups are formed: (1) experimental-match: participants receiving the experimental intervention which they identified as the preferred option; (2) experimental-mismatch: participants receiving the experimental intervention which they identified as the nonpreferred option; (3) comparison-match: participants receiving the comparison treatment which they identified as the preferred option; (4) comparison-mismatch: participants receiving the comparison treatment, which they identified as the nonpreferred option.

(5) *Comparison of the four groups' outcomes is done:* Significant differences in the outcomes between the match and mismatch subgroups, within each of the experimental and the comparison group, reflect the influence of treatment preferences on outcome achievement.

The application of this design is illustrated by the study conducted by Klaber-Moffett et al. (1999). The advantage of this design is the use of randomization to assign participants to study groups, thereby increasing the probability of achieving between-group comparability at baseline. Its major disadvantage is that it ignores participants' preferences when allocating them to treatment, which can contribute to attrition and sense of demoralization, as explained previously. Some researchers consider it unethical to elicit participants' preferences yet ignore them when allocating participants to treatment (Preference Collaborative Review Group, 2009).

Partially randomized clinical trial. The PRCT, as originally devised by Bradley (1993), involves the following:

(1) Informing participants of the treatment options under evaluation, having them rate their acceptability, and asking them to indicate the option of choice, as described in the previous section.
(2) For participants having a clear preference, that is, identifying a treatment option of choice, allocating them to the selected option.
(3) For participants expressing no preference for either treatment option, randomizing them to treatment.

This pattern of assignment, illustrated in Figure 15.1, in a trial involving one experimental group and one comparison group yields four groups: (1) participants allocated to the experimental group on the basis of preference; (2) participants randomly assigned to the experimental group; (3) participants allocated to the comparison group on the basis of preference; and (4) participants randomly assigned to the comparison group. Comparison of the four groups on outcomes determines the extent to which treatment preferences affect outcome achievement. For instance, significant differences between participants who received the experimental intervention on the basis of preference or chance are indicative of the extent to which preferences contributed to the outcomes: finding greater improvement in outcomes in those receiving

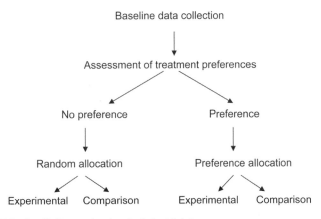

Figure 15.1 Partially randomized clinical trial.

the treatment on the basis of preference, as compared to chance, supports the contribution of preferences to outcome achievement.

The application of the PRCT is illustrated by Coward's (2002) study. The advantage of the PRCT is that it accounts for participants' preferences, thereby reflecting, partially, the collaborative process for treatment related decision-making and the client-centered approach to care. Its disadvantages include the high probability of having unbalanced group sizes, which limits meaningful between-group comparison, and of not achieving group comparability on various client characteristics assessed at baseline due to well-known differences in personal and clinical profiles of clients with and without preferences. Such differences could confound the intervention effects (Sidani et al., 2009). The limitations of the PRCT are addressed in the two-stage PRCT.

Two-stage PRCT. The two-stage PRCT design is proposed to overcome the limitations of the PRCT. The two-stage PRCT consists of the following steps:

(1) Participants are randomized to either of two trial arms, random or preference, after obtaining baseline data.
(2) Participants in the random arm are randomly assigned to treatment, as is usually done in an RCT.
(3) Participants in the preference arm are informed of the treatment options under investigation, are asked to rate their acceptability, and indicate their preferences, as described previously. Participants expressing a preference are allocated to the option of choice. Participants indicating no preference are randomly assigned to treatment.

This design results in four groups in the trial with one experimental and one comparison treatment, as those identified for the PRCT. However, it is believed that randomization, done in Step 1, maintains comparability on baseline characteristics and balanced size of the four groups. Differences in outcomes achieved by the four groups provide evidence of the influence of treatment preferences. The application of the two-stage PRCT is illustrated in some studies included in King et al.'s (2005) systematic review. The group comparability and balanced size makes the PRCT the most advantageous for dismantling the contribution of treatment preferences. Its disadvantage rests in the large sample size required to attain adequate statistical power to detect the combined effects of preferences and the intervention (Sidani et al., 2009).

Accounting for client preferences in an effectiveness study, by allocating clients to the treatment of choice, is useful. It reflects the treatment-related decision-making process applied in day-to-day practice. It yields results of relevance to and potentially reproducible in practice, as they depict responses to the intervention exhibited by clients seen in the practice setting who do and do not find it acceptable and consistent with their preference.

Section 5

Translation of Interventions

Chapter 16
Translation of Interventions

Translation is the last phase of the process for designing, evaluating, and translating interventions. A careful design of the intervention and systematic evaluation of its effects yield cumulative evidence, derived from the results of pilot, efficacy, and effectiveness studies, supporting the appropriateness of the intervention in addressing the presenting problem; the acceptability of the intervention to clients and healthcare professionals; and the effectiveness of the intervention in producing optimal outcomes. Interventions with demonstrated effectiveness are translated, that is, incorporated and implemented into the context of day-to-day practice in order to facilitate the provision of high-quality care across the healthcare continuum, worldwide.

Although different definitions of translation have been advanced (e.g., Bosnian-Herzegovinian American Academy of Arts and Sciences cited by Festic & Gajic, 2009; National Institutes of Health, 2000), the one that is most congruent with the last phase of the process for intervention design, evaluation, and translation, has been generated by the Canadian Institutes of Health Research and adopted by the National Center for the Dissemination of Disability Research in the United States and by the World Health Organization. The definition characterizes translation as a dynamic process that involves the synthesis, exchange, and ethically sound application of knowledge to improve health of clients, provide effective and efficient services, and to strengthen the healthcare system. Knowledge refers to evidence of the success of the intervention in addressing the presenting problem and in achieving beneficial health outcomes. The primary purpose of translation is to minimize or close the gap between evidence, and clinical and policy decision-making (Graham et al., 2006), and hence to promote access to and provision of high-quality care. High-quality care entails the delivery of interventions that are appropriate in addressing the health-related problem with which clients present, acceptable to clients, and effective in yielding optimal outcomes.

The application of the translation process involves the systematic review of evidence pertaining to the intervention, the transformation of the evidence into meaningful guidelines for practice, and the transfer of the guideline into day-to-day practice. The process needs to be applied in collaboration with

Design, Evaluation, and Translation of Nursing Interventions, First Edition.
Souraya Sidani and Carrie Jo Braden.
© 2011 John Wiley & Sons, Inc. Published 2011 by John Wiley & Sons, Inc.

clinical and policy decision-makers in order to enhance the relevance and applicability of the guidelines to the context of practice within local settings. The steps of the translation process are described in this chapter.

16.1 Systematic review of evidence

Systematic review of evidence is a foundational step in the intervention translation process. It consists of searching for, critically appraising, and synthesizing theoretical and empirical evidence pertaining to the intervention targeting the presenting problem of interest. Theoretical evidence relates to the theory of the problem and the theory underlying the intervention. The theory of the problem provides an understanding of the problem requiring remediation in terms of its nature, manifestations or indicators, and determinants. Theory underlying the intervention clarifies the aspects of the problem targeted by the intervention, describes the intervention in terms of its goals, components, activities, mode of delivery, and dose, and explains the mechanisms mediating the intervention effects on the ultimate outcomes. Empirical evidence encompasses results of quantitative (experimental and nonexperimental) and qualitative studies that evaluated the intervention. The studies include those undertaken within a program of research aimed at testing the acceptability, feasibility, efficacy, and effectiveness of the intervention, or those conducted by different researchers to examine the success of the intervention in addressing the presenting problem as experienced by different subgroups of the target population or by various client populations in different settings. In either case, the results are synthesized to (1) determine whether or not the intervention produces the intended outcomes, the magnitude of the observed intervention effects, and the dose–response relationship, and (2) identify intervention components consistently implemented, conceptual and/or methodological factors that moderated the intervention effects, the most significant mediators of the intervention effects, and the mode of delivery found feasible, acceptable to clients, promoting fidelity in the delivery of the intervention's active ingredients, and variations in intervention implementation associated with beneficial outcomes. The synthesized findings address the questions of relevance to practice: Which clients, presenting with which socio-demographic and clinical profile and characteristics (determinants and level of severity) of the problem, benefit to what extent from the intervention or its components, given in what format, at what dose level, and in which settings. The systematic reviews reported by Blue and Black (2005), Fan and Sidani (2009), and Morin et al. (2006) illustrate the synthesis of empirical literature described.

The theoretical and empirical evidence are integrated to highlight elements of the intervention theory that are supported empirically. The integrated knowledge provides a frame of reference for clinical decision-makers or healthcare professionals to: (1) discern the presenting problem addressed by the intervention; (2) select valid and clinically relevant instruments to assess the problem in terms of its determinants, indicators, and level of severity that are specifically targeted by the intervention; (3) distinguish the specific elements or essential ingredients from the nonspecific elements of the intervention; (4) comprehend the rationale of the intervention, that is, how and why the intervention works; (5) recognize client and/or setting or environmental factors that facilitate or hinder the implementation of the intervention as well as client engagement and enactment of treatment recommendations, and subsequently the achievement of beneficial outcomes; and (6) identify the minimal and optimal dose levels associated with improvements in the outcomes. A clear and comprehensive knowledge of the theoretical underpinnings of the intervention, combined with awareness of variability in client, setting, and intervention characteristics that still results in intended changes in the outcomes, are necessary to carefully operationalize the intervention in the context of practice (Tucker et al., 2007). The operationalization consists of translating the evidence into meaningful guidelines.

16.2 Translation of evidence

The second step in the translation process consists of "translating" or transforming the integrated theoretical and empirical evidence into meaningful guidelines that offer clear and useful directions for practice. Whether labeled "clinical practice guidelines" or "best practice guidelines," the guidelines have been described as systematically developed statements to assist healthcare professional and client decision about appropriate care for specific clinical circumstances (Moreira et al., 2006). The content of available guidelines varies. Most commonly, the guidelines include a list of interventions and/or specific strategies for managing a particular problem; some guidelines incorporate summarized evidence of the effectiveness of the listed interventions, whereas others provide references for useful resources related to the listed interventions (Coopey et al., 2006; Ledbetter & Stevens, 2000). Still, other guidelines present specific recommendations derived from evidence and experts' judgment, for the assessment and the management of the presenting problem; the recommendations indicate which instrument to use in the assessment and which specific, combination, or sequence of interventions to use to address the presenting problem. The recommendations are synthesized in pictorial algorithms, as illustrated by the work of Schutte-Rodin et al. (2008). The utility of these guidelines in directing clinical decision-making has been questioned. They provide information on what interventions to use but fall short of explaining the why (i.e., rationale), the how (i.e., implementation) of the listed intervention (Frank et al., 2002; Tucker et al., 2007), and for whom (i.e., characteristics of presenting problem and of clients). Accordingly, the content of the guidelines has to identify the client population most likely to benefit from the intervention, the step-by-step protocol on how to carry out the intervention, and evaluation guide to monitor the process and outcome of implementing the intervention, as proposed by Titler et al. (1999). Specifically, the guidelines consist of a package covering the following information, derived from the integrated theoretical and empirical evidence that is synthesized in the first step of the translation process:

(1) *Presenting problem:* The scientific and lay terms used to refer to the presenting problem are presented. The problem is defined conceptually (i.e., what it is) and operationally (i.e., what are its manifestations or indicators). The determinants of the problem that are amenable to change and targeted by the intervention are identified.

(2) *Instrument to assess the presenting problem:* The instrument is used to assess the presenting problem prior to the implementation of the intervention with the purpose of determining if clients experience the problem at a prespecified level of severity and as related to the determinant targeted by the intervention, and following delivery of the intervention at prespecified points in time with the purpose of monitoring the effectiveness of the intervention. The instrument is described in terms of its name, content covered, scoring procedure, and interpretation of the scores.

(3) *Client population:* The socio-demographic and clinical characteristics of the subgroups of the target population found to benefit from the intervention, to various extent, are identified.

(4) *Intervention:* Several characteristics of the intervention are specified including (1) name of the intervention, which is necessary for verbal communication related to treatment/care among healthcare professionals and between professionals and clients, and for documenting what was provided to clients in pertinent records; (2) goal of the intervention, which represents what the intervention is set to achieve relative to the presenting problem and/or general functioning; (3) resources, that is, the material and human resources required for delivering the intervention are specified; (4) the components and activities that operationalize the active ingredients of the intervention and that should be carried out to claim that the intervention is delivered and to yield the intended beneficial outcomes; (5) the range of nonspecific elements of the intervention and their operationalization in mode or format for delivering the intervention; (6) the dose range at which the intervention can be given to achieve beneficial outcomes; and (7) the mechanisms responsible for producing the outcomes. In addition, a log is appended that lists the activities of which the intervention is comprised. The log provides a means for guiding healthcare professionals' implementation of the intervention, for evaluating fidelity of its implementation, and for documenting its delivery to clients.

Table 16.1 illustrates the content of an intervention implementation guideline. Once developed, the guideline is transferred to direct practice.

Table 16.1 Guideline for intervention implementation

Item	Description
Presenting problem	
Scientific term	Physical fatigue
Lay term	Feeling of tiredness
Definition	Sense of lack of energy and decreased capacity for activity or physical work
Indicators	Feeling tired in whole body; weary; worn out; having no energy; weakness or lack of strength
Determinants	Illness condition resulting in physiological alterations; experience of other symptoms such as pain and insomnia; physical inactivity
Instrument to assess presenting problem	
Name and content	One item, 10-point numeric rating scale, capturing overall experience of tiredness
Interpretation of scores	Score reflects level of fatigue severity
	Interpretation: 1–3: mild; 4–6: moderate; 7–10: severe
	Change of 1 point indicates clinically important difference in level of fatigue severity
Client population	Clients experiencing moderate-to-severe physical fatigue associated with cancer and multiple sclerosis
	Adult, English-speaking, cognitively intact
Intervention	
Name	Energy conservation and activity management
Goal	To assist clients in managing physical fatigue and maintaining engagement in usual physical activity
Resources	Private room; handout summarizing recommendations; paper; pen
Components and activities	Component 1: Education
	Inform clients of skills to prioritize their usual activities and develop a daily routine that includes periods of rest and activities
	Recommendations to be followed: (1) set priority for usual activities, (2) delegate activities if possible, (3) schedule prioritized activities at times of peak energy, (4) postpone nonessential activities, (5) pace activities, (6) develop a structured daily routine that involves periods of rest and activities, (7) limit naps to 20–30 minutes, avoid naps in late afternoon and evening
	Component 2: Coaching
	Assist clients in prioritizing their usual activities and preparing a list of important activities
	Support clients in generating an energy conservation plan to engage in prioritized activities at time of peak energy
	Instruct clients to monitor level of fatigue to identify peak and low energy times
Mode of delivery	Face-to-face discussion with clients

(Continued)

Table 16.1 (*Continued*)

Item	Description
Dose	One 15–30 minute session
Rationale	Planning engagement in valued activities at times of peak energy minimizes interference of fatigue with performance of these activities
	Engagement in physical activities reduces feeling of tiredness, promotes sense of control, and prevents inactivity that contributes to physical fatigue

16.3   Transfer of guideline to practice

Transfer of the guidelines to the practice setting is the last step of the translation process that has to be undertaken in collaboration with clinical decision-makers (i.e., healthcare professionals and clinical leaders) and policy decision-makers (i.e., managers and healthcare payers) in order to enhance the relevance and the applicability, and hence the uptake and implementation, of the guideline to the context of practice. Transfer involves two main activities: (1) adaptation of the guideline to fit the particular practice context in which it will be implemented, and (2) dissemination of the guideline for implementation by healthcare professionals responsible for providing the intervention to clients.

16.3.1   Adaptation of guideline

Although adaptation of the guideline is considered critical for facilitating its uptake and implementation, the methods and procedures for performing this activity and its anticipated result are not clearly described. Drawing on the combined approach for understanding the problem and the experiential approach for designing and examining the acceptability of interventions described in the previous chapters, the following steps are proposed for adapting the guidelines:

(1) Identify key clinical and policy decision-makers in the practice context in which the guidelines are to be implemented. Clinical decision-makers include clinical directors of programs, clinical leaders, and healthcare professionals who will ultimately be responsible for implementing the intervention. Involving this range of clinical decision-makers ensures representation of various perspectives in the adapted guideline and consensus on its content, which instills a sense of "ownership" of and commitment to the implementation of the guideline; as well as the clarification of the role of each group of decision-makers in the dissemination of the guideline and in the application of the intervention. The presence of policy decision-makers, primarily management representatives, during the discussion promotes the consistency of the guideline with the vision, philosophical

orientation, and standards of care adapted by the organization, and the organizational support for initiatives to change practice.

(2) Invite the selected clinical and policy decision-makers to a group session focused on discussing the guideline. The invitation has to clarify the purpose of the discussion and inform participants of the need to make available any data or experiential observations they may have about the prevalence of the presenting problem, the characteristics of the client population experiencing the problem, the dominant view about the problem and its treatment among clients and healthcare professionals, and the type and effects of treatments currently used to address the presenting problem.

(3) Facilitate the group discussion with the aims of identifying elements of the guidelines that are relevant and applicable to the practice setting and those that require modifications to fit the characteristics of the client population served and of the practice settings; and of reaching an agreement on the modifications to be made while maintaining fidelity to the intervention theory, specifically the active ingredients that define the intervention. The discussion is structured and entails reviewing one element of the guideline at a time; engaging participants in critical review of what it connotes, as stated, and of how relevant and applicable it is to their practice; requesting participants to suggest how the element can be modified to enhance its consistency with the reality of practice; reviewing the suggested modifications to ensure their congruence with the intervention's active ingredients and their feasibility in the practice context; and moderating the group discussion to each consensus on the modifications to be made. For instance, the characteristics of the client population most likely to benefit from the intervention, as specified in the guideline, are compared to those of the client population served in the practice setting. Comparability of the characteristics points to the relevance of the intervention, whereas dissimilarity in some characteristics indicates the need to modify some elements of the guidelines. For example, if the client population served is non-English speaking primarily, then the language used to relay intervention-related information (e.g., printed list of treatment recommendations) is to be changed, or the target population is modified to include clients' significant others who speak English and are capable of translating the information into the clients' native language. The characteristics of the intervention described in the guideline are carefully reviewed with a particular attention to each component and related activities as these operationalize the intervention's active ingredients. After reading pertinent information, participants are asked about their understanding of the nature of the activities constituting the component (which is necessary to determine comprehension of what is to be done), the feasibility of carrying out the activities within the constraints of the practice context, the perceived acceptability of the activities to healthcare professionals who will assume the responsibility of engaging in the intervention activities, and the specific activities to be modified. Participants are informed of modifications made and found to be still contributing to

favorable outcomes in an effectiveness study using a pragmatic clinical trial design, or are encouraged to explain the nature of the modifications. The latter modifications are meticulously analyzed to determine if:

(1) they are proposed in essential activities that operationalize the active ingredients and they deviate from the essential activities—these changes may not be accepted as they may threaten the validity or accuracy of the adapted guideline in reflecting the intended intervention;

(2) they are proposed in nonessential activities and they may dilute the purity or fidelity with which the intervention's active ingredients are carried out—these modifications are also not accepted; or

(3) they are proposed in nonessential activities and they do not jeopardize the fidelity of implementing the intervention's active ingredients—these modifications are accepted and incorporated in an adapted guideline.

16.3.2 Dissemination and implementation of guideline

The adapted guideline, approved by decision-makers, is disseminated to healthcare professionals with the primary responsibility of providing the intervention to clients, and strategies are devised to monitor the healthcare professionals' implementation of the guideline. Various simple (e.g., in-service education), multicomponent (e.g., education, skill training workshop, reminders), and multilevel (e.g., healthcare professional performance evaluation, facilitative administrative practices targeting individual and groups of healthcare professionals, management, and healthcare system) strategies have been used in guideline dissemination efforts. Systematic reviews of the strategies' effectiveness in promoting healthcare professionals' awareness, uptake, and actual implementation of guidelines have shown that multicomponent, multilevel approaches are more successful than simple ones (e.g., Fixsen et al., 2005; Russell & Walsh, 2009). Nonetheless, the magnitude of the strategies' effects was at best moderate.

The emerging perspective is to frame the healthcare professionals' practice relative to the uptake and application of the guideline as a form of human behavior (Eccles et al., 2005). As such, theories that explain behavior in terms of determinants that are amenable to change, such as knowledge, attitudes, and social influences (Godin et al., 2008) could be used to design and/or select the most appropriate or congruent strategies to address the identified determinants and hence to promote performance of the intended behavior related to the implementation of the guideline, as illustrated with the work of Hrisos et al. (2008).

With the lack of compelling evidence to support the effectiveness and efficiency of specific strategies, it would be recommended to collaborate with clinical and policy decision-makers to select and apply the strategies that are feasible, acceptable, appropriate, and consistent with the characteristics of the particular practice setting for the purpose of disseminating and implementing the guideline. No matter what dissemination strategies are employed, the challenge is to maintain the continued use of the guideline over time!

References

Abraham, C. & Michie, S. (2008) A taxonomy of behavior change techniques used in interventions. *Health Psychology*, 27, 379-387.

Adolfson, E.T., Starring, B., Smide, B., & Wikblad, K. (2008) Type 2 diabetes patients' experiences of two different educational approaches – A qualitative study. *International Journal of Nursing Studies*, 45, 986-994.

Ahern, K. & Le Brocque, R. (2005) Methodological issues in the effects of attrition. Simple solutions for social scientists. *Field Methods*, 17, 53-69.

Ajzen, I. (1991) The theory of planned behavior. *Organizational Behavior & Human Decision Processes*, 50, 179-211.

American Nurses Association (2003) *Nursing's Social Policy Statement*, 2nd edn. American Nurses Association, Washington, DC.

Ames, S.C., Rock, E., Hurt, R.D., et al. (2008) Development and feasibility of a parental support intervention for adolescent smokers. *Substance Use and Misuse*, 43, 497-511.

Andrykowski, M.A. & Manne, S.L. (2006) Are psychological interventions effective and accepted by cancer patients? I. Standards and levels of evidence. *Annals Behavioral Medicine*, 32, 93-97.

Arega, A., Birkmeyer, N.J.O, Lurie, J.D.N., et al. (2006) Racial variation in treatment preferences and willingness to randomize in the Spine Patient Outcomes Research Trial (SPORT). *Spine*, 31, 2263-2269.

Armstrong, T.S., Cohen, M.Z., Erikson, L., & Cleeland, C. (2005) Content validation of self-report measurement instruments: An illustration from the development of a brain tumor module of the M.D. Anderson Symptom Inventory. *Oncology Nursing Forum*, 3, 669-676.

Artieta-Pinedo, J., Paz-Pascual, C., Grandes, G., et al. (2010) The benefits of antenatal education for the childbirth process in Spain. *Nursing Research*, 59, 194-202.

Awad, M.A., Shapiro, S.H., Lund, J.P., & Feine, J.S. (2000) Determinants of patients' treatment preferences in a clinical trial. *Community Dental Oral Epidemiology*, 28, 119-125.

Bakas, T., Farran, C.J., Austin, J.K., et al. (2009) Content validity and satisfaction with a stroke caregiver program. *Journal of Nursing Scholarship*, 41, 368-375.

Baldwin, S.A., Wampold, B.E., & Imel, Z.E. (2007) Untangling the alliance-outcome correlation: Exploring the relative importance of therapist and patient variability in the alliance. *Journal of Consulting & Clinical Psychology*, 75, 842-852.

Bamberger, M. & White, H. (2007) Using strong evaluation designs in developing countries: Experience and challenges. *Journal of Multi Disciplinary Evaluation*, 4, 58-73.

Design, Evaluation, and Translation of Nursing Interventions, First Edition.
Souraya Sidani and Carrie Jo Braden.
© 2011 John Wiley & Sons, Inc. Published 2011 by John Wiley & Sons, Inc.

Bandura, A. (1997) *Self-Efficacy: The Exercise of Control.* Freeman, New York.

Barkauskas, V.H., Lusk, S.L., & Eakin, B.L. (2005) Selecting control interventions for clinical outcome studies. *Western Journal of Nursing Research,* 27, 346-363.

Barlow, J., Wright, C., Sheasby, J., et al. (2002) Self-management approaches for people with chronic conditions: A review. *Patient Education & Counseling,* 48, 177-187.

Baron, R.M. & Kenny, D.A. (1986) The moderator-mediator variable distinction in social psychological research: Conceptual, strategic, and statistical considerations. *Journal of Personality and Social Psychology,* 51, 1173-1182.

Bartholomew, L.K., Parcel, G.S., & Kok, G. (1998) Intervention mapping: A process for developing theory- and evidence-based health education programs. *Health Education & Behavior,* 25, 545-563.

Baskin, T.W., Tierney, S.C., Minami, T., & Wampold, B.E. (2000) Establishing specificity in psychotherapy: A meta-analysis of structural equivalence of placebo-controls. *Journal of Consulting & Clinical Psychology,* 71, 973-979.

Becker, C., Davis, E., & Schaumberg, K. (2007) An analog study of patient preferences for exposure versus alternative treatments of posttraumatic stress disorder. *Behavior Research & Therapy,* 45, 2861-2873.

Bedi, N., Chilvers, C., Churchill, R., et al. (2000) Assessing effectiveness of treatment of depression in primary care. Partially randomized preference trial. *British Journal of Psychiatry,* 177, 312-318.

Bellg, A.J., Borrelli, B., Resnick, B., et al. (2004) Enhancing treatment fidelity in health behavior change studies: Best practices and recommendations from the NIH Behavior Change Consortium. *Health Psychology,* 23(5), 443-451.

Bennett, J.A. (2000) Mediator and moderator variables in nursing research: Conceptual and statistical differences. *Research in Nursing & Health,* 23, 415-420.

Blue, C.L. & Black, D.R. (2005) Synthesis of intervention research to modify physical activity and dietary behaviours. *Research and Theory for Nursing Practice,* 9(1), 25-61.

Bock, B.C., Marcus, B.H., Pinto, B.M., & Forsyth, L.H. (2001) Maintenance of physical activity following an individualized motivationally tailored intervention. *Annals of Behavioral Medicine,* 23, 79-87.

Bollinger, C.T., van Biljon, X., & Axelsson, A. (2007) A nicotine mouth spray for smoking cessation: A pilot study of preference, safety and efficacy. *Respiration,* 74, 196-201.

Bootzin, R.R., Franzen, P.L., & Shapiro, S.L. (2004) Behavioral treatments for insomnia. In: M.R. Pressman (ed) *Understanding Sleep: The Evaluation and Treatment of Sleep Disorders,* 2nd edn. American Psychological Association, Washington, DC.

Borglin, G. & Richards, D.A. (2010) Bias in experimental nursing research: Strategies to improve the quality and explanatory power of nursing science. *International Journal of Nursing Studies,* 47, 123-128.

Borkovec, T.D. (1993) Between-group therapy outcome research: Design and methodology. In: L.S. Onken, J.D. Blaine, & J.J. Oren (eds) *Behavioral Treatments for Drug Abuse and Dependence.* (National Institute on Drug Abuse (NIDA) Research Monograph Series 137). US Department of Health and Human Services, Washington, DC.

Borrego, J., Ibanez, E.S., Spendlove, S.T., & Pemberton, J.R. (2007) Treatment acceptability among Mexican American parents. *Behavior Therapy,* 38, 218-227.

Borrelli, B., Sepinwall, D., Ernst, D., et al. (2005) A new tool to assess treatment fidelity and evaluation of treatment fidelity across 10 years of health behavior research. *Journal of Consulting & Clinical Psychology,* 73, 852-860.

Bottomley, A. (1997) To randomize or not to randomize: Methodological pitfalls of the RCT in psychosocial intervention studies. *European Journal of Cancer*, 6, 222-230.

Bouffard, J.A., Taxman, F.S., & Silverman, R. (2003) Improving process evaluations of correctional programs by using a comprehensive evaluation methodology. *Evaluation & Program Planning*, 26, 149-161.

Bowen, A.M., Horvath, K., & Williams, M.L. (2007) A randomized control trial of internet-delivered HIV prevention targeting MSM. *Health Education Research*, 22, 120-127.

Bowers, T.G. & Clum, G.A. (1998) Relative contribution of specific and nonspecific treatment effects: Meta-analysis of placebo-controlled behavior therapy research. *Psychological Bulletin*, 103, 313-323.

Braden, C.J. (2002) In: G. Lamb & M. Koithan (eds) *Involvement/Participation, Empowerment, and Knowledge Outcome Indicators of Case Management*. State of the Science Paper #2. Case management Society of American, Little Rock, Arkansas.

Bradley, C. (1993) Designing medical and educational intervention studies. *Diabetes Care*, 16, 509-518.

Brandt, P.A., Kirsch, S.D., Lewis, F.M., & Casey, S.M. (2004) Assessing the strength and integrity of an intervention. *Oncology Nursing Forum*, 31, 833-837.

Brown, S.A. (1992) Meta-analysis of diabetes patient education research: Variations in intervention effects across studies. *Research in Nursing & Health*, 15, 409-419.

Brown, S.J. (2002) Nursing intervention studies: A descriptive analysis of issues important to clinicians. *Research in Nursing & Health*, 25, 317-327.

Bruckenthal, P. & Broderick, J.E. (2007) Assessing treatment fidelity in pilot studies assist in designing clinical trials. An illustration from a nurse practitioner community-based intervention for pain. *Advances in Nursing Science*, 30, E72-E84.

Brug, J., Oenema, A., & Ferreira, I. (2005) Theory, evidence and intervention mapping to improve behavior nutrition and physical activity interventions. *International Journal of Behavioral Nutrition & Physical Activity*, 2, 2-8.

Bryman, A. (2001) *Social Research Methods*. Oxford University Press, New York.

Buckwalter, K.C., Grey, M., Bowers, B., et al. (2009) Intervention research in highly unstable environments. *Research in Nursing & Health*, 32, 110-121.

Bulecheck, G.M. & McCloskey, J.C. (1992) *Nursing Interventions: Essential Nursing Treatments*, 2nd edn. Saunders, Philadelphia, PA.

Burke, J.G., O'Campo, P., Peak, G.L., et al. (2005) An introduction to concept mapping as a participatory public health research method. *Qualitative Health Research*, 15, 1392-1410.

Burns, N. & Grove, S.K. (2005) *The Practice of Nursing Research. Conduct, Critique, and Utilization*. Saunders, Philadelphia, PA.

Campbell, M., Fitzpatrick, R., Haines, A., et al. (2000) Framework for design and evaluation of complex interventions to improve health. *British Medical Journal*, 321, 694-696.

Campbell, N.C., Murray, E., Darbyshire, J., et al. (2007) Designing and evaluating complex interventions to improve health care. *British Medical Journal*, 334, 455-459.

Carballo-Diéguez, A., Exner, T., Dolezal, C., et al. (2007) Rectal microbicide acceptability: Results of a volume escalation trial. *Sexually Transmitted Diseases*, 34, 224-229.

Carroll, C., Patterson, M., Wood, S., et al. (2007) A conceptual framework for implementation fidelity. *Implementation Science*, 2, 40-48.

Carter, S.L. (2007) Review of recent treatment acceptability research. *Education & Training in Developmental Disabilities*, 42, 301-316.

Chatterji, M. (2007) Grades of evidence. Variability in quality of findings in effectiveness studies of complex field interventions. *American Journal of Evaluation*, 28, 239-255.

Cheong, J.W., MacKinnon, D.P., & Khoo, S.T. (2003) Investigation of mediational processes using parallel process latent growth curve modeling. *Structural Equation Modeling*, 10, 238-262.

Chung, L.K., Cimprich, B., Janz, N.K., & Mills-Wismeski, S.M. (2009) Breast cancer survivorship program. Testing for cross-cultural relevance. *Cancer Nursing*, 32, 236-245.

Cochran, B.N., Pruitt, L., Fukuda, S., & Feeny, N.C. (2008) Reasons underlying treatment preferences. *Journal of Interpersonal Violence*, 23, 276.

Cohen, B.E., Kamaya, A.M., Macer, J.L., et al. (2007) Feasibility and acceptability of restorative yoga for treatment of hot flushes: A pilot trial. *Maturitas*, 56, 198-204.

Collie, K., Kreshka, A., Ferrier, S., et al. (2007) Videoconferencing for delivery of breast cancer support groups to women living in rural communities: A pilot study. *Psycho-Oncology*, 16, 778-782.

Concato, J., Shah, N., & Horwitz, R.I. (2000) Randomized, controlled trials, observational studies, and the hierarchy of research designs. *New England Journal of Medicine*, 342(25), 1887-1892.

Concato, J. & Horwitz, R.I. (2004) Beyond randomized versus observational studies. *The Lancet*, 363, 1660-1661.

Conn, V.S., Rantz, M.J., Wipke-Tevis, D.D., & Maas, M.L. (2001) Designing effective nursing interventions. *Research in Nursing & Health*, 24, 433-442.

Cook, T.D. & Campbell, D.T. (1979) *Quasi-Experimentation: Design and Analysis Issues for Field Settings*. Houghton Mifflin, Boston.

Cook, T.D., Scriven, M., Coryn, C.L.S., & Evergreen, S.D.H. (2010) Contemporary thinking about causation in evaluation: A dialogue with Tom Cook and Michael Scriven. *American Journal of Evaluation*, 31, 105-117.

Cooper, H. (1998) *Synthesizing Research: A Guide for Literature Reviews*, 3rd edn. Sage, Thousand Oaks, CA.

Cooper, L.A., Gonzales, J.J., Gallo, J.J., et al. (2003) The acceptability of treatment of depression among African-American, Hispanic and White primary care patients. *Medical Care*, 41, 479.

Coopey, M., Nix, M.P., & Clancy, C.M. (2006) Translating research into evidence-based nursing practice and evaluating effectiveness. *Journal of Nursing Care Quality*, 21, 195-202.

Corrigan, P.W. & Salzer, M.S. (2003) The conflict between random assignment and treatment preference: Implications for internal validity. *Evaluation and Program Planning*, 26, 109-121.

Coward, D. (2002) Partial randomized design in a support group intervention study. *Western Journal of Nursing Research*, 24, 406-421.

Coyler, H. & Kamath, P. (1999) Evidence base practice: A philosophical and political analysis: Some matters for consideration by professional practitioners. *Journal of Advanced Nursing*, 29, 188-193.

Crano, W.D. & Messe, L.A. (1985) Assessing and redressing comprehension artifacts in social intervention research. *Evaluation Review*, 9, 144-172.

Crits-Christoph, P. & Mintz, J. (1991) Implications of therapist effects for the design and analysis of comparative studies of psychotherapies. *Journal of Consulting and Clinical Psychology*, 59, 20-26.

Crits-Christoph, P., Baranackie, K., Kurcias, J., et al. (1991) Meta-analysis of therapist effects in psychotherapy outcome studies. *Psychotherapy Research*, 1, 81–91.

Cupertino, A.P., Richter, K.P., Cox, L.S., Nazir, N., Greiner, K.A., Ashluwalia, J.S., & Ellerbeck, E.F. (2008) Smoking cessation pharmacotherapy preferences in rural primary care. *Nicotine & Tobacco Research*, 10, 301–307.

D'Agostino, R.B. (2009) The delayed-start study design. *New England Journal of Medicine*, 361, 1304-1306.

Dana, N. & Wambach, K.A. (2003) Patient satisfaction with an early discharge home visit program. *Journal of Obstetrics & Gynecology and Neonatal Nursing*, 32, 190-198.

Davidson, E.J. (2006) The RCTs-only doctrine: Brakes on the acquisition of knowledge? *Journal of MultiDisciplinary Evaluation*, 6, ii-v.

Davies, H.T.O. (1999) Bias in treatment trials. *Hospital Medicine*, 60, 599-601.

Deacon, B.J. & Abramowitz, J.S. (2005) Patients' perceptions of pharmacological and cognitive-behavioral treatments for anxiety disorders. *Behavior Therapy*, 36, 139-145.

De Maat, S., Dekker, J., Schoevers, R., & de Jonghe, F. (2007) The effectiveness of long-term psychotherapy: Methodological research issues. *Psychotherapy Research*, 17, 59-65.

De Vries, H. & Brug, J. (1999) Computer-tailored interventions motivating people to adopt health promoting behaviors: Introduction to a new approach. *Patient Education & Counseling*, 36, 99-105.

Dijkstra, A. (2005) Working mechanisms of computer-tailored health education: Evidence from smoking cessation. *Health Education Research*, 20, 527-539.

Dijkstra, A. & DeVries, H. (1999) The development of computer-generated tailored intervention. *Patient Education & Counseling*, 36, 193-203.

DiMatteoa, M.R., Sherbourne, C.D., Hays, R.D., et al. (1993) Physicians' characteristics influence patient adherence to medical treatment: Results from the medical outcomes study. *Health Psychology*, 12, 93-102.

Dinger, U., Strack, M., Leichsenrig, F., et al. (2008) Therapist effects on outcome and alliance in inpatient psychotherapy. *Journal of Clinical Psychology*, 64, 344-354.

Dirksen, S.R. & Epstein, D.R. (2008) Efficacy of an insomnia intervention on fatigue, mood and quality of life in breast cancer survivors. *Journal of Advanced Nursing*, 61, 664-675.

Dodd, M. J., Janson, S., Facione, N., Fawcett, J., Froelicher, E.S., Humphreys, J., Lee, K., Miaskowski, C., Puntillo, K., Rankin, S., & Taylor, D. (2001) Advancing the science of symptom management. *Journal of Advanced Nursing*, 33(5), 668-676.

Dodd, M.J. & Miaskowski, C. (2000) The Pro-Self Program: A self-care intervention program for patients receiving cancer treatment. *Seminars in Oncology Nursing*, 16, 300-308.

Donaldson, S.I. & Christie, C.A. (2004) Determining causality in program evaluation and applied research: Should experimental evidence be the gold standard? *Journal of MultiDisciplinary Evaluation*, 3, 60-77.

Dumas, J.E., Lynch, A.M., Laughlin, J.E., et al. (2001) Promoting intervention fidelity. Conceptual issues, methods, and preliminary results from the EARLY ALLIANCE Prevention trial. *American Journal of Preventive Medicine*, 20, 38-47.

Dumbridgue, H.B., Al-Bayat, M.I., Ng, C.C.H., & Wakefield, C.W. (2006) Assessment of bias in methodology for randomized controlled trials published on implant dentistry. *Journal of Prostodontics*, 15, 257-263.

Dumville, J.C., Torgerson, D.J., & Hewitt, C.E. (2006) Reporting attrition in randomized controlled trials. *British Medical Journal*, 332, 969-971.

Dwight-Johnson, M., Unutzer, J., Sherbourne, C., et al. (2001) Can quality improvement programs for depression in primary care address patient preferences for treatment? *Medical Care*, 39, 934-944.

Dzewaltowski, D.A., Estabrooks, P.A., Klesges, L.M., et al. (2004) Behavior change intervention research in community settings: How generalizable are the results. *Health Promotion International*, 19, 235-245.

Eakin, B.L., Brody, J.S., & Lusk, S.L. (2001) Creating a tailored, multi-media, computer-based intervention. *Computers in Nursing*, 19, 152-160.

Eccles, M., Grimshaw, J., Walker, A., et al. (2005) Changing the behavior of health-care professionals: The use of theory in promoting the uptake of research findings. *Journal of Clinical Epidemiology*, 58, 107-112.

Eckert, T.L. & Hintze, J.M. (2000) Behavioral conceptions and applications of acceptability: Issues related to service delivery and research methodology. *School Psychology Quarterly*, 15, 123-149.

Edinger, J.D., Wohlgemuth, W.K., Radtke, R.A., et al. (2007) Dose-response effects of cognitive-behavioral insomnia therapy: A randomized clinical trial. *Sleep*, 30, 203-212.

Einhorn, H.J. & Hogarth, R.M. (1986) Judging probable cause. *Psychological Bulletin*, 99, 3-19.

Elkin, I., Falconnier, L., Martinovich, Z., & Mahoney, C. (2006) Therapist effects in the National Institute of Mental Health Treatment of Depression Collaborative Research Program. *Psychotherapy Research*, 16, 144-160.

Ellis, P.M. (2000) Attitudes towards and participation in randomized clinical trials in oncology. A review of the literature. *Annals of Oncology*, 11, 939-945.

Epstein, D.R. & Bootzin, R.R. (2002) Insomnia. *Nursing Clinics of North America*, 37, 611-631.

Eremenco, S., Cella, D., & Arnold, B. (2005) A comprehensive method for the translation and cross-cultural validation of health status questionnaires. *Evaluation and the Health Professions*, 28, 212-232.

Etter, M. & Etter, J-F. (2007) Acceptability and impact of a partial smoking ban in a psychiatric hospital. *Preventive Medicine*, 44, 64-69.

Evers, G. (2003) Developing nursing science in Europe. *Journal of Nursing Scholarship*, 35, 9-13.

Fan, L. & Sidani, S. (2009) Effectiveness of diabetes self-management education intervention elements: A meta-analysis. *Canadian Journal of Diabetes*, 33, 18-26.

Fernandez, A.F., Patten, C.A., Schroeder, D.R., et al. (2006) Characteristics of six-month tobacco use outcomes of black patients seeking smoking cessation intervention. *Journal of Health Care for the Poor & Underserved*, 17, 413-424.

Fernández, M.E., Gonzales, A., Tortolero-Luna, G., Partida, S., & Bartholomew, L.K. (2005) Using intervention mapping to develop a breast and cervical cancer screening program for Hispanic farmworkers: Cultivando La Salud. *Health Promotion Practice*, 6, 394-404.

Ferriter, M. & Huband, N. (2005) Does the non-randomized controlled study have a place in the systematic review? A pilot study. *Criminal Behavior & Mental Health*, 15, 111-120.

Festic, E. & Gajic, O. (2009) Translational science research: Towards better health. *Bosnian Journal of Basic Medical Sciences*, 9(Suppl. 1), S1-S2.

Finn, C.A. & Sladeczek, I.E. (2001) Assessing the social validity of behavioral interventions: A review of treatment acceptability measures. *School Psychology Quarterly*, 16, 176-206.

Finnis, D.G., Kaptchuk, T.J., Miller, F., & Benedetti, F. (2010) Biological, clinical, and ethical advanced of placebo effects. *Lancet*, 375, 686-695.

Fishbein, M. (2000) The role of theory in HIV prevention. *AIDS Care*, 12, 273-278.

Fishbein, M. & Yzer, M.C. (2003) Using theory to design effective health behavior interventions. *Communication Theory*, 13, 164-183.

Fisher, P., McCavrey, R., Hosford, C., & Vickers, A. (2006) Evaluation of specific and non-specific effects in homeopathy: Feasibility study for a randomized trial. *Homeopathy*, 95, 215-222.

Fixsen, D.L., Naoom, S.F., Blase, K.A., et al. (2005) *Implementation Research: A Synthesis of the Literature*. University of South Florida, Tampa.

Fleming, T.R. (2010) Clinical trials: Discerning hype from substance. *Annals Internal Medicine*, 153, 400-406.

Foley, J. (2005) Nitrous oxide inhalation sedation: What do patients, carers and dentists think about it? *European Journal of Pediatric Dentistry*, 1, 23-29.

Folstein, M., Folstein, S., & McHugh, P. (1975) Mini-mental state: A practical method for grading the cognitive state of patients for the clinician. *Journal of Psychiatric Research*, 12, 189-198.

Forbes, A. & While, A. (2009) The nursing contribution to chronic disease management: A discussion paper. *International Journal of Nursing Studies*, 46, 119-130.

Forgatch, M.S., Patterson, G., & DeGarmo, D.S. (2005) Evaluating fidelity: Predictive validity for a measure of competent adherence to the Oregon Model of Parent Management Training. *Behavior Therapy*, 36, 3-13.

Foy, R., Francis, J.J., Johnston, M., et al. (2007) The development of a theory-based intervention to promote appropriate disclosure of a diagnosis of dementia. *BMC Health Services Research*, 7, 207-215.

Frank, E., Rush, J., Blehar, M., et al. (2002) Skating to where the puck is going to be: A plan for clinical trials and translation research in mood disorders. *Biological Psychiatry*, 52, 631-654.

Fremont, A.M., Cleary, O.D., Hargraves, J.L., et al. (2001) Patient-centered processes of care and long-term care outcomes of myocardial infarction. *Journal of General Internal Medicine*, 16, 800-808.

French, B. (2005) The process of research use in nursing. *Journal of Advanced Nursing*, 49, 125-134.

Fuertes, J.N., Mislowack, A., Bennett, J., et al. (2007) The physician-patient working alliance. *Patient Education & Counseling*, 66, 29-36.

Germain, A., Moul, D.E., Franzen, P.L., et al. (2006) Effects of a brief behavioral treatment for late-life insomnia. Preliminary findings. *Sleep Medicine*, 2, 403-406.

Gerrish, K. (2000) Individualized care: Its conceptualization and practice within a multiethnic society. *Journal of Advanced Nursing*, 32, 91-99.

Given, B.A., Keilman, L.J., Collins, C., & Given, C.W. (1990) Strategies to minimize attrition in longitudinal studies. *Nursing Research*, 39, 184-186.

Givens, J.L, Houston, T.K., van Voorhees, B.W., et al. (2007) Ethnicity and preferences for depression treatment. *General Hospital Psychiatry*, 29, 182-191.

Glasgow, R.E., Magid, D.T., Beck, A., et al. (2005) Practical clinical trials for translating research to practice. Design and measurement recommendations. *Medical Care*, 43, 551-557.

Glasziov, P., Chalmers, I., Rowlins, M., & McCulloch, P. (2007) When are randomized trials unnecessary? Picking signal from noise. *British Medical Journal*, 334, 349-351.

Godin, G., Bélanger-Gravel, A., Eccles, M., & Grimshaw, J. (2008) Healthcare professionals' intentions and behaviours: A systematic review of studies based on social cognitive theories. *Implementation Science*, 3, 36-47.

Graham, I.D., Logan, J., Harrison, M.B., et al. (2006) Lost in knowledge translation: Time for a map? *The Journal of Continuing Education in the Health Professions*, 26, 13-24.

Grapow, M.T.R., von Watternwyl, R., Guller, U., et al. (2006) Randomized controlled trials do not reflect reality: Real-world analyses are critical for treatment guidelines! *The Journal of Thoracic & Cardiovascular Surgery*, 132, 5-7.

Green, J. (2000) The role of theory in evidence-based health promotion practice. *Health Education Research*, 15, 125-129.

Griffiths, K.M. & Christensen, H. (2006) Review of randomized controlled trials of Internet interventions for mental disorders and related conditions. *Clinical Psychologist*, 10, 16-29.

Gross, D. & Fogg, L. (2001) Clinical trials in the 21st century: The case for participant-centered research. *Research in Nursing & Health*, 24, 530-539.

Gum, A.M., Arean, P.A., Hunkeler, E., et al. (2006) Depression treatment preferences in older primary care patients. *The Gerontologist*, 4, 14-22.

Guruge, S., Shirpak, K.R., Hyman, I., et al. (2010) A meta-synthesis of post-migration changes in marital relationships in Canada. *Canadian Journal of Public Health*, 101, 327-331.

Guyatt, G.H., Haynes, B., Jaeschke, R., et al. (2002) Introduction: The philosophy of evidence-based medicine. In: G. Guyatt & D. Rennie (eds) *Users' Guides to the Medical Literature: A Manual for Evidence-Based Clinical Practice*. AMA Press, Chicago.

Gwadry-Sridher, F., Guyatt, G.H., Arnold, M.O., et al. (2003) Instruments to measure acceptability of information and acquisition of knowledge in patients with heart failure. *The European Journal of Heart Failure*, 5, 783-791.

Haaga, D.A.F. (2004) A healthy dose of criticism for randomized trials: Comment on Westen, Novotny, and Thompson-Brenner (2004). *Psychological Bulletin*, 130, 674-676.

Hacklett, G.K.B., Arbon, P., Scuttere, S.D., & Borg, M. (2005) The experience of making treatment decisions for women with early stage breast cancer: A diagrammatic representation. *European Journal of Cancer Care*, 14, 249-255.

Haerens, L., Deforche, B., Vandelanotte, C., et al. (2007) Acceptability, feasibility and effectiveness of a computer - tailored physical activity intervention in adolescents. *Patient Education & Counseling*, 66, 303-310.

Hale, J.F. (1998) Application of the PRECEDE-PROCEED model for comprehensive community assessment, education programming, and evaluation in a combat hospital community during the Gulf War. *Home Health Care Management Practice*, 11, 52-65.

Hallberg, I.R. (2009) Moving nursing research forward towards a stronger impact on health care practice? *International Journal of Nursing Studies*, 46, 407-412.

Halpern, S.D. (2003) Evaluating preference effects in partially unblended, randomized clinical trials. *Journal of Clinical Epidemiology*, 56, 109-115.

Hamunen, K. & Kalso, E. (2005) A systematic review of trial methodology, using the placebo groups of randomized controlled trials in paediatric postoperative pain. *Pain*, 116, 146-158.

Hark, T.T. & Stump, D.A. (2008) Statistical significance versus clinical significance. *Seminars Cardiothoracic Vascular Anesthesiology*, 12, 5-6.

Harris, R. & Dyson, E. (2001) Recruitment of frail older people to research: Lessons learnt through experience. *Journal of Advanced Nursing*, 36, 643-651.

Hart, E. (2009) Treatment definition in complex rehabilitation interventions. *Neuropsychological Rehabilitation*, 19, 824-840.

Hazlett-Stevens, H., Craske, M.G., Roy-Byrne, P.P., et al. (2002) Predictors of willingness to consider medication and psychosocial treatment for panic disorder in primary care patients. *General Hospital Psychiatry*, 24, 316–321.

Heaman, M. (2001) Conducting health research with vulnerable women: Issues and strategies. *Canadian Journal of Nursing Research*, 33, 81–86.

Heinsman, D.T. & Shadish, W.R. (1996) Assignment methods in experimentation: When do nonrandomized experiments approximate answers from randomized experiments? *Psychological Methods*, 1, 154–169.

Heit, M., Rosenquist, C., Culligan, P., et al. (2003) Predicting treatment choice for patients with pelvic organ prolapse. *The American College of Obstetrics & Gynecology*, 101, 1279.

Hertzog, M.A. (2008) Considerations in determining sample size for pilot studies. *Research in Nursing & Health*, 31, 180–191.

Hibbard, J.H., Greene, J., & Tusler, M. (2009) Improving the outcomes of disease management by tailoring care to the patient's level of activation. *American Journal of Managed Care*, 15, 353–360.

Hill, A.B. (1965) The environment and disease: Association or causation? *Proceedings of the Royal Society of Medicine*, 58, 295–300.

Hitchcock Noël, P., Marsh, G., Larme, A.C., et al. (1998) Patient choice in diabetes education curriculum. *Diabetes Care*, 21, 896–901.

Holmbeck, G.N. (1997) Toward terminological, conceptual, and statistical clarity in the study of mediators and moderators: Examples from the child-clinical and pediatric psychology literatures. *Journal of Consulting & Clinical Psychology*, 65, 599–610.

Holtz, A. (2007) Comparative effectiveness of health interventions: Strategies to change policy and practice. Report from ECRI Institute's 15th Annual Conference. Conference Report.

Howard, L. & Thornicroft, G. (2006) Patient preference and randomized controlled trials in mental health research. *British Journal of Psychiatry*, 188, 303–304.

Hrisos, S., Eccles, M., Johnston, M., et al. (2008) An intervention modeling experiment to change GPs' intentions to implement evidence-based practice: Using theory-based interventions to promote GP management of upper respiratory tract infection without prescribing antibiotics # 2. *BMC Health Services Research*, 8, 10–21.

Huibers, M.J.H., Bleijenberg, G., Beurskens, A.J.H.M., et al. (2004) An alternative trial design to overcome validity and recruitment problems in primary care research. *Family Practice*, 21, 213–218.

Hupcey, J.E. & Penrod, J. (2005) Concept analysis: Examining the state of the science. *Research and Theory for Nursing Practice: An International Journal*, 19, 197–208.

Huppert, J.D., Bufka, L.F., Barlow, D.H., et al. (2001) Therapists, therapist variables, and cognitive-behavioral therapy outcome in a multicenter trial for panic disorder. *Journal of Consulting & Clinical Psychology*, 69, 747–755.

Hyde, P. (2004) Fool's gold: Examining the use of gold standards in the production of research evidence. *British Journal of Occupational Therapy*, 67, 89–94.

Institute of Medicine (2001) *Crossing the Quality Chasm: A New Health System for the 21st Century*. National Academy Press, Washington, DC.

Jackson, K.M. & Trochim, W.M.K. (2002) Concept mapping as an alternative approach for the analysis of open-ended survey responses. *Organizational Research Methods*, 5, 307–336.

Jacobs, G.D., Pace-Schott, E.F., Stickgold, R., & Otto, M.W. (2004) Cognitive behavior therapy and pharmacotherapy for insomnia. A randomized controlled trial and direct comparison. *Archives of Internal Medicine*, 164, 1888-1986.

Jacobson, N.S., Roberts, L.J., Berns, S.B., & McGlinchey, J.B. (1999) Methods for defining and determining the clinical significance of treatment effects: Description, application, and alternatives. *Journal of Consulting & Clinical Psychology*, 67, 300-307.

Janevic, M.R., Janz, M.K., Dodge, J.A., et al. (2003) The role of choice in health education intervention trials: A review and case study. *Social Science & Medicine*, 56, 1581-1594.

Jansen, S.J.Y., Kievit, J., Nooij, M.A., et al. (2001) Patients' preferences for adjuvant chemotherapy in early-stage breast cancer: Is treatment worthwhile? *British Journal of Cancer*, 84, 1577-1585.

Jenkins, V. & Fallowfield, L. (2000) Reasons for accepting or declining to participate in randomized clinical trials for cancer therapy. *British Journal of Cancer*, 82, 1783-1788.

Jennings, B.M. & Loan, L.A. (2001) Misconceptions among nurses about evidence-based practice. *Journal of Nursing Scholarship*, 33, 121-127.

Jo, B. (2002) Statistical power in randomized intervention studies with noncompliance. *Psychological Methods*, 7, 178-193.

Jo, B. (2008) Causal inference in randomized experiments with mediational processes. *Psychological Methods*, 13, 314-336.

Johnson, C.A., Cen, S., Gallaher, P., et al. (2007) Why smoking prevention sometimes fail. Does effectiveness depend on sociocultural context and individual characteristics? *Cancer Epidemiology Biomarkers Prevention*, 16, 1043-1049.

Johnson, M.O. & Remien, R.H. (2003) Adherence to research protocols in a clinical context: Challenges and recommendations from behavioral intervention trials. *American Journal of Psychotherapy*, 57, 348-360.

Joyce, A.S., Ogradniczuk, J.S., Piper, W.E., & McCallum, M. (2003) The alliance as mediator of expectancy effects in short-term individual therapy. *Journal of Clinical & Consulting Psychology*, 71(4), 672-679.

Judge Santacrocce, S., Maccarelli, L.M., & Grey, M. (2004) Intervention fidelity. *Nursing Research*, 53, 63-66.

Kaptchuk, T.J. (2001) The double-blind, randomized, placebo-controlled trial: Gold standard or golden calf? *Journal of Clinical Epidemiology*, 54, 541-549.

Kaul, S. & Diamond, G.A. (2010) Trial and error. How to avoid commonly encountered limitations of published clinical trials. *Journal of the American College of Cardiology*, 55, 415-427.

Kazdin, A.E. (1980) Acceptability of alternative treatments for deviant child behavior. *Journal of Applied Behavior Analysis*, 13, 259-273.

Kazdin, A.E. (2003) *Research Design in Psychology*. Allyn and Bacon, Boston.

Keirse, M.J.N.C. & Hansens, M. (2000) Control of error in randomized clinical trials. *European Journal of Obstetrics & Gynecology and Reproductive Biology*, 92, 67-74.

Keller, C., Fleury, J., Sidani, S., & Aisnworth, B. (2009) Fidelity to theory in PA intervention research. *Western Journal of Nursing Research*, 31, 289-311.

Kelly, C.M., Baker, E.A., Brownson, R.C., & Schootman, M. (2007) Translating research into practice: Using concept mapping to determine locally relevant intervention strategies to increase physical activity. *Evaluation & Program Planning*, 30, 282-293.

Kelly, P.J., Lesser, J., Cheung, A-L., et al. (2010) A prospective randomized controlled trial of an interpersonal violence prevention program with a Mexican American community. *Family & Community Health*, 33(3), 207-215.

Kiesler, D.J. & Auerbach, S.M. (2006) Optimal matches of patient preferences for information, decision-making and interpersonal behavior: Evidence, models, and interventions. *Patient Education & Counseling*, 61, 319-341.

Kim, D-M., Wampold, B.E., & Bolt, D.M. (2006) Therapist effects in psychotherapy: A random-effects modeling of the National Institute of Mental Health Treatment of Depression Collaborative Research Program data. *Psychotherapy Research*, 16, 161-172.

Kim, M.J. (2002) Priorities for advancing nursing knowledge. *Journal of Nursing Scholarship*, 34, 211-212.

King, M., Nazareth, I., Lampe, F., et al. (2005) Impact of participant and physician intervention preferences on randomized trials. A systematic review. *Journal of the American Medical Association*, 293, 1089-1099.

Klaber-Moffett, J.K, Torgerson, D., Bell-Syer, S., et al. (1999) Randomised controlled trial of exercise for low back pain: Clinical outcomes, costs, and preferences. *British Medical Journal*, 319, 279-283.

Kleinman, P.H., Woody, G.E., Todd, T.C., et al. (1990) Crack and cocaine abusers in outpatient psychotherapy. In: L.S. Onken & J.D. Blaine (eds) *Psychotherapy and Counseling in the Treatment of Drug Abuse*. National Institute on Drug Abuse (NIDA) Research Monograph Series 104. National Institute on Drug Abuse, Washington, DC.

Klem, M.L., Viteri, J.E., & Wing, R.R. (2000) Primary prevention of weight gain for women aged 25-34: The acceptability of treatment formats. *International Journal of Obesity*, 24, 219-225.

Kok, G., Schaalma, H., Ruiter, R.A.C., et al. (2004) Intervention mapping: A protocol for applying health psychology theory to prevention programmes. *Journal of Health Psychology*, 9, 85-98.

Kotwall, C.A., Mahoney, L.J., Myers, R.E., & Decoste, L. (1992) Reasons for non-entry in randomized clinical trials for breast cancer: A single institutional study. *Journal of Surgical Oncology*, 50, 125-129.

Kovach, C.R. (2009) Some thoughts on the hazards of sloppy science when designing and testing multicomponent interventions, including the Kitchen Skin phenomenon. *Research in Nursing & Health*, 32, 1-3.

Kowinsky, A., Greenhouse, P.K., Zombek, V.L., et al. (2009) Care management redesign: Increasing care manager time with patients and providers while improving metrics. *Journal of Nursing Administration*, 39, 388-392.

Kraemer, H.C., Wilson, T., Fairburn, C.G., & Agras, S. (2002) Mediators and moderators of treatment effects in randomized clinical trials. *Archives General Psychiatry*, 59, 877-883.

Kraemer, M.S., Martin, R.M., Sterne, J.A.C., et al. (2009) The double jeopardy of clustered measurement and cluster randomization. *British Medical Journal*, 339, 503-505.

Kreuter, M.W., Bull, F.C., Clark, E.M., & Oswald, D.L. (1999a) Understanding how people process health information: A comparison of tailored and nontailored weight-loss materials. *Health Psychology*, 18, 487-494.

Kreuter, M.W., Stretcher, V.J., & Glassman, B. (1999b) One size doesn't fit all: The case for tailoring print materials. *Annals Behavioral Medicine*, 21, 276-283.

Kreuter, M.W., Sugg-Skinner, C., Holt, C.L., et al. (2005) Cultural tailoring for mammography and fruit and vegetable intake among low-income African-American women in urban public health centers. *Preventive Medicine*, 41, 53-62.

Kroezer, W., Werkman, A., & Brug, J. (2006) A systematic review of randomized trials on the effectiveness of computer-tailored education on physical activity and dietary behaviors. *Annals Behavioral Medicine*, 31, 205-223.

Labonte, R. (1993) *Health Promotion and Empowerment Practice Frameworks.* Centre for Health Promotion, University of Toronto, ParticipACTION, Toronto, Ontario, Canada.

Lam, W.W.T., Fielding, R., Ho, E.Y.Y., et al. (2005) Surgeon's recommendation, perceived operative efficacy and age dictate treatment choice by Chinese women facing breast cancer surgery. *Psycho-Oncology*, 14, 585-593.

Lambert, M.F. & Wood, J. (2000) Incorporating patient preferences into randomized trials. *Journal of Clinical Epidemiology*, 53, 163-166.

Lambert, N., Rowe, G., Bowling, A., et al. (2004) Reasons underpinning patients' preferences for various angina treatments. *Health Expectations*, 6, 246-256.

Lancaster, G.A., Dodd, S., & Williamson, P.R. (2004) Design and analysis of pilot studies: Recommendations for good practice. *Journal of Evaluation in Clinical Practice*, 10, 307-312.

Landy, S.H., McGinnis, J.E., & McDonald, S.A. (2005) Pilot study evaluating preference for 3-mg versus 6-mg subcutaneous sumatriphan. *Headache*, 45, 346-349.

Lang, A.J. (2005) Mental health treatment preferences of primary care patients. *Journal of Behavioral Medicine*, 28, 581-586.

Larson, P.J., Miaskowski, C., McPhail, L., et al. (1998) The PRO-SELF mouth aware program: An effective approach for reducing chemotherapy-induced mucositis. *Cancer Nursing*, 21, 263-268.

Lauver, D.R., Ward, S.E., Heidrich, S.M., et al. (2002) Patient-centered interventions. *Research in Nursing & Health*, 25, 246-255.

Laverack, G. & Labonte, R. (2000) A planning framework for community empowerment goals within health promotion. *Health Policy and Planning*, 15, 255-262.

Lebow, J.L. (1987) Acceptability as a simple measure in mental health program evaluation. *Evaluation & Program Planning*, 10, 191-195.

Ledbetter, C.A. & Stevens, K.R. (2000) Basics of evidence-based practice part 2: Unscrambling the terms and processes. *Seminars in Perioperative Nursing*, 9, 98-104.

Lehman, A.F. & Steinwachs, D.M. (2003) Evidence-based psychosocial treatment practices in schizophrenia: Lessons from the Patient Outcomes Research Team (PORT) Project. *Journal of the American Academy of Psychoanalysis & Dynamic Psychiatry*, 31, 141-154.

Leigh, J.P., Ward, M.M., & Fries, J.F. (1993) Reducing attrition bias with an instrumental variable in a regression model: Results from a panel of rheumatoid arthritis patients. *Statistics in Medicine*, 12, 1-14.

Leung, C.M., Ho, G.K.H., Foong, M., et al. (2005) Small-group hypertension health education programme: A process and outcome evaluation. *Journal of Advanced Nursing*, 52(6), 631-639.

Leventhal, H. & Friedman, M.A. (2004) Does establishing fidelity of treatment help in understanding treatment efficacy? Comment on Bellg et al. (2004). *Health Psychology*, 23, 452-456.

Lindsay, B. (2004) Randomized controlled trials of socially complex nursing interventions: Creating bias and unreliability? *Journal of Advanced Nursing*, 45, 84-94.

Lindsay Davis, L., Broome, M.E., & Cox, R.P. (2002) Maximizing retention in community-based clinical trials. *Journal of Nursing Scholarship*, 34, 47-53.

Lippke, S. & Ziegelman, J.P. (2008) Theory-based health behavior change: Developing, testing, and applying theories for evidence-based interventions. *Applied Psychology: An International Review*, 57, 698-716.

Lipsey, M.W. (1990) *Design Sensitivity. Statistical Power for Experimental Research*. Sage, Thousand Oaks, CA.

Lipsey, M.W. (1993) Theory as method: Small theories of treatments. *New Directions for Program Evaluation*, 57, 5-38.

Lipsey, M.W. & Wilson, D.B. (2001) The way in which intervention studies have "personality" and why it is important to meta-analysis. *Evaluation & The Health Professions*, 24, 236-254.

Luborsky, L., McLellan, A.T., Diguer, L., et al. (1997) The psychotherapist matters: Comparison of outcomes across twenty two therapists and seven patient samples. *Clinical Psychology: Science & Practice*, 4, 53-65.

Lugtenberg, M., Burgers, J.S., & Westert, G.P. (2009) Effects of evidence-based clinical practice guidelines on quality of care: A systematic review. *Quality Safety Health Care*, 18, 385-392.

Lutz, W., Leon, S.C., Martinovich, Z., et al. (2007) Therapist effects in outpatient psychotherapy: A three-level growth curve approach. *Journal of Counseling Psychology*, 54, 32-39.

Lutzen, K. (2000) A global perspective on domestic and international tensions in knowledge development. *Journal of Nursing Scholarship*, 32, 335-337.

Lynn, M.R. (1986) Determination and quantification of content validity. *Nursing Research*, 35, 382-385.

MacDonald, S., Rothwell, H., & Moore, L. (2007) Getting it right: Designing adolescent-centered smoking cessation services. *Addiction*, 102, 1147-1150.

Macias, C., Barreira, P., Hargreaves, W., et al. (2005) Impact of referral source and study applicants' preference for randomly assigned service on research enrollment, service engagement, and evaluative outcomes. *American Journal of Psychiatry*, 162, 781-787.

MacKinnon, D.P. & Fairchild, A.J. (2009) Current directions in mediation analysis. *Current Directions in Psychological Science*, 18, 16-20.

Maclure, M. (2009) Explaining pragmatic trials to pragmatic policymakers. *Journal of Clinical Epidemiology*, 62, 476-478.

Mahon, N.E., Yarcheski, A., Yarcheski, T.J., & Hanks, M.M. (2010) A meta-analytic study of predictors of anger in adolescents. *Nursing Research*, 59, 178-184.

Mahoney, E.K., Trudeau, S.A., Penyack, S.E., & MacLeod, C.E. (2006) Challenges to intervention implementation. Lessons learned in the bathing persons with Alzheimer's disease at home study. *Nursing Research*, 55, S10-S16.

Manojlovich, M. & Sidani, S. (2008) Nurse dose: What's in a concept? *Research in Nursing & Health*, 31, 310-319.

Marteau, T.M. & Johnston, M. (1990) Health professionals: A source of variance in health outcomes. *Psychology & Health*, 5, 47-58.

Martin, D.J., Garske, J.P., & Davis, M.K. (2000a) Relation of the therapeutic relation with outcome and other variables: A meta-analytic review. *Journal of Consulting & Clinical Psychology*, 68, 438-450.

McClelland, G.H. (2000) Increasing statistical power without increasing sample size. *American Psychologist*, 55, 963-964.

McCloskey, J.C. & Bulecheck, G.M. (2000) *Nursing Intervention Classification*, 3rd edn. Mosby, St Louis, MO.

McCommon, Ā., Kirk, S.F.L., & Ramsley, J.K. (2009) Process evaluation of an internet-based resource for weight control: Use and views of an obese sample. *Journal of Nutrition Education & Behavior*, 41, 261-267.

McCormack, B. (2003) Researching nursing practice: Does person-centredness matter? *Nursing Philosophy*, 4, 179-188.

McCormack, B. & McCance, T.V. (2006) Development of a framework for person-centered nursing. *Journal of Advanced Nursing*, 56, 472-479.

McCormack, J.P., Dolovich, L., Levine, M., et al. (2003) Providing evidence-based information to patients in general practice and pharmacies: What is the acceptability, usefulness and impact on drug use? *Health Expectations*, 6, 281-289.

McEwen, A. & West, R. (2009) Do implementation issues influence the effectiveness of medications? The case of nicotine replacement therapy and bupropion in UK Stop Smoking Services. *BMC Public Health*, 9, 28-36.

McGilton, K., Fox, M.T., & Sidani, S. (2005) A theory-driven approach to evaluating a communication intervention. *Canadian Journal of Program Evaluation*, 20, 27-48.

McGrew, J.H., Bond, G.R., Dietzen, L., & Salyers, M. (1994) Measuring the fidelity of implementation of a mental health program model. *Journal of Consulting & Clinical Psychology*, 62, 670-678.

McGuire, D.B., DeLoney, V.G., Yeager, K.A., et al. (2000) Maintaining study validity in a changing clinical environment. *Nursing Research*, 49, 231-235.

McKee, M., Britton, A., Black, N., et al. (1999) Interpreting the evidence: Choosing between randomised and non-randomised studies. *British Medical Journal*, 19, 312-315.

McKnight, P.E., McKnight, K.M., Sidani, S., & Figueredo, A.J. (2007) *Missing Data: A Gentle Introduction*. Guilford Publications, New York.

McLaughlin, C.P. & Kaluzny, A.D. (2000) Building client centered systems of care: Choosing a process direction for the next century. *Health Care Management Review*, 25, 73-82.

McPherson, K. & Britton, A. (2001) Preferences and understanding their effects on health. *Quality in Health Care*, 10, i61-i66.

Melder, C., Esbensen, A.-A., & Tusinski, K. (2006) Addressing program fidelity using onsite observations and program provider descriptions of program delivery. *Evaluation Review*, 30, 714-740.

Messer, S.B. & Wampold, B.E. (2002) Let's face facts: Common factors are more potent than specific therapy ingredients. *Clinical Psychology Practice*, 9, 21-25.

Michie, S. & Abraham, C. (2004) Interventions to change health behaviors: Evidence-based or evidence-inspired? *Psychology & Health*, 19, 29-49.

Michie, S., Johnston, M., Francis, J., et al. (2008) From theory to intervention: Mapping theoretically derived behavioral determinants to behavior change techniques. *Applied Psychology: An International Review*, 57, 660-680.

Millat, B., Borie, F., & Fingerhut, A. (2005) Patients' preference and randomization: New paradigm of evidence-based clinical research. *World Journal of Surgery*, 29, 596-600.

Mills, N., Metcalfe, C., Ronsmans, C., et al. (2006) A comparison of socio-demographic and psychological factors between patients consenting to randomisation and those selecting treatment (the ProtecT study). *Contemporary Clinical Trials*, 27, 413-419.

Miranda, J. (2004) An exploration of participants' treatment preferences in a partial RCT. *Canadian Journal of Nursing Research*, 36, 100-114.

Mirtz, T.A., Thompson, M.A., Green, L., et al. (2005) Adolescent idiopathic scoliosis screening for school, community, and clinical health promotion practice utilizing the PRECEDE-PROCEED model. *Chiropractic & Osteopathy*, 13, 25-35.

Moreira, T., May, C., Mason, J., & Eccles, M. (2006) A new method of analysis enabled a better understanding of clinical practice guideline development processes. *Journal of Clinical Epidemiology*, 59, 1190-1206.

Morin, C.M. (1993) *Insomnia: Psychological assessment and management*. Guilford, New York.

Morin, C.M. (2006) Combined therapeutics for insomnia: Should our first approach be behavioral or pharmacological? *Sleep Medicine*, 7(Suppl. 1), S15-S19.

Morin, C.M., Bootzin, R.R., Buysse, D.J., et al. (2006) Psychological and behavioral treatment of insomnia: Update of the recent evidence (1998-2004). *Sleep*, 29, 1398-1414.

Morin, C.M., Gaulier, B., Barry, T., & Kowatch, R.A. (1992) Patients' acceptance of psychological and pharmacological therapies for insomnia. *Sleep*, 15, 302-305.

Morrow, D.G., Weiner, M., Steinley, D., et al. (2007) Patient's health literacy and experience with instructions: Influence preferences for heart failure medication instructions. *Journal of Aging and Health*, 19, 575-593.

Moser, D.K., Dracup, K., & Doering, L.V. (2000) Factors differentiating dropouts from completers in a longitudinal, multicenter clinical trial. *Nursing Research*, 49, 109-116.

Mowbray, C.T., Holter, M.C., Teague, G.B., & Bybee, D. (2003) Fidelity criteria: Development, measurement, and validation. *American Journal of Evaluation*, 24, 315-340.

Mulhall, J.P. & Montorsi, F. (2006) Evaluating preference trials of oral phosphodiesterase 5 inhibitors for erectile dysfunction. *European Urology*, 49, 30-37.

Mykhalovskiy, E. & Weir, L. (2004) The problem of evidence-based medicine: Directions for social science. *Social Science & Medicine*, 59, 1059-1069.

Naber, D. & Kasper, S. (2000) The importance of treatment acceptability to patients. *International Journal of Psychiatry in Clinical Practice*, 4(Suppl. 1), S25-S34.

Najavits, L.M. & Weiss, R.D. (1994) Variations in therapist effectiveness in the treatment of patients with substance use disorders: An empirical review. *Addiction*, 89, 679-688.

Nallamothu, B.K., Hayward, R.A. & Bates, E.R. (2008) Beyond the randomized clinical trial. The role of effectiveness studies in evaluating cardiovascular therapies. *Circulation*, 118, 1294-1303.

Nápoles-Springer, A.M., Santayo-Olsson, J., O'Brien, H., & Stewart, A.L. (2006) Using cognitive interviews to develop surveys in diverse populations. *Medical Care*, 44(Suppl. 1), S21-S30.

National Institutes of Health, National Cancer Institute (2000) *Theory at a Glance. A Guide for Health Promotion Practice*. U.S. Department of Health and Human Services, National Institutes of Health, Washington, DC.

Naylor, M.D. (2003) Nursing intervention research and quality of care: Influencing the future of healthcare. *Nursing Research*, 52, 380-385.

Nock, M.K. (2007) Conceptual and design essentials for evaluating mechanisms of change. *Alcoholism: Clinical & Experimental Research*, 31(Suppl. 3), 4S-12S.

Oakley, A., Strange, V., Bornell, C., et al. (2006) Process evaluation in randomized controlled trials of complex interventions. *British Medical Journal*, 332, 413-416.

Oakley, A., Strange, V., Toroyan, T., et al. (2003) Using random allocation to evaluate social interventions: Three recent U.K. examples. *Annals of the AAPSS*, 589, 170-189.

Okiishi, J., Lambert, M.J., Nielson, S.L., & Ogles, B.M. (2003) Waiting for supershrink: An empirical analysis of therapist effects. *Clinical Psychology & Psychotherapy*, 10, 361-373.

Oremus, M., Cosby, J.L., & Wolfson, C. (2005) A hybrid qualitative method for pretesting questionnaires: The example of a questionnaire to caregivers of Alzheimer's disease patients. *Research in Nursing & Health*, 28, 419-430.

Oxman, A.D., Lombard, C., Treweek, S., et al. (2009) Why we will remain pragmatists: Four problems with the impractical mechanistic framework and a better solution. *Journal of Clinical Epidemiology*, 62, 485-488.

Oxman, T.E., Schulberg, H.C., Greenberg, R.L., et al. (2006) A fidelity measure for integrated management of depression in primary care. *Medical Care*, 44, 1030-1037.

Padhye, N.S., Cron, S.G., Gusik, G.M., et al. (2009) Randomization for clinical research: An easy-to-use spreadsheet method. *Research in Nursing & Health*, 32, 561-566.

Padsakoff, P.M., MacKenzie, S.B., Lu, J-Y., & Padsakoff, N.P. (2003) Common method biases in behavioral research: A critical review of the literature and recommended remedies. *Journal of Applied Psychology*, 88, 879-903.

Painter, J.E., Borba, C.P.C., Hynes, M., et al. (2008) The use of theory in health behavior research from 2000-2005: A systematic review. *Annals of Behavioral Medicine*, 35, 358-362.

Pallesen, S., Nordhus, I.H., Kvale, G., et al. (2003) Behavioral treatment of insomnia in older adults: An open clinical trial comparing two interventions. *Behavior Research & Therapy*, 41, 31-48.

Pawson, R. & Tilley, N. (1997) *Realistic Evaluation*. Sage, London, UK.

Pearson, M.L., Wu, S., Schaefer, J., et al. (2005) Assessing the implementation of the chronic care model in quality improvement collaboratives. *Health Services Research*, 40, 978-996.

Peduzzi, P., Henderson, W., Hartigan, P., & Lavori, P. (2002) Analysis of randomized controlled trials. *Epidemiologic Reviews*, 24, 26-38.

Pillemer, K., Suitor, J.J., & Wethington, E. (2003) Integrating theory, basic research, and intervention: Two case studies from caregiving research. *The Gerontologist*, 43(Special issue 1), 19-28.

Pincus, T. (2002) Limitations of randomized clinical trials in chronic diseases: Explanations and recommendations. *Advances*, 18, 14-21.

Polit, D.F. & Beck, C.T. (2006) The content validity index: Are you sure you know what's being reported? Critique and recommendations. *Research in Nursing & Health*, 29, 489-497.

Porter, R., Frampton, C., Joyce, P.R., & Mulder, R.T. (2003) Randomized controlled trials in psychiatry. Part 1: Methodology and critical evaluations. *Australian and New Zealand Journal of Psychiatry*, 37, 257-264.

Preference Collaborative Review Group (2009) Patients' preferences within randomized trials: Systematic review and patient level meta-analysis. *British Medical Journal Online* (downloaded on February 3, 2009).

Project MATCH Research Group (1998) Therapist effects in three treatments for alcohol problems. *Psychotherapy Research*, 8, 455-474.

Pruitt, R.H. & Privette, A.B. (2001) Planning strategies for the avoidance of pitfalls in intervention research. *Journal of Advanced Nursing*, 35, 514-520.

Radwin, L.E. (2003) Cancer patients' demographic characteristics and ratings of patient-centered nursing care. *Journal of Nursing Scholarship*, 35, 365-370.

Radwin, L.E., Cabral, H.J., & Wilkes, G. (2009) Relationships between patient-centered cancer nursing interventions and desired health outcomes in the context of the health care system. *Research in Nursing & Health*, 32, 4-17.

Raudenbush, S.W. (2001) Comparing personal trajectories and drawing causal inferences from longitudinal data. *Annual Reviews Psychology*, 52, 501-525.

Raudenbush, S.W. & Bryk, A.S. (2002) *Hierarchical Linear Models. Applications and Data Analysis Methods*, 2nd edn. Sage, Thousand Oaks, CA.

Reid Ponte, P.R., Conlin, G., Conway, J.B., et al. (2003) Making patient-centered care come alive. *Journal of Nursing Administration*, 33, 82-90.

Reimers, T.M. & Wacker, D.P. (1988) Parents' ratings of the acceptability of behavioral treatment recommendations made in an outpatient clinic: A preliminary analysis of the influence of treatment effectiveness. *Behavioral Disorders*, 14, 7-15.

Resnick, B., Bellg, A.J., Borelli, B., et al. (2005) Examples of implementation and evaluation of treatment fidelity in the BCC studies: Where we are and where we need to go. *Behavioral Medicine*, 29(Special suppl.), 46-54.

Resnicow, K., Baranowski, T., Ahluwalia, J.S., & Baranowski, R.L. (1999) Cultural sensitivity in public health: defined and demystified. *Ethnicity & Disease*, 9, 10-21.

Revere, D. & Dunbar, P.J. (2001) Review of computer-generated outpatient health behavior interventions: Clinical encounters "in absentia". *Journal American Medical Informatics Association*, 8, 62-79.

Ribisl, K.M., Walton, M.A., Mowbray, C.T., et al. (1996) Minimizing participant attrition in panel studies through the use of effective retention and tracking strategies: Review and recommendations. *Evaluation & Program Planning*, 19, 1-25.

Richardson, J. (2000) The use of randomized controlled trials in complementary therapies: Exploring the issues. *Journal of Advanced Nursing*, 32, 398-406.

Riedel-Heller, S.G., Matschinger, H., & Angermeyer, M.C. (2005) Mental disorders - Who and what might help? Help-seeking and treatment preferences of the lay public. *Social Psychiatry Psychiatric Epidemiology*, 40, 167-174.

Robitaille, Y., Laforest, S., Fournier, M., et al. (2005) Moving forward in fall prevention: An intervention to improve balance among older adults in real-world settings. *American Journal of Public Health*, 95(11), 1-8.

Rolfe, G. (2009) Complexity and uniqueness in nursing practice: Commentary on Richards and Hamers (2009). *International Journal of Nursing Studies*, 46, 1156-1158.

Rosal, M.C., Goins, K.V., Carbone, E.T., & Cortes, D.E. (2004) Views and preferences of low-literate Hispanics regarding diabetes education: Results of formative research. *Health Education & Behavior*, 31, 388-405.

Rossi, P.H., Freeman, H.E., & Lipsey, M.W. (2004) *Evaluation: A Systematic Approach*, 7th edn. Sage, Thousand Oaks, CA.

Rothman, A.J. (2004) "Is there nothing more practical than a good theory?": Why innovations and advances in health behavior change will arise if interventions are used to test and refine theory. *International Journal of Behavioral Nutrition & Physical Activity*, 1, 11-17.

Rothwell, P.M. (2005) External validity of randomized controlled trials: "To whom do the results of this trial apply?" *Lancet*, 365, 82-93.

Rowe, G., Lambert, N., Bowling, A., et al. (2005) Assessing patients' preferences for treatment for angina using a modified repertory grid method. *Social Science & Medicine*, 60, 2585-2595.

Ruggeri, M., Lasalvia, A., Bisoffi, G., et al. (2003) Satisfaction with mental health services among people with schizophrenia in five European sites: Results from the EPSILON Study. *Schizophrenia Bulletin*, 29, 229-245.

Russell, K. & Walsh, D. (2009) Can the use of behavioural intervention studies support change in professional practice behaviours? A literature review. *Evidence Based Midwifery*, 7, 54-59.

Ryan, P. (2009) Integrated theory of health behavior change: Background and intervention development. *Clinical Nurse Specialist*, 23, 161-170.

Rycroft-Malone, J., Harvey, G., Seers, K., et al. (2004) An exploration of the factors that influence the implementation of evidence into practice. *Journal of Clinical Nursing*, 13, 913–924.

Sackett, D.L., Richardson, W.S., Rosenberg, W.M., & Haynes, R.B. (1997) *Evidence-Based Medicine: How to Practice and Teach EBM*. Churchill Livingstone, New York.

Sales, A., Smith, J., Curran, G., & Kochevar, L. (2006) Models, strategies, and tools. Theory in implementing evidence-based findings into health care practice. *Journal of General Internal Medicine*, 21(Suppl. 1), S43–S49.

Sandelowski, M. & Barraso, J. (2007) *Handbook for Synthesizing Qualitative Research*. Springer Publishing Company, New York.

Saunders, R.P., Evans, M.H., & Joshi, P. (2005) Developing a process-evaluation plan for assessing health promotion program implementation: A how-to guide. *Health Promotion Practice*, 6, 134–147.

Savard, J., Simard, S., Hervouet, S., et al. (2005) Insomnia in men treated with radical prostatectomy for prostate cancer. *Psycho-Oncology*, 14, 147–156.

Schafer, J.L. & Kang, J. (2008) Average causal effects from nonrandomized studies: A practical guide and simulation example. *Psychological Methods*, 13, 279–313.

Schumacher, K.L., Koresawa, S., West, C., Dodd, M., Paul, S.M., Tripathy, D., Koo, P., & Miaskowski, C. (2005) Qualitative research contribution to a randomized clinical trial. *Research in Nursing & Health*, 28, 268–280.

Schutte-Rodin, S., Broch, L., Buysse, D., et al. (2008) Clinical guideline for the evaluation and management of chronic insomnia in adults. *Journal of Clinical Sleep Medicine*, 4, 487–504.

Scott, A.G. & Sechrest, L. (1989) Strength of theory and theory of strength. *Evaluation and Program Planning*, 12, 329–336.

Scriven, M. (2008) A summative evaluation of RCT methodology: & An alternative approach to causal research. *Journal of MultiDisciplinary Evaluation*, 5, 11–24.

Sehon, S.R. & Stanley, D.E. (2003) A philosophical analysis of the evidence-based medicine debate. *BMC Health Services Research*, 3, 14–22.

Severy, L.J., Tolley, E., Woodsong, C., & Guest, G. (2005) A framework for examining the sustained acceptability of microbicides. *AIDS & Behavior*, 9, 121–131.

Shadish, W.R. (2010) Campbell and Rubin: A primer and comparison of their approaches to causal inference in field settings. *Psychological Methods*, 15, 3–17.

Shadish, W.R., Cook, T.D. & Campbell, D.T. (2002) *Experimental and Quasi-Experimental Design for Generalized Causal Inference*. Houghton-Mifflin, Boston, MA.

Shapiro, J.R., Reba-Harrelson, L., Dymek-Valentine, M., et al. (2007) Feasibility and acceptability of CD-ROM-based cognitive-behavioral treatment for binge-eating disorder. *European Eating Disorder Review*, 15, 175–184.

Shapiro, S.L., Figeredo, A.J., Caspi, O., et al. (2002) Going quasi: The premature disclosure effect in a randomized clinical trial. *Journal of Behavioral Medicine*, 25, 605–621.

Sheiner, L.B. & Rubin, D.B. (1995) Intention-to-treat analysis and the goals of clinical trials. *Clinical Pharmacology Therapy*, 57, 6–15.

Sidani, S. (2003) Symptom management. In: D.M. Doran (ed) *Nursing-Sensitive Outcomes. State of the Science*. Jones and Bartlett Publishers, Sudbury, MA, pp. 115–176.

Sidani, S. (2006) Random assignment: A systematic review. In: R.R. Bootzin & P.E. McKnight (eds) *Strengthening Research Methodology. Psychological Measurement and Evaluation*. American Psychological Association Books, Washington, DC.

Sidani, S. (2008) Effects of patient-centered care on patient outcomes: An evaluation. *Research and Theory for Nursing Practice. An International Journal*, 21, 22-35.

Sidani, S. & Braden, C.J. (1998) *Evaluating Nursing Interventions. A Theory-Driven Approach*. Sage, Thousand Oaks, CA.

Sidani, S., Epstein, D.R., Bootzin, R.R., et al. (2007) Alternative Methods for Clinical Research (NP 05075). Final report submitted to the National Institute of Nursing Research, Washington, DC.

Sidani, S., Epstein, D.R., Bootzin, R.R., et al. (2009) Assessment of preferences for treatment: Validation of a measure. *Research in Nursing & Health*, 32, 419-431.

Sidani, S., Epstein, D.R., & Miranda, J. (2006) Eliciting patient treatment preferences: A strategy to integrate evidence-based and patient-centered care. *Worldviews on Evidence-Based Nursing*, 3, 116-123.

Sidani, S., Epstein, D.R., & Moritz, P. (2003) An alternative paradigm for clinical nursing research: An exemplar. *Research in Nursing & Health*, 26, 244-255.

Sidani, S. & Irvine, D. (1999) A conceptual framework for evaluating the acute care nurse practitioner role. *Journal of Advanced Nursing*, 30, 58-66.

Sidani, S., Miranda, J., Epstein, D., & Fox, M. (2009) Influence of treatment preferences on validity: A review. *Canadian Journal of Nursing Research*, 41, 52-67.

Sidani, S. & Sechrest, L. (1999) Putting theory into operation. *American Journal of Evaluation*, 20, 227-238.

Sidani, S. & Stevens, B.J. (2000) Alternative therapies and placebos: Conceptual clarification and methodological implications. *Canadian Journal of Nursing Research*, 31, 73-86.

Sidani, S., Streiner, D.L. & LeClerc, C.M. (2010a) Mitigating the impact of external forces. In: D.L. Streiner & S. Sidani (eds) *When Research Goes Off the Rails. Why It Happens and What You Can Do about It*. The Guilford Press, New York.

Sidani, S., Streiner, D.L., & LeClerc, C.M. (2010b) When a beautiful intervention meets ugly reality: Implementing an intervention in the real world. In: D.L. Streiner & S. Sidani (eds) *When Research Goes Off the Rails. Why It Happens and What You Can Do about It*. The Guilford Press, New York.

Simmons, R. & Elias, C. (1994) The study of client-provider interactions: A review of methodological issues. *Studies in Family Planning*, 25, 1-17.

Sobieraj, G., Bhatt, M., LeMay, S., et al. (2009) The effect of music on parental participation during pediatric laceration repair. *Canadian Journal of Nursing Research*, 41, 68-82.

Sox, H.C., Helfand, M., Grimshaw, J., et al. (2010) Comparative effectiveness research: Challenges for medical journals. *Trials*, 11, 45-50.

Speight, J. (2005) Assessing patient satisfaction: Concepts, applications, and measurement. *International Society for Pharmaeconomics & Outcomes Research*, 8(Suppl. 1), S6-S8.

Spenceley, S.M., 'OLeary, K.A., Chizawsky, L.L.K., et al. (2008) Sources of information used by nurses to inform practice. An integrative review. *International Journal of Nursing Studies*, 45, 954-970.

Spencer, S.J., Zanna, M.P., & Fong, G.T. (2005) Establishing a causal chain: Why experiments are often more effective than mediational analyses in examining psychological processes. *Journal of Personality & Social Psychology*, 89, 845-851.

Spielman, A., Saskin, P., & Thorpy, M.J. (1987) Treatment of chronic insomnia by restriction of time in bed. *Sleep*, 10, 45-56.

Spillnane, V., Byrne, M.C., Byrne, M., et al. (2007) Monitoring treatment fidelity in a randomized controlled trial of a complex intervention. *Journal of Advanced Nursing*, 60, 343-352.

Spittaels, H., De Bourdeaudhuij, I., & Vandelanotte, C. (2007) Evaluation of a website-delivered computer-tailored intervention for increasing physical activity in the general population. *Preventive Medicine*, 44, 209-217.

Staines, G.L., Cleland, C.M., & Blankertz, L. (2006) Counselor confounds in evaluations of vocational rehabilitation methods in substance dependency treatment. *Evaluation Review*, 30, 139-170.

Stalmeier, P.F.M., van Tol-Geerdink, J.J., van Lin, E.N.J.T., et al. (2007) Doctors' and patient's preferences for participation and treatment in curative prostate cancer radiotherapy. *Journal of Clinical Oncology*, 25, 3096-3100.

Stanford Encyclopedia of Philosophy (2008) *Counterfactual Theories of Causation*. Available on: http://plato.stanford.edu/ (accessed in January, 2010).

Stein, K.F., Sargent, J.T., & Rafaels, N. (2007) Establishing fidelity of the independent variable in nursing clinical trials. *Nursing Research*, 56, 54-62.

Stevens, T. & Ahmedzai, S.H. (2004) Why do breast cancer patients decline entry into randomized trials and how do they feel about their decision later: A prospective, longitudinal, in-depth interview study. *Patient Education & Counseling*, 52, 341-338.

Stewart, M., Brown, J.B., Donner, A., et al. (2000) The impact of patient-centered care on outcomes. *Journal of Family Practice*, 49, 796-804.

Stewart-Williams, S. & Podd, J. (2004) The placebo effect: Dissolving the expectancy versus conditioning debate. *Psychological Bulletin*, 130, 324-340.

Stirman, S.W., DeRubeis, R.J., Crits-Christoph, P., & Rothman, A. (2005) Can the randomized controlled trial literature generalize to nonrandomized patients? *Journal of Consulting & Clinical Psychology*, 73, 127-135.

Stone, G.W. & Pocock, S.J. (2010) Randomized trials, statistics, and clinical inference. *Journal of the American College of Cardiology*, 55, 428-431.

Streiner, D.L. & Sidani, S. (eds) (2010) *When Research Goes Off the Rails. Why It Happens and What You Can Do about It*. The Guilford Press, New York.

Stretcher, V.J., Marcus, A., Bishop, K., et al. (2005) A randomized controlled trial of multiple tailored messages for smoking cessation among callers to the cancer information service. *Journal of Health Communication*, 10, 105-118.

Sullivan, C.M., Rumptz, M.H., Campbell, R., et al. (1996) Retaining participants in longitudinal community research: A comprehensive protocol. *Journal of Applied Behavioral Science*, 32, 262-276.

Swift, J.K. & Callahan, J.L. (2009) The impact of client treatment preferences on outcome: A meta-analysis. *Journal of Clinical Psychology*, 65, 368-381.

Tacher, J.A., Morey, E., & Craighead, W.E. (2005) Using patient characteristics and attitudinal data to identify depression treatment preference groups: A latent-class model. *Depression and Anxiety*, 21, 47-54.

Taljaard, M., Weijer, C., Grimshaw, J.M., et al. (2009) Ethical and policy issues in cluster randomized trials: Rationale and design of a mixed methods research study. *Trials*, 10, 61-70.

Tanaka, E., Inove, E., Kawaguchi, Y., et al. (2006) Acceptability and usefulness of mizoribine in the management of rheumatoid arthritis in methotrexate-refractory patients and elderly patients, based on analysis of data from a large-scale observational cohort study. *Mod Rheumatology*, 16, 214-219.

Tarrier, N., Liversidge, T. & Gregg, L. (2006) The acceptability and preference for the psychological treatment of PTSD. *Behaviour Research & Therapy*, 44, 1643-1656.

Tataryn, D.J. (2002) Paradigms of health and disease: A framework for classifying and understanding complementary and alternative medicine. *The Journal of Alternative & Complementary Medicine*, 8, 877-892.

Temple, W.J., Russell, M.L., Parsons, L.L., et al. (2006) Conservation surgery for breast cancer as the preferred choice: A prospective analysis. *Journal of Clinical Oncology*, 24, 3367–3373.

TenHave, T.R., Coyne, J., Salzer, M., & Katz, I. (2003) Research to improve the simple randomized clinical trial. *General Hospital Psychiatry*, 25, 115–123.

Becker, P.T. (2008) Publishing pilot intervention studies. *Research in Nursing & Health*, 31, 1–3.

Thompson, D., Baranowski, J., Cullen, K., & Baranowski, T. (2007) Development of a theory-based internet program promoting maintenance of diet and physical activity change to 8-year old African American girls. *Computers & Education*, 48, 446–459.

Thorpe, K.E., Zwarenstein, M., Oxman, A.D., et al. (2009) A pragmatic-explanatory continuum indicator summary (PRECIS): A tool to help trial designers. *Journal of Clinical Epidemiology*, 62, 464–475.

Titler, M.G., Mentes, J.C., Rakel, B.A., et al. (1999) From book to bedside: Putting evidence to use in the care of the elderly. *Journal of Quality Improvement*, 25, 545–556.

Towne, L. & Hilton, M. (eds) (2004) Implementing Randomized Field Trials in Education: Report of a Workshop. Committee on Research in Education, National Research Council. National Academy of Science (downloaded from: http://www/nap.edu).

Travaodo, L., Grassi, L., Gil, F., et al. (2005) Physician-patient communication among southern European cancer physicians: The influence of psychosocial orientation and burnout. *Psycho-Oncology*, 14, 661–670.

Tripp-Reimer, T., Woodworth, G., McCloskey, J.C., & Bulechek, G. (1996) The dimensional structure of nursing interventions. *Nursing Research*, 45, 10–17.

Trochim, W.M.K. (1989) An introduction to concept mapping for planning and evaluation. *Evaluation & Program Planning*, 12, 1–16.

Trochim, W. & Kane, M. (2005) Concept mapping: An introduction to structured conceptualization in health care. *International Journal for Quality in Health Care*, 17, 187–191.

Tucker, A.L., Newbland, I.M., & Edmondson, A.C. (2007) Implementing new practices: An empirical study of organizational learning in hospital intensive care units. *Management Science*, 53, 894–907.

Tunis, S.R., Stryer, D.B., & Clancy, C.M. (2003) Practical clinical trials. Increasing the value of clinical research for decision making in clinical and health policy. *Journal of the American Medical Association*, 290, 1624–1632.

United States Government Accountability Office (2009) *Program Evaluation. A Variety of Rigorous Methods Can Help Identify Effective Interventions.* GAO-10-30, Washington, DC.

University of California, San Francisco, School of Nursing Symptom Management Faculty Group (1994) A model for symptom management. *Image: Journal of Nursing Scholarship*, 26, 272–275.

Valentine, J.C. & McHugh, C.M. (2007) The effects of attrition on baseline comparability in randomized experiments in education: A meta-analysis. *Psychological Methods*, 12, 268–282.

Vallance, J.K., Courneya, K.S., Taylor, L.M., et al. (2008) Development and evaluation of a theory-based physical activity guidebook for breast cancer survivors. *Health Education & Behavior*, 35, 174–189.

Van Dam, H.A., van der Horst, F., van den Borne, B., et al. (2003) Provider-patient interaction in diabetes care: Effects on patient self-care and outcomes. A systematic review. *Patient Education & Counseling*, 51, 17–28.

Vandelanotte, C. & De Bourdeaudhuij, I. (2003) Acceptability and feasibility of a computer-tailored physical activity intervention using stages of change: Project FAITH. *Health Education Research*, 18, 304-317.

Vandelanotte, C., De Bourdeaudhuij, I., & Brug, J. (2004) Acceptability and feasibility of an interactive computer-tailored fat intake intervention in Belgium. *Health Promotion International*, 19, 463-470.

Vandenbroucke, J.P. (2004) When are observational studies as credible as randomized trials? *The Lancet*, 363, 1728-1731.

Van Der Berg, M., Timmermans, D.R.M., Knol, D.L., et al. (2008) Understanding regnant women's decision making concerning prenatal screening. *Health Psychology*, 27, 430-437.

Van Die, M.D., Bone, K.M., Burger, H.G., & Teede, H.J. (2009) Are we drawing the right conclusions from randomized placebo-controlled trials? A post-hoc analysis of data from a randomized controlled trial. *BMC Medical Research Methodology*, 9, 41-47.

Van Sluijs, E.M.F., Van Poppel, M.N.M., Twisk, J.W.R., et al. (2005) The positive effect on determinants of physical activity of a tailored, general practice-based physical activity intervention. *Health Education Research*, 20, 345-356.

Victora, C.C., Habricht, J.-P., & Bryce, J. (2004) Evidence-based public health: Moving beyond randomized trials. *American Journal of Public Health*, 94, 400-405.

Villarruel, A.M., Jemmott, L.S., & Jemmott, J.B. (2005) Designing a culturally based intervention to reduce HIV sexual risk for Latino adolescents. *Journal of the Association of Nurses in AIDS Care*, 16(2), 23-31.

Vincent, N. & Lionberg, C. (2001) Treatment preference and patient satisfaction in chronic insomnia. *Sleep*, 24, 411-417.

Visovsky, C. & Schneider, S.M. (2003) Cancer-related fatigue. *Online Journal of Issues in Nursing*, 8(3).

Vogt, D.S., King, D.W., & King, L.A. (2004) Focus groups in psychological assessment: Enhancing content validity by consulting members of the target population. *Psychological Assessment*, 16, 231-243.

Vuorma, S., Teperi, J., Hurskainen, R., et al. (2003) Correlates of women's preferences for treatment of heavy menstrual bleeding. *Patient Education Counseling*, 49, 125-132.

Walker, L.O. & Avant, K.C. (2001) *Strategies for Theory Construction in Nursing*, 2nd edn. Appleton & Lange, Norwalk, Connecticut.

Walker, L.O., Santor, M.K., & Sands, D. (1989) Designing and testing self-help interventions. *Applied Nursing Research*, 2, 96-102.

Waller, G. (2009) Evidence-based treatment and therapist drift. *Behaviour Research and Therapy*, 47, 119-127.

Waltz, J., Addis, M.E., Koerner, K., & Jacobson, N.S. (1993) Testing the integrity of a psychotherapy protocol: Assessment of adherence and competence. *Journal of Consulting & Clinical Psychology*, 61, 620-630.

Wampold, B.E. & Brown, G.S. (2005) Estimating variability in outcomes attributable to therapists: A naturalistic study of outcomes in managed care. *Journal of Consulting & Clinical Psychology*, 73, 914-923.

Watson, B., Procker, S., & Cochrane, W. (2004) Using randomized controlled trials (RCTs) to test service interventions: Issues of standardization, selection and generalisability. *Nurse Researcher*, 11, 28-42.

Weaver, M., Patrick, D.L., Markson, L.E., et al. (1997) Issues in the measurement of satisfaction with treatment. *American Journal of Managed Care*, 3, 579-594.

Weinert, C., Cudney, S., & Hills, W. (2008) Retention in a computer-based outreach intervention for chronically ill rural women. *Applied Nursing Research*, 21, 23-29.

Wensig, M. & Elwyn, G. (2003) Methods for incorporating patients' views in health care. *British Medical Journal*, 326, 877-879.

Wensig, M. & Grol, R. (2000) Patients' view on health care. A driving force for improvement in disease management. *Disease Management & Health Outcomes*, 7, 117-125.

West, S.G. & Thoemmes, F. (2010) Campbell's and Rubin's perspectives on causal inference. *Psychological Methods*, 15, 18-37.

Whittemore, R. & Grey, M. (2002) The systematic development of nursing interventions. *Journal of Nursing Scholarship*, 34, 115-120.

Whittemore, R. & Knafl, K. (2005) The integrative review: Updated methodology. *Journal of Advanced Nursing*, 52, 546-553.

Wolf, D.M., Lehman, L., Quinlin, R., Zullo, T., & Hoffman, L. (2008) Effect of patient-centered care on patient satisfaction and quality of care. *Journal of Nursing Care Quality*, 23, 316-321.

Worrall, J. (2002) What evidence in evidence-based medicine? *Philosophy of Science*, 69(Suppl. 3), S316-S330.

Zwarenstein, M. & Oxman, A. (2006) Why are so few randomized trials useful, and what can we do about it? *Journal of Clinical Epidemiology*, 59, 1125-1126.

Zwarenstein, M. & Treweek, S. (2009) What kind of randomized trials do we need? *Journal of Clinical Epidemiology*, 62, 461-463.

Index

Design, Evaluation, and Translation of Nursing Interventions, First Edition.
Souraya Sidani and Carrie Jo Braden.
© 2011 John Wiley & Sons, Inc. Published 2011 by John Wiley & Sons, Inc.